Pearls in Medicine
for Students

"Dream is not that which you see while sleeping, it is something that does not let you sleep"
&
"Excellence is a continuous process and not an accident"

—**APJ Abdul Kalam (1931–2015)**
Ex-President (India), Author, Inspirational Speaker,
Scientist and Researcher

By the same author:

- Bedside Clinics in Medicine, Part I & II
- MCQs in Internal Medicine
- Chapter in 'API Textbook of Medicine', 8th Edition
- Chapter in 'Postgraduate Medicine', 2009
- Chapters in 'Rheumatology: Principles and Practice', 2010
- Chapters in 'Medicine Update': 2010–5
- Chapter in 'Progress in Medicine', 2016
  and
- Section on Online Appendix of "Kumar & Clark's" Textbook, 'Clinical Medicine'—6th, 7th & 8th Editions

Biography (author):

Included in Marquis Who's Who in the World 2014, 2015 & 2016
and
Who's Who in Science and Engineering 2016–17

Pearls in Medicine
for Students

A Knowledge-bank in Internal Medicine

Second Edition

Arup Kumar Kundu MD FICP MNAS
Professor, Department of Medicine and
In-charge, Division of Rheumatology
IQ City Medical College, West Bengal, India
Formerly,
Professor of Medicine and
In-charge, Division of Rheumatology
NRS MC, RG Kar MC & KPC Medical College, Kolkata, India

JAYPEE *The Health Sciences Publisher*
New Delhi | London | Philadelphia | Panama

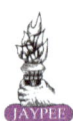

Jaypee Brothers Medical Publishers (P) Ltd

Headquarters

Jaypee Brothers Medical Publishers (P) Ltd.
4838/24, Ansari Road, Daryaganj
New Delhi 110 002, India
Phone: +91-11-43574357
Fax: +91-11-43574314
Email: jaypee@jaypeebrothers.com

Overseas Offices

J.P. Medical Ltd.
83, Victoria Street, London
SW1H 0HW (UK)
Phone: +44-20 3170 8910
Fax: +44-(0)20 3008 6180
Email: info@jpmedpub.com

Jaypee Medical Inc.
The Bourse
325 Chestnut Street, Suite 412
Philadelphia, PA 19106, USA
Phone: +1 267-519-9789
Email: support@jpmedus.com

Jaypee Brothers Medical Publishers (P) Ltd.
Bhotahity, Kathmandu, Nepal
Phone: +977-9741283608
Email: kathmandu@jaypeebrothers.com

Jaypee-Highlights Medical Publishers Inc.
City of Knowledge, Bld. 237, Clayton
Panama City, Panama
Phone: +1 507-301-0496
Fax: +1 507-301-0499
Email: cservice@jphmedical.com

Jaypee Brothers Medical Publishers (P) Ltd.
17/1-B, Babar Road, Block-B, Shaymali
Mohammadpur, Dhaka-1207
Bangladesh
Mobile: +08801912003485
Email: jaypeedhaka@gmail.com

Website: www.jaypeebrothers.com
Website: www.jaypeedigital.com

© 2016, Jaypee Brothers Medical Publishers

The views and opinions expressed in this book are solely those of the original contributor(s)/author(s) and do not necessarily represent those of editor(s) of the book.

All rights reserved. No part of this publication may be reproduced, stored or transmitted in any form or by any means, electronic, mechanical, photocopying, recording or otherwise, without the prior permission in writing of the publishers.

All brand names and product names used in this book are trade names, service marks, trademarks or registered trademarks of their respective owners. The publisher is not associated with any product or vendor mentioned in this book.

Medical knowledge and practice change constantly. This book is designed to provide accurate, authoritative information about the subject matter in question. However, readers are advised to check the most current information available on procedures included and check information from the manufacturer of each product to be administered, to verify the recommended dose, formula, method and duration of administration, adverse effects and contraindications. It is the responsibility of the practitioner to take all appropriate safety precautions. Neither the publisher nor the author(s)/editor(s) assume any liability for any injury and/or damage to persons or property arising from or related to use of material in this book.

This book is sold on the understanding that the publisher is not engaged in providing professional medical services. If such advice or services are required, the services of a competent medical professional should be sought.

Every effort has been made where necessary to contact holders of copyright to obtain permission to reproduce copyright material. If any have been inadvertently overlooked, the publisher will be pleased to make the necessary arrangements at the first opportunity.

Inquiries for bulk sales may be solicited at: jaypee@jaypeebrothers.com

Pearls in Medicine for Students

First Edition: **2008**
Second Edition: **2016**
ISBN: 978-93-85891-58-8

Dedicated to

My daughter Ushasi
My son Dr Abhishek
My beloved students
for their constant inspiration and moral support
and
to my sick patients who have taught me the beauty of medicine

Preface to the Second Edition

By the grace of Almighty, I have been able to bring out the second edition of the book in a new getup. I have appreciably revised and updated each and every chapter, maintaining the previous style and old tradition intact. Many old photographs have been replaced with new photographs of clinical importance. There are altogether 80 chapters after inclusion of 5 new chapters over and above the first edition, where every individual chapter may be regarded as a *window of medicine* as before. The *contents are arranged alphabetically* for easy reading.

The new edition deals with different must-know areas in clinical medicine which a medical student is expected to know at the end of his/her clinical training. There is an exhaustive coverage on different pearls in the arena of clinical medicine. The problem-solving attitude of this monograph will help the students in their viva and practical as well as theoretical examination, and also in their professional life in future. This type of book, I strongly believe, has become the need of the hour. This book remains an invaluable resource for the undergraduates, postgraduates, junior teachers, and practitioners to reach a high level of clinical competence. My endeavor will be successful if it helps the medical students to become successful doctors in future by making them more knowledgeable.

In this new edition, each and every chapter at its end has been enriched with 'The Pearls'.

I would like to record my appreciation for Mr Jitendar P Vij (Group Chairman), Mr Ankit Vij (Group President), Ms Chetna Malhotra Vohra (Associate Director–Content Strategy) Jaypee Brothers Medical Publishers (P) Ltd., and Mr Sushil Shaw (Branch in-charge of Kolkata office), who took immense pain in publishing and distributing the book. This work has only been possible with the constant support and encouragement of my wife Bijoya, son Dr Abhishek, daughter Ushasi, and, lastly, my late father, who showered his blessings from the heaven.

As the book has been written single-handedly, there may be some inadvertent mistakes which must have crept in. So, I welcome healthy suggestions and constructive criticisms from the thoughtful readers to me or to the publishers.

Arup Kumar Kundu
arup2158@gmail.com
arup_kundu@hotmail.com

Preface to the First Edition

I think myself a student even after learning medicine for more than two and half decades. Teaching a large number of students made me realize the need for such kind of book which deals with common medical presentations, and is lucid, handy, concise, updated as well as truly student-oriented. The aim of this book is to provide guidance for undergraduate and postgraduate students, and young physicians doing private practice or serving villages. This book is a distillation of my experience while answering questions for patients and health professionals over 25 years of practice. The manual consists of short descriptions of facts frequently encountered at the bedside, and I do believe that the cumulative symptomatology with differential diagnoses give a glimpse of real-life story of our day to day clinical practice. There are altogether 75 chapters in the book and each chapter may be regarded as a *window of medicine*; individual chapter also contains many jig-saw puzzles.

The contents are arranged alphabetically while the index gives a wider idea about the matters or topics present in the book. To write a book as a single-handed author is a challenging task, and I am fully aware of this. 'Pearls' help us to crystallize knowledge in our memory very easily. I hope as well as expect that the book will be used as a quick-reference ready-reckoner handbook and a learning-revision tool to increase the core knowledge during early years of medical training. The problem-solving attitude will help the students in their theoretical as well as practical examination, and also in their professional life in future. I hope the extensive and beautiful color photographs will boost the students while confronting with the patients at the bedside.

This work would not have been possible without the constant support and encouragement from my family members, especially to speak of my wife Bijoya Kundu, my daughter Ushasi and son Abhishek, which ultimately made the book a reality. I would like to appreciate the attitude of my colleagues Dr SK Pal, Associate Professor and Dr P Chattopadhyay, Assistant Professor who helped by giving some interesting clinical photographs for presentation in the book. I am grateful to all my patients whose photographs are printed here, and to the MSVP, NRS Medical College and Hospital for permitting me to take the photographs.

I would also like to record my appreciation for Mr Sandip Gupta, General Manager (Sales) and Mr Sushil Shaw, Branch in-charge of Kolkata office for extending their cooperation in every step. My sincere thanks are extended to Mr JP Vij, CMD and Mr Tarun Duneja, General Manager (Publishing), of M/S Jaypee Brothers Medical Publishers (P) Ltd, who have helped me throughout and also taken immense pain in publishing this book.

I welcome healthy suggestions and constructive criticisms from the thoughtful readers through e-mail to me (**arup_kundu@hotmail.com**) or the publishers.

Arup Kumar Kundu

Contents

1. Abnormal Sweating 1
2. Alopecia 6
3. Alteration of Facial Contour 10
4. Angular Stomatitis 14
5. Aseptic Fever 16
6. Bald Tongue 21
7. Bedsores 25
8. Blackish Urine 28
9. Blue Fingers/Toes 30
10. Blue Sclera 34
11. Bradycardia 38
12. Bruxism (Teeth Grinding) 43
13. Bull-neck 46
14. Carpal Tunnel Syndrome 49
15. Claw Foot/Claw Hand 52
16. Coprolalia 58
17. Cough 60
18. Cramps 66
19. Depressed Bridge of the Nose 71
20. Dextrocardia 76
21. Diffuse Aches and Pains 80
22. Diplopia 85
23. Discolored Teeth 88
24. Drop Attacks 90
25. Erectile Dysfunction (Impotence) 93
26. Eyes: A Clue to Diagnosis 98
27. Face Reading 106
28. Facial Pain 120
29. Fatigue 124
30. Flushing of Face 128
31. Foul Breath 132
32. Genital Ulcer 135
33. Gingival Bleeding 139

34. Gum Hypertrophy	142
35. Hardness (Thickening) of Skin	145
36. Head-nodding	148
37. Heel Pain	150
38. Herpes Labialis	154
39. Hiccough	161
40. Hirsutism	164
41. Hoarseness of Voice	169
42. Hyperkeratosis of Palms	173
43. Hypertelorism/Hypotelorism	176
44. Indigestion (Dyspepsia)	180
45. Intermittent Claudication	184
46. Joint Pain	188
47. Leg Ulceration	197
48. Lockjaw	200
49. Lump in Right Iliac Fossa	202
50. Macroglossia	208
51. Nerve Thickening	212
52. Night Blindness	215
53. Nocturnal Enuresis	218
54. Pallor	223
55. Parotid Swelling	225
56. Patch Tonsil	228
57. Photosensitivity	231
58. Polycythemia	235
59. Pruritus	239
60. Ptosis	244
61. Purpuric Spots	248
62. Purse-lip Respiration	254
63. Rectal Bleeding	259
64. Recurrent Oral Ulcers	262
65. Red Urine	266
66. Rings around Cornea	270
67. Shake Hands with the Patient	274
68. Sneezing, Yawning and Snoring	278
69. Splinter Hemorrhage	281

70.	Spoon-shaped Nails	289
71.	Sternal (Bone) Tenderness	292
72.	Sudden Cardiac Death	295
73.	Swollen Legs	297
74.	Tongue: A Clue to Many Diseases	306
75.	Weight Gain/Loss	311
76.	Wheezing/Stridor	316
77.	White Nails	318
78.	White (Milky) Urine	322
79.	Winging of the Scapulae	324
80.	Yellowish Palms/Soles	326
	Index	329

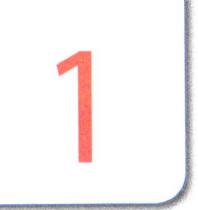

Abnormal Sweating

PROLOGUE

The sweat glands are divided into two classes:
1. Eccrine, and
2. Apocrine glands.

The ***eccrine glands*** are the major sweat glands in the body (99%) and are generally found throughout the surface. The glands present on palms and soles do not respond to temperature but secrete at the time of emotional stress. The ***apocrine glands*** are larger sweat glands and are found in axilla, areola of the nipples, mons pubis, labia majora, ear, eyelid and mammary gland.

The eccrine glands are supplied anatomically by sympathetic fibers, yet they are functionally cholinergic (e.g. pilocarpine increases the flow of sweat and atropine abolishes sweating). The apocrine sweat glands respond to circulating adrenaline (these glands are of sexual significance and remain inactive until puberty).

The daily total amount of sweat secreted by a human is approximately 480–600 mL, which may even rise to 10 liters in extremely hot weather.

TYPES OF SWEATING

There are two types of sweating:
1. **Sensible:** When sweating is increased and evaporation stops, drops of sweat appear on skin surface.
2. **Insensible (approximately 500 mL/day):** The loss of water from skin surface is neither visible nor perceptible; it is not due to active secretion but occurs as a result of passage of water by diffusion of tissue fluid through the epidermis.

Synonym of sweating is perspiration or diaphoresis.

Sweating may be Classified into (Normal Physiological Response)

- Thermal sweating → due to rise of external temperature and is controlled by thermoregulatory centre at hypothalamus

- Emotional (mental) sweating → chiefly palms, soles and axillae are involved
- Sweating due to muscular exercise/exertion → factors involved are thermal sweating + emotional sweating
- Gustatory sweating → eating of spicy food may stimulate sweating in head and neck region
- Miscellaneous → as a result of sympathetic overactivity, nausea/vomiting, syncopal attack, hypoglycemia and asphyxia.

COMPOSITION OF HUMAN SWEAT

- A clear colorless fluid which contains mainly water
- Specific gravity—1.001–1.006; pH 4.5 to 7.0
- Osmolality—120 mosmol/kg (i.e. hyposmotic to plasma)
- Solid present in sweat are lactic acid, carbolic acid, urea, creatinine, sugar, uric acid, nitrogen and non-protein nitrogen, calcium, iodine, iron, sulfur, copper, amino acids, sodium, chloride, potassium and others
- Sodium: 0.9 g/L and potassium: 0.2 g/L.

HYPERHIDROSIS (GENERALIZED)

- Exercise, anxiety, pyrexia, hot climate; familial or idiopathic
- Thyrotoxicosis, hyperpituitarism, acromegaly, carcinoid syndrome, pheochromocytoma, menopause, pregnancy, obesity
- Hypoglycemia
- Acute myocardial infarction, heart failure, shock
- Tuberculosis, other infections/pyrogens, lymphoma, malignancy, rheumatoid arthritis
- Alcohol intoxication, antidepressant drugs, pilocarpine, arecholine hypersensitivity (present in betel nut) and opiates
- Intense pain, syncope
- Rickets, infantile scurvy
- Neurological lesions of cerebral cortex, basal ganglia, spinal cord and sympathetic nervous system; familial dysautonomia.

Constant sweating with heat intolerance is experienced in thyrotoxicosis, while sweating with hot flushes are characteristic of women reaching menopause.

HYPERHIDROSIS (LOCALIZED)

- Organic neurological lesions—brain tumor, spinal cord injury (may help to localize site of lesion), syringomyelia
- Localized sweating of palms, soles and axillae—hot weather, anxiety, psychoneurosis and embarrassment
- Dermatological disorders—dyshidrotic eczema, vitiligo, epidermolysis bullosa, palmoplantar keratoderma, nail-patella syndrome

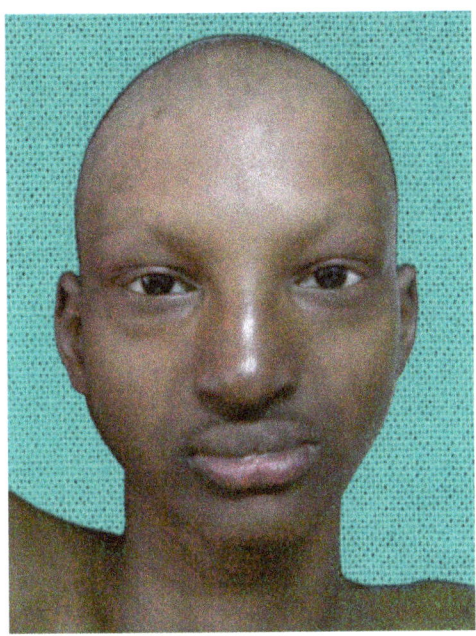

Fig. 1.1: Abnormalities of ectodermal structures like hair, teeth, nail, sweat glands are seen in ectodermal dysplasia. Scalp hair, eyebrows, moustache, beard, teeth and sweat gland are absent here

- Pachydermoperiostotis (or primary hypertrophic osteoarthropathy with grade IV clubbing + leonine face)—affects skinfolds of forehead and extremities
- Granulosis rubra nasi—rare genetic disorder; sweating of tip of the nose with a diffuse erythema associated with.

ANHIDROSIS/HYPOHIDROSIS (GENERALIZED)

It is less common than hyperhidrosis.
- Heat stroke
- Ectodermal dysplasia (Fig. 1.1)
- Scleroderma
- Organic brain damage, especially of the hypothalamus
- Ichthyosis
- Anderson-Fabry's disease
- Miscellaneous—myxedema, atopic eczema, psoriasis, lichen planus.

ANHIDROSIS/HYPOHIDROSIS (LOCALIZED)

- Horner's syndrome (involves half of the face, neck, front and back of upper chest, arm)
- Diabetic or leprosy neuropathy.

Autonomic neuropathy may lead to anhidrosis and/or gustatory sweating.

COLD AND CLAMMY SKIN

A classical physical finding in shock, and is due to sweating associated with cutaneous vasoconstriction; commonly found in:
- Hypoglycemia
- Acute myocardial infarction
- Shock and syncopal states
- Alcohol withdrawal
- Dumping syndrome.

Note: First two conditions give rise to ***drenching perspiration***.

NIGHT SWEATS IN CLINICAL MEDICINE

- Tuberculosis
- Lymphoma
- Chronic myeloid leukemia
- Brucellosis
- Giant cell arteritis
- Acquired immune deficiency syndrome (AIDS)
- Nocturnal (sleeping) hypoglycemia
- Menopausal syndrome
- Amoebic liver abscess
- Rheumatoid arthritis (rare).

OSMIDROSIS (FOUL SMELLING SWEAT)

The personal body odor is basically determined by apocrine gland secretion. Eccrine sweat is usually odorless.
- Substances excreted in the sweat, e.g. garlic, drugs like dimethyl sulphoxide, arsenic, urea in renal failure (urhidrosis)
- Hyperhidrosis of sole, complicated by bacterial overgrowth may give rise to foul odor in some persons with extreme social embarrassment
- Imaginary foul odor is perceived in paranoid delusion
- Others (as a result of bacterial overgrowth after sweat excretion)—acute rheumatic fever, scurvy, gout, diabetes mellitus, pneumonia, enteric fever.

CHROMHIDROSIS (COLORED SWEAT)

- Pigment produced by chromogenic bacteria
- Ten percent of normal people may have colored apocrine sweat (yellow/green/blue)—due to the pigment ***lipofuscins***
- Drugs excreted through sweat, e.g. rifampicin.

MILIARIA

These are vesicles (sudamina)/papules (prickly heat) resulting from blockage and rupture of sweat ducts. These are commonly seen in tropical conditions of heat and high humidity. The clear vesicles contain sweat and are often found on the trunk during febrile illness (especially, when the body is covered by blanket during pyrexia), and is known as *sudaminal rash*.

SWEAT TEST

Pilocarpine iontophoresis test done to diagnose cystic fibrosis by giving injection pilocarpine to the patient and measuring the chloride concentration of the sweat → which is very high (> 60 mEq/L) in cystic fibrosis.

THE PEARLS

Drenching perspiration even in a comfortable temperature makes the clinician suspicious of acute myocardial infarction and hypoglycemia (in a diabetic subject).

History of *night sweats* needs immediate attention and investigation. Gustatory sweating (Frey's syndrome) is uncomfortable and embarrassing, but usually makes no sense.

2

Alopecia

SYNONYM

Partial or complete loss of hair, especially on the scalp.

TYPES

There are two types of hair loss:
1. *Scarring or cicatrical:* Permanent loss of hair follicle with replacement by scar tissue
2. *Non-scarring:* Temporary loss of hair follicle and the scalp skin looks normal.

BASICS

- *Hair growth* is influenced by → genetic, racial, nutritional and hormonal factors
- *Hair loss* may result from → changes in hair follicle due to follicular destruction/dysfunction or fracture of fibers.

CAUSES

Scarring or Cicatrical

- Inflammatory—bacterial folliculitis
- Discoid lupus erythematosus (DLE)
- Tinea capitis with inflammation (kerion)
- Lichen planus
- Idiopathic—pseudopelade
- Folliculitis decalvans
- Scleroderma
- X-irradiation
- Trauma or chemical damage (acid or alkali)
- Neoplasm
- Congenital (aplasia cutis)
- Miscellaneous—furuncle, carbuncle, lupus vulgaris, burn.

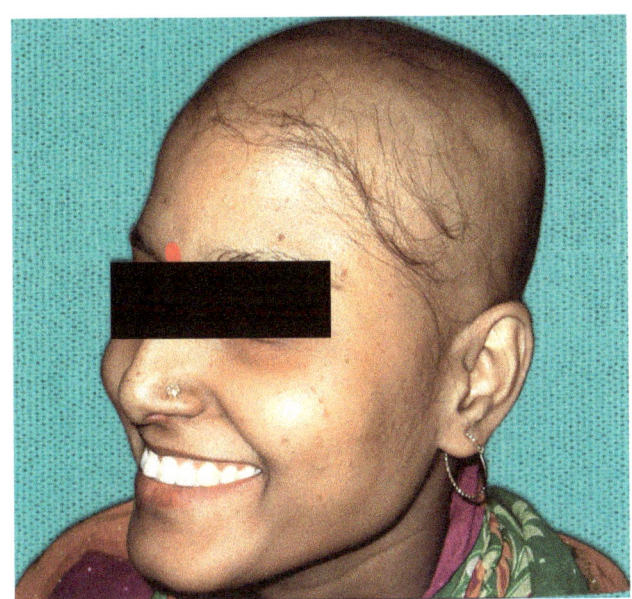

Fig. 2.1: Chemotherapy-induced non-scarring alopecia *(temporary relief of symptoms at the cost of hairs!)*

Non-scarring

- Androgenetic alopecia (male-pattern baldness)
- Alopecia areata
- Telogen effluvium
- Traction alopecia
- Tinea capitis
- Trichotillomania (self-induced hair-pulling)
- Lymphoma, leukemias
- Cosmetic treatment
- Bullous pemphigoid
- Systemic lupus erythematosus (SLE)
- Metabolic—iron deficiency anemia, hypothyroidism, diabetes mellitus
- Drugs—anticancer chemotherapy (Fig. 2.1), oral contraceptive pills, heparin, isotretinoin, lithium
- Miscellaneous—malnutrition, deficiency of protein/zinc/iron, pregnancy.

TRACTION ALOPECIA

Mechanical damage type of hair loss; from repeated tugging and pulling of the hair back into a bun or tight plating, and is usually caused by hair dressing styles or special headgear (e.g. turban wearing Sikhs in India).

PSEUDOPELADE

No cause known. Atrophic, adherent, depressed scarred areas or irregular plaques are seen; stray hair present without any sign of inflammation → may gradually enlarge leaving a shiny scalp without any visible follicular orifice.

TRICHOTILLOMANIA (HAIR PULLING TICS)

Compulsive desire of twisting and pulling of scalp hair; partially alopecic area is formed with irregularly broken, twisted hair growing in different directions.

TELOGEN EFFLUVIUM

Diffuse hair loss occurring 3 months after pregnancy or a severe illness (e.g. septicemia, typhoid meningism) → due to stress, putting all the hairs into the telogen phase of hair shedding at the same time. Full recovery with normal hair growth occurs within a few months.

ALOPECIA AREATA

Localized or patchy hair loss in scalp (Fig. 2.2) which is sharply defined; immune-mediated → commonly seen in children or young adults with patches of baldness

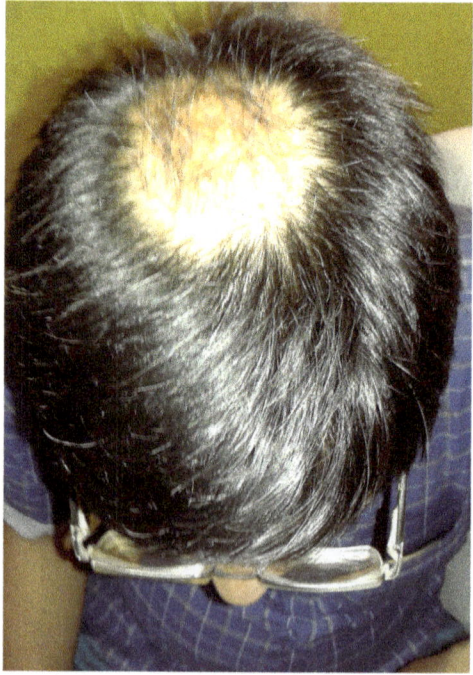

Fig. 2.2: Alopecia areata in scalp

→ broken 'exclamation mark' hair (i.e. narrow at the scalp, and wider and more pigmented at the tip) seen at the periphery of bald area is diagnostic → rare progression to total scalp *(alopecia totalis)* or the entire body *(alopecia universalis)*. Regrowth may occur which is initially replaced by white hairs and may take months to cover the patchy area of baldness in alopecia areata.
- Three types of alopecia, i.e. alopecia areata, alopecia totalis and alopecia universalis
- Differential diagnosis of alopecia areata are trichotillomania, tinea capitis, and alopecia due to SLE or secondary syphilis.

MALE-PATTERN BALDNESS

This type of hair loss is seen primarily at vertex and bitemporal region of scalp in males. The thinning of the hair is asymptomatic and gradual. This type of baldness is seen in females after menopause.

MANAGEMENT

- Reassurance as alopecia puts the person under social and psychological stress
- Wig, camouflage, creative hair style or hair prosthesis, autologous hair transplantation or hair grafting may be of help
- ***Topical immunotherapy:*** Allergic contact sensitization with dinitrochlorbenzene (DNCB), diphencyprone or PUVA (Psoralen and ultraviolet A therapy) may be beneficial
- ***Steroids:*** topical steroids or intralesional injection of steroids (e.g. triamcinolone in alopecia areata) may be given
- Topical 2% minoxidil application or systemic finasteride may be of some help in androgenetic alopecia
- 308 nm xenom chloride excimer laser has been reported to be beneficial after 11-12 sessions, when used in alopecia areata.

THE PEARLS

Examine the scalp, often with the help of a magnifying glass. Examine the patient overall, especially eyebrows and eyelashes.

Initial investigations after history-taking and thorough clinical examination are full blood count, serum ferritin and total protein, thyroid profile, antinuclear antibody (ANA) and serum testosterone.

3
Alteration of Facial Contour

ASYMMETRY OF FACE

- Hemiatrophy (e.g. linear scleroderma-en-coup de sabre)
- Hemihypertrophy
- Residual Bell's palsy (Fig. 3.1)
- Lipodystrophy
- Unilateral facial edema (angioneurotic edema, postural)
- Paget's disease (osteitis deformans)—face seems to be an inverted triangle
- Fibrous dysplasia
- Absence of condyle of mandible (congenital)
- Massive swelling of parotid gland (e.g. mixed parotid tumor, Mikulicz's syndrome)
- Acromegaly with prognathism
- Micrognathia (small mandible or receding chin), e.g. Pierre-Robin syndrome or Treacher Collins syndrome
- Hemifacial spasm (irregular, painless, clonic contraction involving one half of face, and is commonly due to sequelae of Bell's palsy, compressive lesion of facial nerve, trauma or demyelination)
- Plexiform neurofibromatosis
- Absence of teeth or bad (ill-fitted) dentures.

In Parry-Romberg syndrome, the facial hemiatrophy may be associated with atrophy of skin, tongue, gingiva, soft palate, subcutaneous fat, muscle, bone and cartilage of nose/ear; it is a variety of lipodystrophy (Fig. 3.2).

COMMON CAUSES OF BILATERAL FACIAL PALSY OF LOWER MOTOR NEURON TYPE (FACIAL DIPLEGIA)

- Acute infective polyneuritis (Guillain-Barré syndrome)
- Leprosy
- Sarcoidosis
- Forceps delivery
- Leukemia or lymphoma (deposits in parotids)

Chapter 3 Alteration of Facial Contour

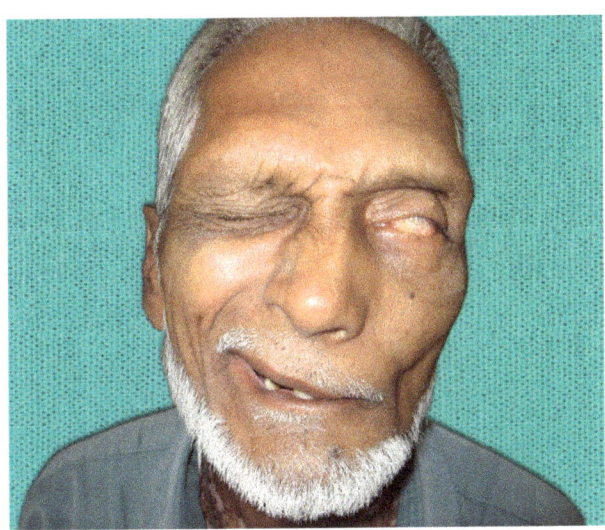

Fig. 3.1: Left sided Bell's palsy producing alteration of facial contour by deviation of face to the right side on showing the teeth. Bell's phenomenon is noted on forced closure of eyes.

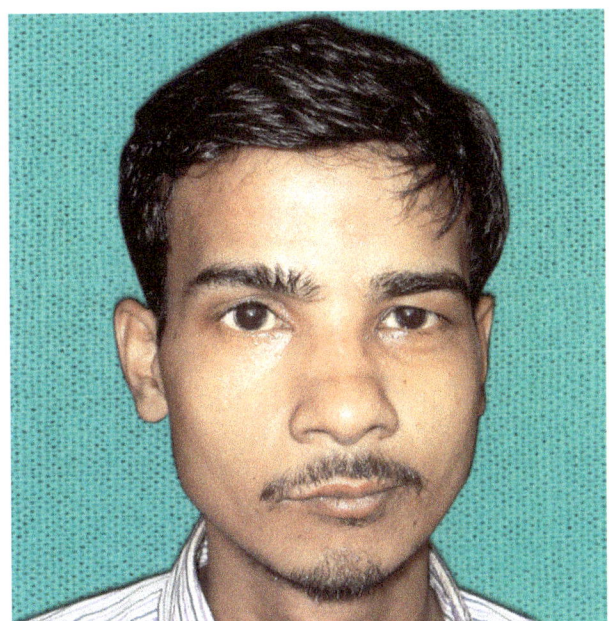

Fig. 3.2: Facial hemiatrophy (left): A patient of Parry-Romberg syndrome

- Bilateral Bell's palsy
- Bilateral otitis media
- Diphtheria.

> Myasthenia gravis and myopathy develop into facial weakness; there is no involvement of facial nerve.

PROGNATHISM (BULL-DOG JAW OR LANTERN JAW)

It is the prominence of mandible and is diagnosed clinically by inspection and observing the lower incisors (mandible) protruding in front of the upper incisors (maxilla); it is seen in:
- Acromegaly
- Fragile-X syndrome
- Nemaline myopathy
- A particular variety of osteopetrosis.

LIMB LENGTH INEQUALITY

- Achondroplasia
- Fibrous dysplasia
- Congenital asymmetry (coxa vara, short femur/tibia) (Fig. 3.3)
- Epiphyseal trauma
- Dislocation of hip joint
- Arteriovenous malformations in one limb
- Osteitis.

HEMIHYPERTROPHY

It is commonly known as ***Klippel-Trenaunay syndrome*** which is internally associated with a spinal cord vascular malformation and externally featured by

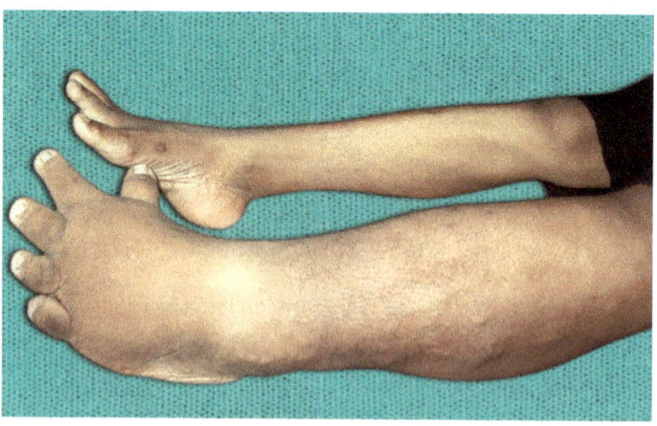

Fig. 3.3: Hypertrophied, deformed and asymmetrical left lower extremity (congenital)—unilateral

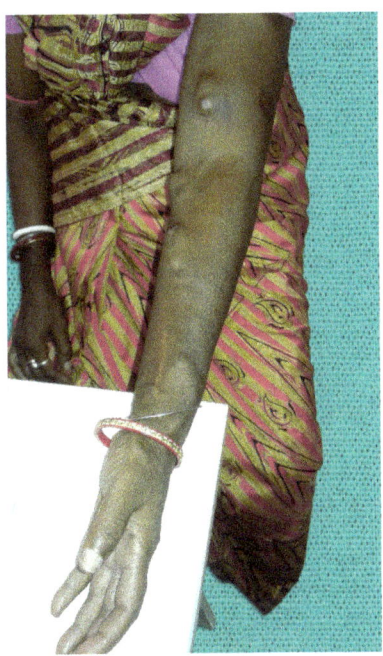

Fig. 3.4: Hemihypertrophy of left upper extremity in a patient of chronic renal failure with continuous hemodialysis done through Brescia-Cimino (artificially made arteriovenous shunt) fistula made in left hand

hemangioma of the trunk or upper or lower extremity + hypertrophy of hemangiomatous limb. The cord lesion may bleed and leads to spinal sensorimotor paralysis.

Hemihypertrophy is also found in congenital arteriovenous fistula or acquired arteriovenous fistula (Brescia-Cimino fistula artificially made for hemodialysis) (Fig. 3.4) in a limb, neurofibromatosis, Russell-Silver syndrome or is idiopathic.

THE PEARLS

Alteration of facial contour may be developmental which may have no importance but many a time a close inspection of face may pin-point some clinical entity. Thus, it may be regarded as a 'window in clinical medicine'.

4

Angular Stomatitis

DEFINITION

Cracking with inflammation of the skin at the angle or corner of mouth. To start with, there is redness → fissuring → crusting (Fig. 4.1).

Stomatitis is inflammation involving oral mucous membranes.

CLINICAL ASSOCIATIONS

- Excessive use of betel-leaf, tobacco, alcohol or chewing masala
- Improperly-fitted denture
- Iron deficiency anemia (associated with glossitis and koilonychia)
- Riboflavin, nicotinic acid, folic acid or pyridoxine deficiency
- Starvation or malnutrition
- Herpes labialis, candidiasis or streptococcal infection at the angle of mouth
- Habitual lip-licking, especially in children.

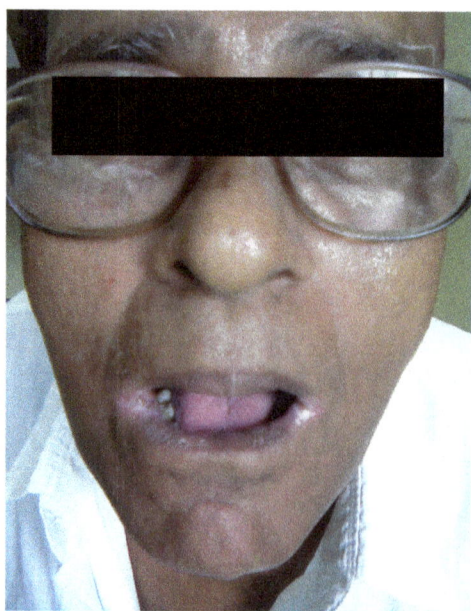

Fig. 4.1: Angular stomatitis due to deficiency of vitamin B-complex and iron

Angular stomatitis leaves no scar on healing.

PERLECHE

- Painful small fissures at the angle of mouth (angular cheilitis)
- Often covered with yellow crusts
- Associated with candidiasis or secondary syphilis.

RHAGADES

- Linear scars at the angles of mouth and nose
- Commonly seen in congenital syphilis.

SWOLLEN LIPS

- Injury
- Angioneurotic edema
- Herpetic infection
- Urticarial rash
- Acromegaly.

GLOSSITIS

- ***Bald tongue:*** There is loss or atrophy of papillae, and is found in iron deficiency anemia, pernicious anemia, tropical sprue and syphilis
- ***Raw-beefy tongue:*** Red, swollen and painful tongue found in vitamin B12 deficiency and pellagra
- ***Median rhomboid glossitis:*** A lozenge-shaped denuded area in the middle of the tongue posteriorly; congenital and of no value clinically
- ***Miscellaneous:*** Chronic superficial glossitis, leukoplakia, fungal infection of tongue, geographic tongue, folic acid deficiency.

 THE PEARLS

Angular stomatitis is common in the community. Usually it indicates iron and/or vitamin deficiency, or malnutrition, which may indicate malabsorption, or lethal disease like occult carcinoma or lymphoma.

5

Aseptic Fever

NON-INFECTIVE (ASEPTIC) CAUSES OF FEVER

- Drug fever—virtually any drug may produce unexplained pyrexia but the main drugs in the list are rifampicin, sulphonamides, methyldopa, procainamide, different vaccines, following anticancer chemotherapy
- Connective tissue diseases, e.g. systemic lypus erythematosus (SLE), rheumatoid arthritis, polymyalgia rheumatica, temporal arteritis, polyarteritis nodosa
- Malignancies
  - Carcinomas (especially of lung, liver and kidney)
  - Lymphomas
  - Leukemias and other hematological malignancies
- Thyroid storm
- Pontine hemorrhage
- Heat stroke
- Crush injury
- Over-atropinisation or dhatura poisoning
- Acute myocardial infarction
- Gout
- Radiation sickness
- Malignant hyperthermia (halothane-induced) or neuroleptic malignant syndrome (haloperidol-induced).

FEVER ASSOCIATED WITH MACULOPAPULAR RASH

- ***Measles:*** Usually appears on the fourth day of illness, maculopapular in type. Rash first appears at the back of the ears, and at the junction of skin and hair on the forehead; ultimately face, neck, trunk, limbs upto palms and soles may be affected. The density of rash is greatest on the forehead. They are discrete, pink and blanch on pressure. Later, the rashes become confluent and give rise to characteristic blotchy appearance (morbilliform rash)
- ***Infectious mononucleosis:*** Rash in this disease usually follows administration of penicillin or ampicillin for a presumed pharyngitis. Associated suggestive features are generalized lymphadenopathy along with splenomegaly
- ***Meningococcemia:*** Usually the rash is hemorrhagic but for the first 12–24 hours it may occasionally be erythematous and maculopapular simulating rash of measles.

Usually it is a disease of children and young adults with characteristic short prodrome (unlike measles and scarlet fever), a rapidly changing rash, pallor and toxicity

- **Toxic shock syndrome:** This is a disease of females with staphylococcal infection, commonly associated with the use of tampons. The patient is acutely ill with vomiting and diarrhea, headache and myalgia which progresses towards shock and rapidly developing maculoerythematous rash
- **Scarlet fever:** The rash first appears behind the ears on the second day and rapidly becomes generalized punctate erythema which is mostly abundant in flexures of the arms and legs. The affected children usually have a flushed face due to fever; the rash does not affect the face. The 'strawberry' and 'raspberry' tongue may give some clue
- **Rubella:** The rash (pink macules) usually begins on the second or third day on face and neck (like measles) but progresses much more rapidly than measles, and become generalized within 24–48 hours. Postauricular and occipital lymphadenopathy are characteristic
- **Enteric fever:** Rose spots are sparse, small rose-red, blanching, slightly raised macules mainly present over upper abdomen and chest during the end of the first week of illness. It is usually visible only on fair-skinned persons. Rarely, these rashes can evolve into non-blanching small hemorrhages
- **Dengue:** Primary rashes appear on the third day of illness, which are erythematous (diffuse flushing) and present over face (Fig. 5.1), neck and shoulder. Secondary or true rash are measly or morbilliform which appears on the sixth day of illness and is usually present over the dosrum of hands and feet. Ultimately, the rash becomes generalized (mostly over the trunk) except the face. The rash may persist from 2 hours to several days and terminates by desquamation. Classically, there is associated saddle-back pyrexia

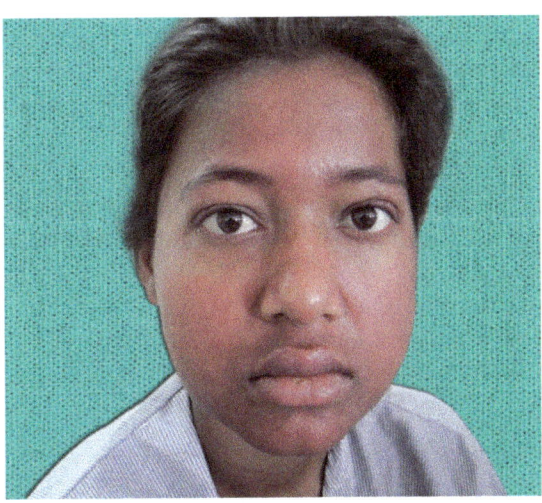

Fig. 5.1: Facial erythematous (diffuse flushing) rash in dengue fever

- ***Acquired immune deficiency syndrome (AIDS):*** A mononucleosis-like syndrome may be seen 2-6 weeks after acquisition of human immunodeficiency virus (HIV) infection. The rash (occurs in 50% patients) is macular, erythematous, and predominantly affects the trunk. The illness is associated with pyrexia, perspiration, lethargy, arthralgia, myalgia and generalized lymphadenopathy.
- ***Typhus:*** Different varieties of typhus like epidemic and endemic typhus, Rocky Mountain spotted fever, scrub typhus and rickettsialpox are associated with pyrexia and rash
- ***Kawasaki disease:*** The affected children may have a polymorphous rash along with fever, conjunctivitis, red lips and red tongue, red indurated hands and cervical lymphadenopathy.

These are the causes of fever with morbilliform rash too.

APPEARANCE OF RASH IN A FEBRILE PATIENT

Mnemonic: 'Very sick person must take double tea', which stands for—
1st day: Varicella (chickenpox)
2nd day: Scarlet fever
3rd day: Pox (smallpox; eradicated globally)
4th day: Measles
5th day: Typhus
6th day: Dengue
7th day: Typhoid or enteric fever.

PYREXIA OF UNKNOWN ORIGIN (PUO)

Definition (by Petersdorf and Beeson, 1961):
- Fever more than 101°F on several occasions
- A duration of fever more than 3 weeks
- Failure to reach a provisional diagnosis after 1 week of inpatient investigations or by 3 outpatient visits.

Later on, PUO has been classified into four different types (Durack and Street, 1991):
1. ***Classic PUO*** (as previous definition except the time frame which is 3 outpatient department [OPD] visits or 3 days in hospital)—hidden infection, obscure malignancy or collagen vascular diseases
2. ***Nosocomial PUO*** (hospital-acquired)
3. ***Neutropenic PUO*** (when neutrophil count is ≤ 500/mm^3)
4. ***HIV-associated PUO*** (e.g. tuberculosis, non-Hodgkin's lymphoma [NHL], drug fever).

DISEASES INITIALLY PRESENT AS PUO

- Collagen vascular diseases or autoimmune rheumatic diseases, e.g. SLE, rheumatoid arthritis

- Lymphomas, leukemias, carcinomas or multiple myeloma
- Tuberculosis, liver abscess, AIDS, brucellosis
- Factitious fever, drug fever, habitual hyperthermia.

CLINICAL EXAMINATION OF PUO WHICH NEEDS SPECIAL ATTENTION

- *Oral cavity:* Teeth and gum for sepsis
- *Thyroid:* Enlargement and tenderness → thyroiditis
- *Eye:* Phlyctenular conjunctivitis and other manifestations of systemic disease
- *Lymph nodes:* With special attention to cervical and epitrochlear nodes
- *Bone:* Sternal tenderness, gibbus with tenderness
- *Musculoskeletal system:* Still's disease, systemic onset juvenile idiopathic arthritis.
- *Skin:* Rashes and nodules
- *Blood vessels:* Evidences of vasculitis/arteritis (temporal arteritis)
- *Cardiovascular system:* Murmurs and pericardial rub
- *Respiratory system:* Pleural rub, basal pneumonia
- *Gastrointestinal tract:* Enlargement of liver, spleen or kidney, tenderness of renal angle
- *Intercostal tenderness:* Amebic liver abscess/empyema thoracis
- *Genitalia:* Phimosis, discharge per urethra, any swelling, epididymitis (filarial/tubercular)
- *Per rectal or vaginal examination:* Abscess, tumors
- *Fundoscopy:* Choroid tubercles (i.e. miliary tuberculosis)
- *Covered area, if any:* Breast abscess, any sepsis under bandages/plasters.

FEVER WITH LEUKOCYTOSIS BUT WITHOUT INFECTION

- Acute pancreatitis
- Diabetic ketoacidosis
- Acute myocardial infarction
- Gout.

POSSIBILITIES IN COMBINATION WITH ARTHRITIS, FEVER AND RASH

- Viral infections (rubella, parvovirus B19)
- Gonococcemia or meningococcemia
- Periodic fever syndrome
- Acute rheumatic fever
- Systemic lupus erythematosus (Fig. 5.2)
- Adult Still's disease
- Sarcoidosis
- Serum sickness

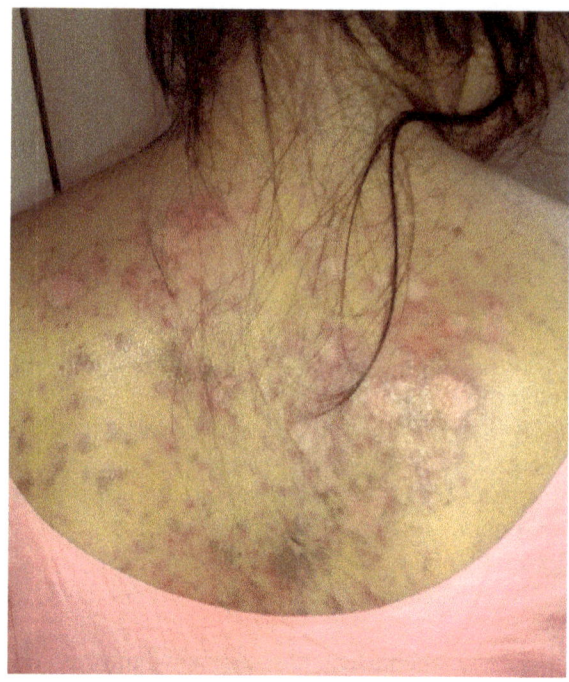

Fig. 5.2: Patient with systemic lupus erythematosus (SLE) having aseptic fever and rash

- Secondary syphilis
- Familial mediterranean fever (FMF)
- Vasculitis
- Lyme disease.

THE PEARLS

Fever is a headache and PUO is a nightmare for the attending doctor. Meticulous history taking and repeated clinical examination many a time, gives clue to the diagnosis in PUO. Pyrexia and pain are two common symptoms which compels the patient to attend a doctor or clinic.

6

Bald Tongue

DEFINITION

Total loss or atrophy of the papillae resulting in a smooth or plane dorsum of the tongue.

CLUE TO DIAGNOSIS

- ***Iron deficiency anemia*** (most common cause) (Fig. 6.1)
  ↓
  History of (H/O) bleeding piles, menorrhagia or melena; intake of NSAIDs (non steroidal anti-inflammatory drug); dietary history is important; enquire ***H/O pica*** (eating of strange substances like mud, ice, etc.); working bare-footed (hookworm infestation)
  ↓
  Look for anemia, glossitis, angular stomatitis, cheilosis, koilonychia, mild splenomegaly (rarely found)
  ↓
  Enquire for dysphagia, specially in middle-aged women (Plummer-Vinson syndrome or Paterson-Kelly syndrome)

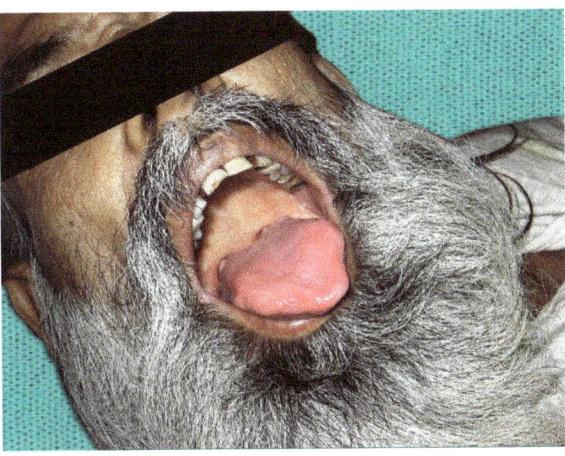

Fig. 6.1: Bald tongue developing due to iron deficiency anemia

↓

Investigate blood for hemoglobin (Hb%), peripheral smear red blood cell (RBC) morphology, color index, serum iron (Fe), total iron binding capacity (TIBC), and stool for occult blood and hookworm ova

↓

Examine per rectally or per vaginally, along with upper and lower gastrointestinal (GI) endoscopy in search for a carcinoma of large gut/peptic ulcer or fibroid of uterus.

- **Pellagra**
  - Dermatitis found in nicotinic acid deficiency.
  - Seen in exposed part with erythema and desquamation.
  - There may be roughening and pigmentation.
  - Dermatitis in the neck (Casal's collar) is pathognomonic.
  - Associated cheilosis, angular stomatitis and raw-beefy tongue.
- **Pernicious anemia**

↓

Strict vegetarian or H/O gastrectomy

↓

H/O glossitis, cheilitis, tingling and numbness, or premature graying of hair

↓

M = F; around age of 60 years

↓

Investigate peripheral blood smear with mean corpuscular volume (MCV), mean corpuscular hemoglobin concentration (MCHC), RBC morphology (it is the most common cause of vitamin B12 deficiency in temperate climate); histamine-fast achlorhydria and positive Schilling's test

- **Tropical sprue (Fig. 6.2)**

↓

Residents or visitors to tropical regions

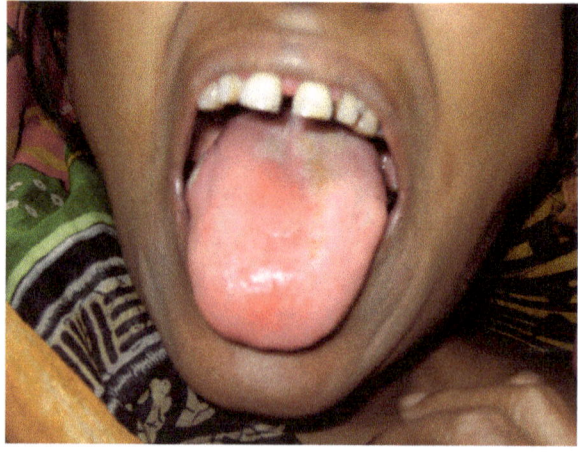

Fig. 6.2: Young girl with glossitis as a result of tropical sprue

↓

H/O malabsorption
↓

Clinical features like anorexia, diarrhea, ↓ weight, anemia and features of different nutritional deficiency like glossitis, cheilosis
↓

Deficiency of Fe, folic acid and vitamin B12
↓

Investigate for ↑ fecal fat, and positive D-xylose absorption test
↓

Positive jejunal biopsy with shortened and thickened villi, ↑ crypt depth, infiltration of mononuclear cells in lamina propria and epithelium.

- **Syphilis**
↓

Young adult with H/O exposure
↓

Clinical features like skin rash, condyloma lata, lymphadenopathy and snail track ulcers in mouth
↓

Along with bald tongue, mucous patches in lips, oral mucosa, palate, pharynx, vulva, vagina, glans penis or inner prepuce may be seen
↓

Investigate VDRL (Venereal Disease Research Laboratory Test), Kahn test, FTA-ABS (fluorescent treponemal antibody-absorption) or TPI (treponema pallidum immobilization) test.

In iron deficiency anemia (microcytic-hypochromic anemia) MCV, MCH and MCHC are low; both serum Fe and ferritin are low but TIBC is increased. Pernicious anemia is a macrocytic anemia with high MCV, MCH and MCHC.
  Remember, in anemia due to chronic systemic diseases like rheumatoid arthritis, systemic lupus erythematosus (SLE), etc. serum Fe is low, TIBC is low but serum ferritin is normal or elevated.

WHITE PATCHES IN TONGUE

- ***Leukoplakia of tongue***
    - Look for sharp teeth, ill-fitting dentures, sepsis (chronic infection), H/O chewing tobacco or smoking or consuming alcohol, syphilis (rare, nowadays)
    - Premalignant condition
    - Superficial layer of tongue shows extensive keratinization and cornification (causes whiteness of the patch)
    - If non-responsive to conservative treatment, biopsy should be done to exclude malignancy.

- Hairy leukoplakia [serrated white areas in margins of tongue; painless and are due to Epstein-Barr virus (EBV) infection in a patient of AIDS]
- Candidiasis of tongue
- Severe and chronic iron deficiency anemia.

Except in candidiasis, all the above white plaques are adherent to tongue.
6 'S' in leukoplakia are sharp teeth, sepsis, smoking, spirits, syphilis and spices.

 THE PEARLS

Treat bald tongue with iron and vitamin B-complex. Often the bald tongue indicates iron deficiency anemia—chronic blood loss or gastric carcinoma in an aged person (or occult carcinoma).

Leukoplakia, many a time, is the forerunner of carcinoma of the tongue. So, examination of the tongue forms an essential part of clinical examination.

7

Bedsores

WHAT ARE BEDSORES?
These are denuded areas of skin, usually over the bony prominences, formed as a result of prolonged bed rest or immobilization. Bedsore is also known as ***pressure sore*** or ***decubitus ulcer***.

PREDISPOSING FACTORS
- Prolonged bed rest or immobilization as a result of deep coma, paraplegia, hemiplegia or fracture in lower limbs, or severe form of arthritis
- Patients with history of urinary (i.e. bed-wetting, especially at night) or fecal incontinence.
- Lengthy stay in bed without change of posture (i.e. without frequent turning)
- Associated with anemia, malnutrition, diabetes mellitus or any immunodeficiency, peripheral vascular disease or peripheral neuropathy.

COMMON SITES (FIGS 7.1 AND 7.2)
- Sacrum (classical bedsore)
- On the lateral malleoli, heels
- Shoulder blades
- Back of the heels or feet
- Occiput
- Elbows
- Hips (skin of buttocks/sides over greater trochanters) or knees
- Pressure exerted by any mechanical device applying shearing force, e.g. skeletal traction point.

ETIOPATHOGENESIS
It is believed that bedsores develop when the skin and the tissue below it becomes damaged due to non-adequate flow of blood. The basic pathogenesis is due to:
- Loss of muscular action upon the circulation
- Vasomotor paralysis due to destruction of the vasoconstrictor fibers and
- Partly due to disuse.

Poor nutrition of the patient is an added factor.

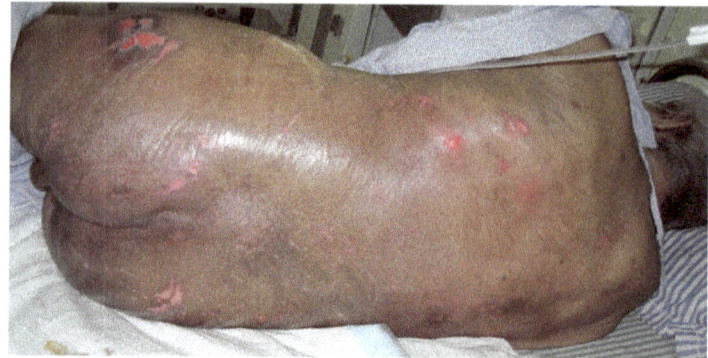

Fig. 7.1: Bedsores—denuded skin over bony prominences at back of a debilitated patient

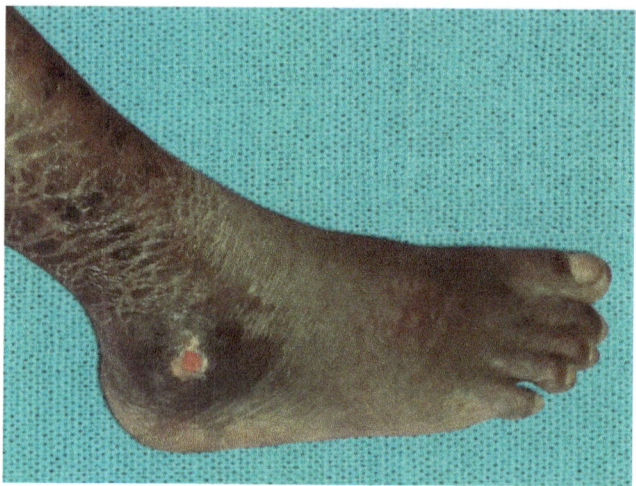

Fig. 7.2: Trophic ulcer over lateral malleolus in a patient of peripheral neuropathy developing from lepromatous leprosy

STAGING

Bedsores may range from mild reddening of the skin to large non-healing, nagging ulcers which, at times, may extend into muscles and bones. They are described on the basis of four stages:
- ***Stage I:*** Red, painful, warmer skin which does not blanch
- ***Stage II:*** Skin breaks open and forms an ulcer, which looks like an abrasion, blister or crater. Painful and tender
- ***Stage III:*** Ulcer gets worse and extends into the subcutaneous tissue, forming a small crater. Subcutaneous fat may be affected but not muscle, tendon or bone
- ***Stage IV:*** Ulcer becomes deep with extensive tissue necrosis and destruction, leading to damage of muscle, tendon and bone. Exposed bone or muscle is visible or directly palpable. Infection may complicate any stage.

PREVENTION AND TREATMENT

Prevention

- Repositioning in a wheelchair
- ***Repositioning in bed:*** Change position in bed in every 2 hours (i.e. frequent turning). Water-beds, foam mattress pad or a water-filled mattress is used to help positioning, relieving pressure and protect vulnerable areas. Adjust the elevation of bed and use cushions to protect bony areas
- ***Skin care:*** Clean the affected skin with mild soap and warm water or a no-rinse cleanser. Protect the skin with talcum powder to avoid excess moisture. Inspect the skin daily for any area of redness, blister, etc. Prevent soiling of the skin by urine (use catheter) or feces (use rectal tube); use protective lotions in healthy skin with frequent change of diaper. A good nursing care is must
- ***Nutrition:*** Good nutritious diet with sufficient water to keep the skin hydrated
- ***Miscellaneous:*** The patient should quit smoking and stay active in bed. Treatment of anemia and diabetes should be done simultaneously. Monitor complete hemogram, blood sugar, serum proteins, creatinine and electrolytes. A daily exercise in bed matched with the ability of the patient is encouraged. A physiotherapist may help in appropriate exercise program.

Treatment

Bedsores increase the morbidity in hospitalized patients. They progress rapidly and often very difficult to treat. Stage I and II bedsores usually heal within weeks to months but stages III and IV refuse to heal. Major outlines of treatment are:
- A primary care physician, specialising in wound care, oversees the treatment plan
- Wound care—regular cleaning and applying dressing (stages III and IV)
- Debridement
- Pain management
- Infection control—swab the wound and treat specific infections by local or systemic antibiotic [with special reference to methicillin-resistant *Staphylococcus aureus* (MRSA) infection]
- Good nutritious diet. Proper hydration of the patient
- If surgery (flap reconstruction) is considered, a team of Neurosurgeon, Orthopedic Surgeon and Plastic Surgeon should be consulted.

THE PEARLS

Bedsores are easier to prevent than to treat. The attending physician should remember that anemia, malnutrition, diabetes mellitus or any immunodeficiency increases the chance of development of bedsores in a susceptible patient. Bedsores may be complicated by superadded infections, which may lead to death of the patient by developing into septicemia.

8

Blackish Urine

POSSIBILITIES

Though very rare, black discoloration of urine often puzzles the clinicians.

- **Alkaptonuria:** The urine becomes black on standing, often after voiding (Fig. 8.1). If collected in a test tube, it starts blackening from above downwards. The urine blackens on alkalinization too. Confirmation of the diagnosis is done by chromatographic and spectophotometric study of urine which demonstrate presence of homogentisic acid. It is due to deficiency of homogentisic acid oxidase in human body. The other name of the disease is **ochronosis**. The brown stain of the napkin of infants makes the parents suspicious of some serious illness; the child may have gray-brown sclera or bluish-black discoloration of ear cartilage. The adults may present with arthritis of big joints while the roentgenography of spine may reveal calcification of intervertebral discs

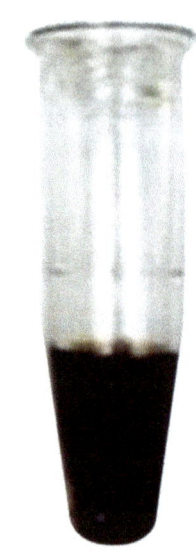

Fig. 8.1: Black urine in a patient of alkaptonuria (ochronosis)

- **Tyrosinosis:** An autosomal recessive disorder of tyrosine aminotransferase deficiency associated with hepatic and renal tubular dysfunction
- **Melanuria:** In disseminated melanoma, melanogen present in urine gives the black discoloration
- **Poisoning with phenol or cresol:** Addition of ferric chloride turns the urine into blue or violet color
- **Drugs:** Quinine, methyldopa or porphyrin therapy.

Blackwater fever due to severe *Plasmodium falciparum* infection produces red urine.

TREATMENT

- Relieve anxiety—reassurance

- Adequate fluid intake to prevent renal insufficiency in cases of drug-induced or poisoning-induced black urine
- Treatment of the specific cause.

DIFFERENT COLOR CHANGES IN URINE

Normally, fresh urine is clear to straw-yellow colored, and the color varies from person to person and from day to day. The color of normal urine is due to urochrome and uroerythrin pigments. In normal condition, urine darkens on standing because of oxidation of colorless urobilinogen to colored urobilin. The different color changes in urine are:
1. **Red urine:** *See* Chapter 65
2. **Pink or dark orange:** Rifampicin, senna
3. **Yellowish-brown:** Nitrofurantoin, furazolidone, sulfasalazine, riboflavin
4. **Milky-white:** *See* Chapter 78
5. **Black urine:** Already described
6. **Deep yellow:** Concentrated urine, jaundice
7. **Cloudy:** Presence of pus cells, blood, cellular debris or crystals (phosphates or urates)
8. **Green urine:** *Pseudomonas* infection in urine, drugs (methylene blue, propofol).

BLACK STOOL

- Melena (***altered blood in stool*** due to production of acid hematin)
- Ingestion of iron as hematinic (produces hard stool in contrast to melena which is semisolid in consistensy)
- Ingestion of bismuth (used in treatment of duodenal ulcer)
- Intake of liquorice, charcoal (used in treating poisoning) or blackberries.

Other than melena all are non-sticky black stools and often known as ***pseudo-melena***.
   Melena stool is black/tarry, semisolid and with offensive odor; red-colored fluid comes out from it after addition of water, and the patient usually complains of vertigo, dizziness or syncopal attack during defecation.

THE PEARLS

The patient himself/herself tells the doctor about the color changes in urine if it deviates from normal color. The diseases developing into black urine are rare and their treatment is unsatisfactory. However, it is another 'window in clinical medicine'.

9

Blue Fingers/Toes

PROLOGUE

Blue fingers or toes are seen in vasospasm due to any condition, commonly as a result of Raynaud's phenomenon. True cyanosis (central or peripheral) is also responsible for blueness in finger/toe-tips and nail-beds.

RAYNAUD'S PHENOMENON (FIG. 9.1)

It is a vasospastic disorder (i.e. intense vasospasm of peripheral arteries), manifested clinically by the classical 'triphasic color response' which is sequential development of digital blanching (pallor due to vasospasm), cyanosis (blue due to sluggish blood flow) and rubor (redness due to vasodilatation or reactive hyperaemia) of the fingers and toes following cold exposure and subsequent rewarming. Some patients may develop only pallor and cyanosis, while others may experience cyanosis only. The changes in the fingers and toes are often diagnosed by nail-fold capillography. The fingers are affected more commonly than the toes. The duration of the attack is variable but may last for hours. Numbness, burning or paraesthesia, and severe pain in the digits are common features. Usually cold and stress are recognized precipitating factors.

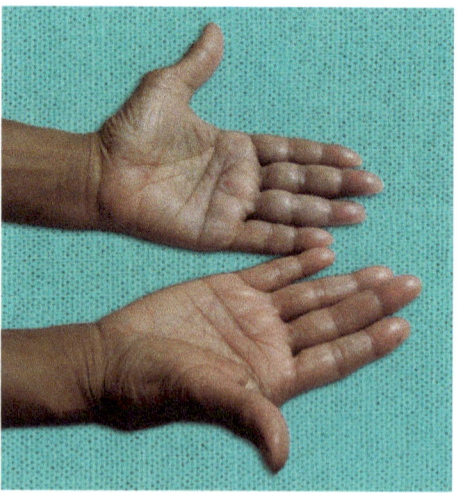

Fig. 9.1: A patient with Raynaud's phenomenon in systemic lupus erythematosus (the rewarming rubor phase just after phase of blueness)

Mechanism

- Exaggerated reflex sympathetic vasoconstriction
- Enhanced digital vascular responsiveness to cold or to normal sympathetic stimuli.

Color	Mechanism	Clinical features
Pallor (white)	Vasospasm (ischemia)	Pain and numbness
Cyanosis (blue)	Subsequent venular spasm (stasis)	Pain and numbness
Rubor (red)	Vasodilatation (reperfusion)	Warmth, throbbing pain

Common Causes

It is of two types—primary and secondary.
1. ***Primary Raynaud's phenomenon:*** Raynaud's disease (F > M, 15–30 years, bilateral and symmetrical, no cause found, fingers > toes); positive family history may be there; over 50% of patients with Raynaud's phenomenon have Raynaud's disease. Rarely, the earlobes and the tip of the nose may be involved. The radial, ulnar and pedal pulses remain normal as it is a disease of arterioles; it does not progress to digital ulceration or infarction. Long-acting preparation of nifedipine may be of some help
2. ***Secondary Raynaud's phenomenon***
    - ***Collagen vascular diseases:*** Scleroderma, systemic lupus erythematosus (SLE), dermatomyositis, CREST (calcinosis, Raynaud's phenomenon, esophageal dysmotility, sclerodactyly, and telangiectasia) syndrome, mixed connective tissue disease (MCTD), rheumatoid arthritis
    - ***Obliterative arterial disease:*** Atherosclerosis, thoracic inlet syndrome, thromboangiitis obliterans
    - ***Occupational:*** Vibration tool injury, electric shock, exposure to cold (e.g. frost bite), piano playing, vinyl chloride, typing
    - ***Blood dyscrasias:*** Myeloproliferative disorders, hyperviscosity syndromes, cryoglobulinaemia
    - ***Neurologic disorders:*** Syringomyelia, carpal tunnel syndrome, spinal cord tumors.
    - ***Drug-induced:*** Ergot derivatives, β-blockers, methysergide, vinblastine or bleomycin
    - ***Miscellaneous:*** Pulmonary hypertension, crutch pressure, carcinoid syndrome.

OTHER VASOSPASTIC DISORDERS

- ***Pernio (chilblains)*** → Swelling of tips of toes with ulceration, often associated with pruritus and burning sensation → associated with cold exposure
- ***Erythromelalgia*** → M > F, feet > hands with burning pain and erythema of the extremities → may precipitate from myeloproliferative disorders, or nifedipine/bromocriptine-induced → precipitated by warm exposure and relieved by exposing to cool air or elevation of the limb

- Livedo reticularis (*see* Chapter 61)
- Frost bite
- Vasculitis due to any cause
- Acrocyanosis → persistent cyanosis of the hands, less frequently, the feet → resulting from arterial vasoconstriction and secondary dilatation of capillaries and venules → cold exposure increases the incidence. F > M and usually below 30 years of age. Asymptomatic with normal pulses and without any skin ulceration → differential diagnosis with Raynaud's phenomenon (acrocyanosis is persistent and not episodic, and blanching does not occur).

MANAGEMENT

- Reassurance. Avoid unnecessary exposure to cold or trauma. To wear gloves and mittens, protect the body with warm clothing and abstain from tobacco smoking. Avoid β-blockers, ergotamine and oral contraceptive pills
- ***Drugs:*** Reserved for severe cases
  - Nifedipine, amlodipine, diltiazem (calcium-channel blockers)
  - Losartan, topical nitroglycerin, low-dose aspirin or dipyridamole, statins (empirical use)
  - Prazosin, doxazocin, terazocin (α_1-adrenergic antagonist)
  - Methyldopa, guanethidine, phenoxybenzamine (sympatholytics)
  - Iloprost (prostacyclin analogue and an endogenous vasodilator)
  - Pentoxyfylline, naftidrofuryl, inositol nicotinate
  - Calcitonin gene-related peptide
  - The phosphodiesterase inhibitor sildenafil and tadalafil are very promising and effective; oral endothelin antagonist bosentan is currently being tried
  - Surgical sympathectomy.

ULCERS (DIGITAL) AT FINGER OR TOE-TIPS

- Raynaud's phenomenon, e.g. scleroderma (Fig. 9.2)
- Thromboangiitis obliterans
- Leprosy
- Diabetes mellitus
- Trauma
- Vasculitis
- Atherothrombosis.

ERYTHEMA OF FINGERS

- Dermatomyositis
- Frost bite
- Chilblains
- Rewarming phase of Raynaud's phenomenon (Fig. 9.1)
- Systemic lupus erythematosus
- Urticaria.

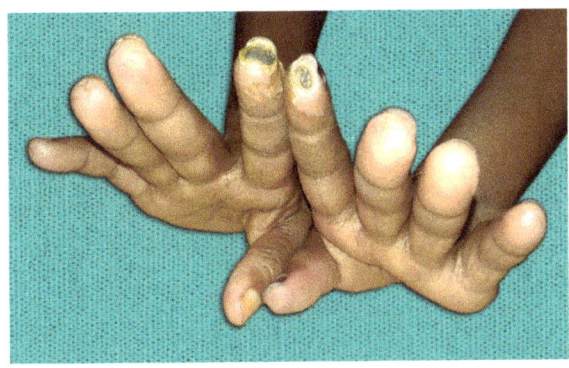

Fig. 9.2: Digital infarction (pitted scars) and digital ulceration in progressive systemic sclerosis (i.e. scleroderma)

REGIONAL CYANOSIS (BLUENESS)

- **One limb:** Arterial embolism or phlebothrombosis of a large vein with little collaterals
- **One finger or toe:** Vasculitis due to any etiology
- **Face and upper extremity:** Superior vena caval syndrome
- **Differential cyanosis**
  - **Blue feet:** Patent ductus arteriosus with reversal of shunt
  - **Blue hands:** Coarctation of aorta with transposition of great vessels
- **Acrocyanosis** (*see* previous page)
- **Erythrocyanosis** (young lady → with short skirts → exposure to cold).

🍐 THE PEARLS

Blue digits are always a medical emergency whether it is due to cyanosis, vasculitis or Raynaud's phenomenon. Thorough clinical examination along with detailed history may be beneficial to have an etiological diagnosis. The patient should be tackled by a rheumatologist or internist.

10

Blue Sclera

CLINICAL INVESTIGATION

Search for multiple fractures (generalized osteopenia makes the bone brittle), loose-jointedness and progressive deafness.
↓
A case of osteogenesis imperfecta (most common cause) (Fig. 10.1)
↓
Due to thinness of sclerae, the underneath choroid with its vessels give rise to blue tinge in the eyes (Fig. 10.2).
↓
Associated features: Pseudoarthrosis, sabre tibia, pectus excavatum or carinatum, kyphoscoliosis, blue-yellow teeth with dental abnormalities (dentinogenesis imperfecta), blue tympanic membrane, aortic incompetence or mitral valve prolapse.
↓
Four types commonly (Type I, II, III and IV), where II and III are severe types.

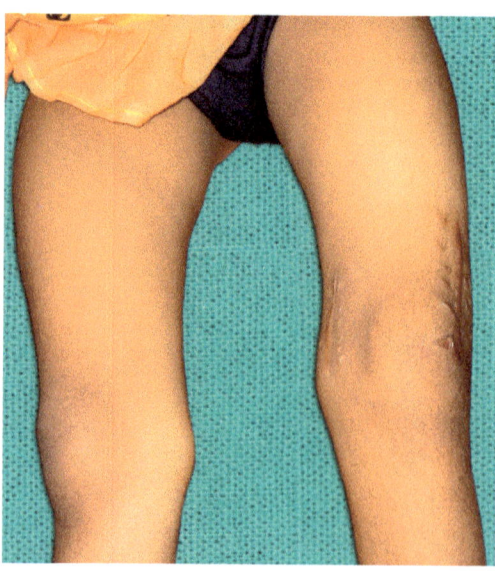

Fig. 10.1: Scar marks for repair of repeated femur fracture in osteogenesis imperfecta

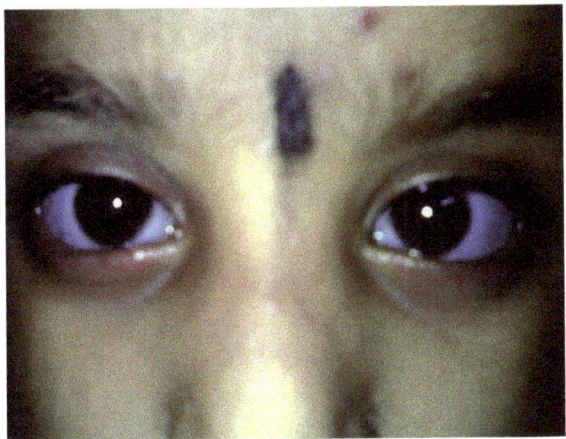

Fig. 10.2: Classical blue sclera in osteogenesis imperfecta

X-ray of skull reveals **Wormian bones** (small irregular bones related to sutures), especially in parietal bones.
Note: Treatment is not satisfactory but bisphosphonates (i.e. intravenous palmidronate) and stem cell therapy are tried.

DIFFERENTIAL DIAGNOSIS OF BLUE SCLERA

- Marfan's syndrome
- Hypophosphatasia
- Pseudohypoparathyroidism
- Brittle corneal syndrome
- Corneal encroachment of sclera
- Staphyloma
- Ehlers-Danlos syndrome (Figs 10.3 and 10.4)
- Pseudoxanthoma elasticum
- Newborn baby (underlying uveal tissue is visible due to thinness and immaturity of scleral collagen fibers)
- Pyknodysostosis
- Paget's disease.

DIFFERENTIAL DIAGNOSIS OF BLUISH DISCOLORATION OF BODY

- Cyanosis (cyanosed skin blanches on pressure)
- Sulfhemoglobinemia or methemoglobinemia
- ***Carbon monoxide poisoning:*** Cherry-red flush due to formation of carboxyhemoglobin
- ***Argyria:*** Deposition of silver salts in the skin due to silver poisoning. The skin does not blanch on pressure
- ***Amiodarone toxicity:*** The skin may take a bluish hue (ceruloderma).

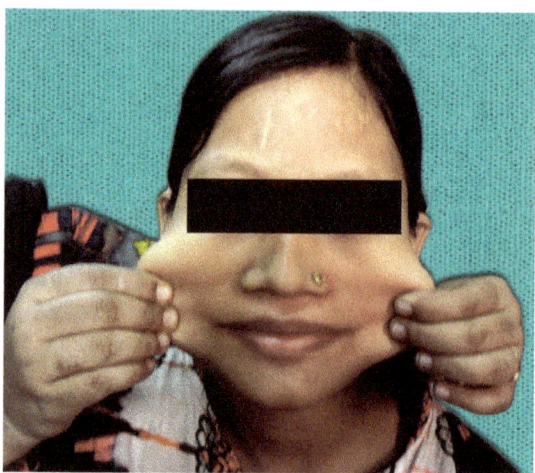

Fig. 10.3: Hyperextensible skin over face in Ehlers-Danlos syndrome

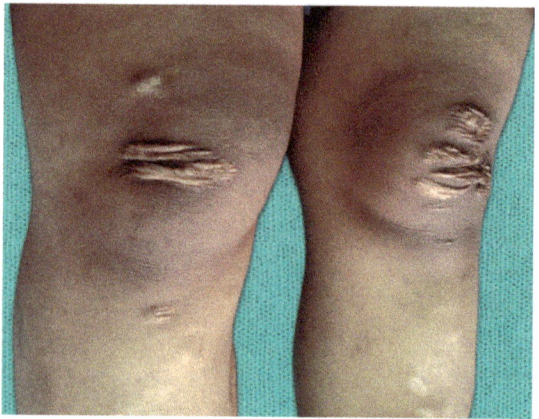

Fig. 10.4: Cigarette-paper scars over skin in Ehlers-Danlos syndrome

Blue vision has been recorded after use of sildenafil.

LOOSE-JOINTEDNESS

This term is sometimes used to describe hypermobile joints (Fig. 10.5). Joint hypermobility, the ability of a joint to move beyond its normal range of motion, is common in children (10–15%). It is a benign condition, which decreases with age. The patient may suffer from pain (e.g. back pain), sprain or scoliosis. Physiotherapy helps to strengthen the joints. Loose-jointedness is often termed as **double-jointedness**, and the major causes are:

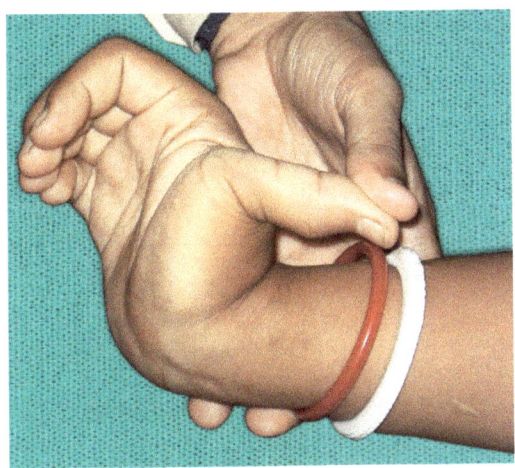

Fig. 10.5: Hypermobile joints in hand (may be found in normal healthy adult)

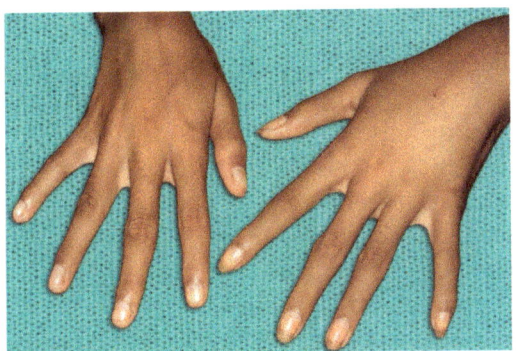

Fig. 10.6: Long and slender fingers in a patient of Marfanoid habitus

- Ehlers-Danlos syndrome
- Marfan's syndrome (Fig. 10.6)
- Down's syndrome
- Cleidocranial dysostosis
- Osteogenesis imperfecta
- Morquio syndrome.

THE PEARLS

Blue tint to the white of eyes (blue sclera) (Fig. 10.2) has created interest to the physicians from ancient days. Majority are heterogeneous group of genetic disorders and thus they are not benefited much with treatment. Utmost the physician can diagnose the disease and reassure the patient or his relatives.

11

Bradycardia

DEFINITION

Normal pulse rate in an adult is 60–100 beats/minute (average 72 beats/minute). When the pulse rate is less than 60 beats/minute, it is labelled as **bradycardia**. Bradycardia may be regular or irregular. 'Bradus' means slow and 'kardia' means heart in Greek.

COMMON CAUSES OF BRADYCARDIA

- *Physiological:* Athletes, meditation, yoga or during sleep.
- *Pathological*
  - Myxedema (hypothyroidism)
  - Obstructive jaundice
  - Increased intracranial tension
  - Drugs like β-blockers, digitalis, verapramil or diltiazem
  - Complete heart block, 2° heart block
  - Sick sinus syndrome (sinoatrial disease)
  - Acute myocardial infarction (specially, recent inferior wall infarction)
  - Vasovagal attack, hypersensitive carotid sinus
  - Hypothermia (core temperature < 95°F)
  - Hyperkalemia
  - Severe hypoxia
  - Organophosphorus poisoning
  - Obstructive sleep apnea syndrome (episodic and usually nocturnal)
  - Aging (i.e. in elderly persons due to idiopathic degeneration).

Regular athletic training and myxedema are the most common causes of bradycardia in clinical practice. Athletes, yoga and meditation give rise to high vagal tone; while during sleep, the sympathetic activity is reduced.

WHAT ARE SINUS BRADYCARDIA AND RELATIVE BRADYCARDIA?

- *Sinus bradycardia:* The pulse rate is less than 60 beats/minute where the impulse is originating from sinoatrial (SA) node. The causes are similar to the causes of

bradycardia mentioned above except complete heart block. In complete heart block, the impulse originates from ventricular wall (i.e. idioventricular rhythm) and not from SA node.
- *Relative bradycardia*: It is known that with per degree (°F) rise in temperature in an adult, the pulse rate is increased by 10 beats/minute (in children it is 12–15 beats/minute). In relative bradycardia, the increase in pulse rate is less than 10 beats/minute with per degree (°F) rise in temperature. For example, the pulse rate will be 90 beats/minute, when the temperature is increased by 3°F (actually, it should be 102 beats/minute). The common examples are:
  - Any viral fever (e.g. dengue, yellow fever)
  - First week of enteric fever
  - Brucellosis, Weil's disease.

SYMPTOMS RECOGNIZED BY THE PATIENT WITH BRADYCARDIA

Commonly the symptoms are dizziness, light-headedness, weakness, worsening fatigue, fainting (syncope) or near-fainting, or palpitations. In very slow pulse rate, patient may experience confusion or seizures.

BRADYCARDIA WITH CONVULSIONS

- Complete heart block (Stokes-Adams syndrome)
- Increased intracranial tension due to meningoencephalitis or brain tumor
- Bradycardia due to any cause with very slow pulse rate
- Prior to development of myxedema coma.

HOW TO CONFIRM THE CAUSE OF BRADYCARDIA?

- *Electrocardiography (ECG):* Confirms bradycardia (R-R interval > 25 small squares with normal P-QRST complexes). ECG also points towards 2° heart block, complete heart block, hypothermia or hyperkalemia.
- *Holter monitoring:* Helpful in diagnosing intermittent slow pulse rate with symptoms.
- *Tilt-table testing:* It is done in suspected neurocardiogenic syncope associated with bradycardia.
- *Exercise testing:* A sub-normal increase in heart rate after exercise (chronotropic incompetence) can be useful in diagnosing sick sinus syndrome.

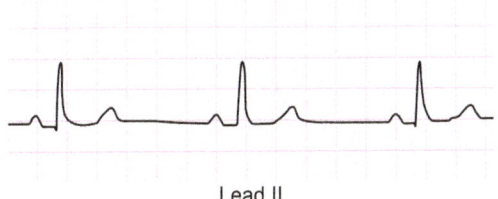

Lead II

Fig. 11.1: Sinus bradycardia—the lead II ECG tracing shows a regular sinus rhythm with SA node discharging at 50 times/minute

- Electrophysiological testing is done in selected cases.
- ***Blood testing:*** Thyroid function tests, liver function tests, serum electrolytes and cardiac enzymes test.

INDICATION OF PACEMAKER IN BRADYARRHYTHMIAS

Temporary

- Reversible heart block in symptomatic patients (e.g. 2° and complete heart block arising out of poisoning, drug overdose or dyselectrolytemias)
- Symptomatic sinus bradycardia
- Atrial fibrillation with slow ventricular response
- Acute myocardial infarction developing into Mobitz type II (2° heart block) or complete heart block.

Permanent

- Sick sinus syndrome
- Mobitz type II atrioventricular (AV) block
- Symptomatic bradyarrhythmia
- Complete heart block (acquired) with very slow pulse rate
- Symptomatic congenital heart blocks.

CAUSES OF TACHYCARDIA (PULSE RATE > 100/MINUTE)

- ***Sinus tachycardia*** (pulse rate > 100 beats/ minute where the impulse is originating from SA node; Takhus means swift in Greek):
    - Exercise, emotion, excitement, anxiety, intense pain and in children
    - Heart failure
    - Thyrotoxicosis
    - Severe anemia
    - Pyrexia
    - Acute hemorrhage
    - Shock (e.g. acute myocardial infarction)
    - Myocarditis
    - Hypoxia
    - Pregnancy
    - Drugs like salbutamol, atropine, nifedipine.

In sinus tachycardia, average heart rate is 100–160 beats/minute.

- ***Relative tachycardia:*** Here, the increase in pulse rate is more than 10 beats/ minute with per degree (°F) rise in temperature. For example, the pulse rate will

be 120/minute, when the temperature is increased by 3°F (actually, it should be 102/minute). The common examples are:
- Acute rheumatic fever
- Tuberculosis
- Diphtheritic myocarditis
- Polyarteritis nodosa.

■ *Paroxysmal tachycardia* (pulse rate > 160 beats/minute)—it is of two types:
- Supraventricular [i.e. paroxysmal atrial tachycardia (PAT) and paroxysmal nodal tachycardia (PNT)]
- Ventricular tachycardia (VT).

Paroxysmal tachycardia is commonly due to rheumatic carditis, ischemic heart disease, thyrotoxicosis, hypertensive heart disease, cardiomyopathy and Wolff-Parkinson-White (WPW) syndrome.

SINUS RHYTHM, NODAL RHYTHM AND IDIOVENTRICULAR RHYTHM

■ *Sinus rhythm:* Normal cardiac rhythm is regular and ranges between 60 and 100 beats/minute (average 72 beats/minute). It is known as sinus rhythm because it is generated by the SA node. SA node is the natural pacemaker of the heart.
■ *Nodal rhythm:* When SA node fails, the AV node originates impulse at the rate of 40–60/minute, resulting in a pulse rate of 40–60 beats/minute. It is nodal rhythm.
■ *Idioventricular rhythm:* When cardiac impulse originates from the ventricles at the rate of 36/minute, the pulse rate at ventricular rhythm will be 36 beats (30–40) per minute, and is known as idioventricular rhythm. The ventricular rhythm in complete heart block is an example of idioventricular rhythm.

ABSENT RADIAL PULSE

■ Anatomical abnormality (aberrant radial artery or congenital)
■ Severe atherosclerosis
■ Takayasu's disease (pulseless disease)
■ Embolization into radial artery (from subacute bacterial endocarditis, atrial fibrillation or left ventricular thrombus)
■ Brachial artery catheterization, or previous tied-off artery at surgery
■ Stenosis of subclavian artery
■ Death.

Always palpate the palm which may be cold, clammy, painful, and may or may not be associated with small ulcers/gangrene at the tip of fingers (e.g. in embolism) when radial pulse is not palpable.

RADIO-RADIAL DELAY (INEQUALITY BETWEEN TWO RADIAL PULSES)

- Normal anatomical variations
- Thoracic inlet syndrome, e.g. cervical rib
- Pre-subclavian coarctation
- Supravalvular aortic stenosis (congenital)
- Takayasu's disease
- Aneurysm of arch of aorta
- Pressure over one-sided axillary artery by lymph nodes.

RADIO-FEMORAL DELAY

In health, there is no radio-femoral delay.
- Coarctation of aorta (important bedside diagnostic clue in a young hypertensive)
- Atherosclerosis of aorta
- Aortoarteritis
- Thrombosis or embolism of aorta.

THE PEARLS

Always try to determine the cause of bradycardia. At the first hand, try to exclude regular athletic training and practice of yoga. Bradycardia should always be investigated.
Prognostically, outcome of bradycardia is worse than tachycardia for the patient.

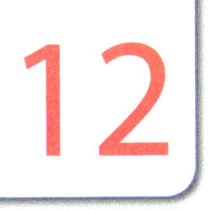

Bruxism (Teeth Grinding)

WHAT IS BRUXISM?

It is an involuntary and forceful teeth grinding during sleep or wakefulness, often leading to damage of the teeth. The classical age of onset is 10–20 years though this may appear in childhood, and may affect 10–20% of the population. It is commonly seen in anxious people.

The person is usually unaware of the problem; (male: female) M:F = 1:1, and the problem usually remits by the age 40. Dental examination may give a clue to diagnosis where the damage is minor. Night time bed partner primarily notices the situation.

Usually no treatment is necessary but in severe cases, a rubber tooth guard is required to prevent disfiguring injury of teeth. Stress management, biofeedback, psychotherapy or benzodiazepines may be of some help. Contrary to common belief, bruxism has no relation with intestinal infestation with helminths.

Teeth chattering is usually seen in fever with chill and rigor, or with shivering due to exposure to very cold weather.

SLEEP-RELATED DISORDERS

- Insomnia (most common complaint in general population and mental disorders)
- Sleep-walking (somnambulism)
- Sleep terrors (occurs during first several hours after onset of sleep)
- Sleep-related epileptic seizures
- Bruxism
- Clusture headache (a variety of migraine)
- Abnormal swallowing, coughing, choking and aspiration of saliva
- Sleep-related gastroesophageal reflux disease (GERD)—often associated with hiatal hernia
- Nocturnal angina
- Sleep enuresis (bed-wetting)
- Sleep-talking
- Nocturnal leg cramps
- Nocturnal paroxysmal dystonia
- Paroxysmal nocturnal hemoglobinuria (sleep-related acidic reaction of the blood produces hemolysis, making the morning urine brownish red)

- Sleep apnea (respiratory dysfunction during sleep disturbing nocturnal sleep with excessive daytime somnolence)
- Restless leg syndrome (or Ekbom's syndrome; causes are idiopathic, peripheral neuropathy, iron deficiency, uremia)
- Periodic limb movement disorder (previously known as **nocturnal myoclonus**)
- Sleep paralysis (totally unable to perform a voluntary movement despite remaining alert and aware)
- Narcolepsy (periods of irresistible sleep) may coexist with cataplexy (sudden loss of lower limb tone and falling with full awareness)—often accompanied by hypnagogic hallucinations (on falling asleep).

Some rare activities experienced by sleep-walkers are sleep dropping (fall from a height), sleep sex (with no recollection of any of the sexual events), sleep art (produces works of art during sleep) and Zzz-mailing (sending emails over internet while sleep-walking).

EXCESSIVE DAYTIME SLEEPINESS (HYPERSOMNIA)

- Chronic sleep disruption at night (insomnia). Inadequate night-time sleep due to fatigue/excessive consumption of caffeine or alcohol are very common causes of daytime sleepiness
- Narcolepsy (recurrent bouts of irresistible sleep)
- Obstructive sleep apnea syndrome
- Sleeping sickness (African trypanosomiasis by *Trypanosoma brucei* complex).
- Depressive illness
- Following infections, e.g. infectious mononucleosis
- Symptomatic hypersomnia—organic brain diseases, e.g. encephalitis, toxic or metabolic encephalopathies; tumor, vascular or traumatic brain damage
- Neurotic hypersomnia—in hysterics or neuroasthenic individual
- Drug-induced—sedatives, antiepileptics
- Kleine-Levin syndrome—episodic hypersomnolence and hyperphagia in adolescent boys; rare
- Idiopathic hypersomnia—hereditary with excessive night-time sleep; also known as **sleep drunkenness**.

INSOMNIA

It is the **difficulty in sleeping** and in general one-third of adults suffer from this ailment. It may be categorized by:
- **Early insomnia**, i.e. difficulty in getting off to sleep (commonly due to anxiety, depression, mania and substance abuse).
- **Middle insomnia**, i.e. waking up from sleep at mid-night (mostly due to sleep apnea, polyuria or nocturia and benign hypertrophy of prostate).
- **Late insomnia**, i.e. early morning waking (commonly due to depression and malnutrition).

- Hypocretin (orexin) neuropeptides are involved in sleep-waking cycle (present between cerebral cortex and reticular formation).
- Electrophysiologic parameters of sleep are recorded by **polysomnography** i.e. electroencephalogram (EEG) + electrooculogram (EOG) → records eye-movements activity) + electromyogram (EMG → measured on chin and neck muscles).

PAIN IN TEMPOROMANDIBULAR REGION

- Bruxism—temporomandibular pain dysfunction syndrome
- Osteoarthritis of temporomandibular joint
- Temporomandibular joint dysfunction or Costen's syndrome
- Temporal arteritis (develops jaw claudication)
- Trismus—involuntary spasm of masseter and temporalis due to tetanus
- Tic douloureux (trigeminal neuralgia)
- Ishemic heart disease (usually does not cross the lower borders of jaw).

THE PEARLS

Bruxism and other sleep-related disorders require neuropsychiatric assistance for relief. Often these entities pose a social problem. Bruxism is common in children with cerebral palsy and mental retardation.

13

Bull-neck

PROLOGUE

The space between the mandibles and the clavicles bulges with enlarged lymph nodes (Fig. 13.1) and edema; commonly from malignant diphtheria.

CAUSES OF CERVICAL LYMPHADENOPATHY

- Infection, malignancy or ulcer within the oral cavity
- Infection of ear, eye and nose
- Scalp infection by louse or dandruff
- Tuberculosis (pulmonary or miliary)
- Lymphoma
- Lymphatic leukemia (acute and chronic)
- Metastasis in cervical lymph nodes
- Infectious mononucleosis
- Sarcoidosis
- Rubella infection.

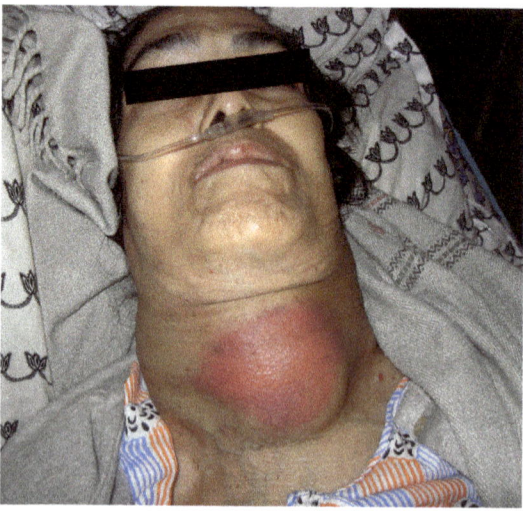

Fig. 13.1: Bull-neck with thyroid hemorrhage

LYMPHADENOPATHY WITH SINUS FORMATION

- Tuberculosis
- Malignancy
- Actinomycosis.

DIFFERENTIAL DIAGNOSIS OF BULL-NECK

- Surgical emphysema (press the stethoscope over the swelling and listen the crepitus)
- Enlarged submandibular glands (Mikulicz's syndrome)
- Ludwig's angina
- Lipomas encircling the front and the nape of neck (Madelung's collar).

AXILLARY LYMPHADENOPATHY

- Infection of the upper extremity
- Breast carcinoma
- Lymphoma, melanoma
- Miliary tuberculosis
- Lymphatic leukemia (acute or chronic)
- Brucellosis
- Cat-scratch disease.

EPITROCHLEAR LYMPHADENOPATHY

- Hand infections
- Lymphoma, especially non-Hodgkin's lymphoma (NHL)
- Sarcoidosis
- Secondary syphilis, human immunodeficiency virus (HIV) infection
- Lymphatic leukemia (acute or chronic)
- Tularemia
- Infectious mononucleosis.

INGUINAL LYMPHADENOPATHY

- Infection or cellulitis of the lower limb
- Filarisis
- Syphilis
- Metastasis from genital malignancy, pelvic carcinoma
- Chancroid, lymphogranuloma venereum (bilateral inguinal 'bubo')
- Lymphoma
- Miliary tuberculosis
- Lymphatic leukemia (acute and chronic).

The importance of epitrochlear lymphadenopathy is highest to a clinician in comparison to inguinal lymphadenopathy, which rates lowest.

MATTED LYMPH NODES

- Signifies periadenitis
- Most commonly in tuberculosis; may be seen in chronic lymphadenitis and NHL.

CONSISTENCY OF LYMPH NODE SWELLING

- Stony hard → malignancy
- Elastic and rubbery → Hodgkin's disease
- Variegated → NHL
- Firm and shotty → secondary syphilis
- Soft and fluctuating → cold abscess, inflammatory abscess.

PATHOLOGICAL SIGNIFICANCE OF ENLARGED NODES

- Nodes are pathologically significant, if:
  - More than 1 cm in diameter
  - Firm in consistency
  - Tender on palpation
  - Matted.
- Following factors should always be kept in mind in assessing the pathological nature of nodes:
  - Age of the patient
  - The physical characteristics (described above)
  - Anatomical sites involved
  - The total clinical setting.

VIRCHOW'S NODE

- Also known as **Ewald's node** or **sentinel node**.
- **Position:** Medial group of left-sided supraclavicular nodes which lie in between two heads of left sternomastoid muscle; always palpated from back of the patient.
- Receive lymphatics from:
  - Upper limb (left)
  - Breast (left)
  - Lung (left)
  - Stomach (Troisier's sign)
  - Testes.
- Bronchogenic carcinoma commonly produces **scalene node enlargement**.

THE PEARLS

It is the duty of the physician to examine the patient for generalized lymphadenopathy (involvement of three or more non-contiguous lymph node areas) if cervical adenopathy is found. One has to remember that lymph node enlargement is commonly due to reactive hyperplasia, infections, inflammatory/autoimmune or malignancy.

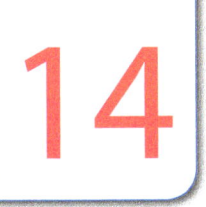

Carpal Tunnel Syndrome

WHAT IS CARPAL TUNNEL SYNDROME (CTS)?

It is the entrapment neuropathy caused by compression of the median nerve in the carpal tunnel at wrist. **Carpal tunnel** is formed at wrist by carpal bones behind and flexor retinaculum in front. The patient, commonly a *female*, complains of pain in the hand *during night* which wakes her up; to ameliorate the pain, the patient shakes her hand ('wake and shake'). Pain and paresthesia (tingling, numbness and burning sensation) over palmar surfaces of radial three-and-a-half fingers (i.e. thumb, index, middle and radial half of the ring finger) are complained. There may be weakness of abductor pollicis brevis (at thenar eminence) with or without wasting, and the patient may face difficulty in flexion, abduction and opposition of the thumb.

A thorough systematic clinical examination (see the causes mentioned below), many a time, clinches the diagnosis. Always look for old scar mark at wrist (of both the sides) indicating previous surgery. The common tests performed at the bedside are:

- ***Tinel's sign:*** Tapping over the median nerve over the volar aspect of wrist will produce paresthesia (i.e. shock-like pain or tingling) along the cutaneous distribution of the nerve (i.e. in thumb, index, middle and radial half of ring finger). The specificity of this clinical test is high.
- ***Phalen's sign:*** Gentle, passive, unforced, maximal wrist flexion to 90° induces pain or paresthesia in the distribution of median nerve.
- ***Carpal compression test (Durkan's test):*** Pressure with the examiner's thumb over the patient's carpal tunnel for 30 seconds induces symptoms. This test is more specific and sensitive than previous two tests.
- ***Tourniquet test:*** Raising the blood pressure over systolic pressure by inflating the cuff for 2 minutes produces paresthesia along the cutaneous distribution of median nerve.

ETIOLOGY

- Idiopathic (probably the most common cause)
- Myxedema
- Acromegaly
- Rheumatoid arthritis
- Pregnancy (third trimester) or patient on oral contraceptives; premenstrual edema

- Compression of median nerve by edema, tenosynovitis, fibrosis or fasciitis, or Colles' fracture (recent or malunited)
- Amyloidosis (primary)
- Patient on chronic hemodialysis (due to deposition of β_2-microglobulin, an amyloid)
- Sarcoidosis
- Exposure to vibration (works involved in chipping, grinding), work-related (computer operators), traumatic injury to wrist, eosinophilic fasciitis, systemic sclerosis
- Osteoarthritis, rarely
- Obesity
- Diabetes mellitus.

DIFFERENTIAL DIAGNOSIS

- Cervical radiculopathy
- Chronic tendititis or tenosynovitis
- Reflex sympathetic dystrophy syndrome
- Osteoarthritis
- Arthritides other than rheumatoid arthritis
- Occlusion of vessels at wrist.

CONFIRMATION OF DIAGNOSIS

X-ray and ultrasonography are not very helpful. Electrodiagnostic studies like nerve conduction velocity (NCV; delayed in CTS) and electromyography (EMG; recording of muscle action potential from abductor pollicis brevis is helpful in diagnosis) confirm CTS and rule out other possibilities.

DIFFERENT ENTRAPMENT NEUROPATHIES

- *Upper extremity*
  - Carpal tunnel syndrome (at wrist)—median nerve. Most common cause in the upper extremity
  - Elbow tunnel syndrome (cubital tunnel at elbow)—ulnar nerve
  - At spiral groove of humerus after a fracture—radial nerve
  - Trapped in spinoglenoid notch—suprascapular nerve.
- *Lower extremity*
  - Meralgia paresthetica (trapped under inguinal ligament)—lateral femoral cutaneous nerve. Most common cause in the lower extremity
  - At head of fibula—common peroneal nerve
  - Tarsal tunnel syndrome (at the flexor retinaculum at ankle joint, the tarsal tunnel)—posterior tibial nerve
  - Morton's metatarsalgia (between 2nd/3rd and 3rd/4th metatarsal heads)—trapped medial and lateral plantar nerves.

MANAGEMENT

Prognosis of CTS is variable and some cases may resolve spontaneously. The outline of management are:
- Avoid precipitating activities. Eliminate repetitive trauma.
- Drugs like nonsteroidal anti-inflammatory drugs (NSAIDs) or diuretics with variable results.
- Low-dose oral corticosteroids (10–20 mg for 4 weeks) in selected patients.
- Wrist splint or braces in neutral position used at night.
- Ultrasound therapy at wrist may be of some help.
- Local steroid injection proximal to carpal tunnel avoiding median nerve—often beneficial though some cases may recur.
- Surgical decompression may result in permanent relief (a day care procedure). Result of surgery is usually excellent.
- Simultaneous treatment of the underlying cause, e.g. myxedema, acromegaly or amyloidosis.
- Alternative therapies like acupuncture, stretching, chiropractic therapy may be helpful in some of the patients. Vitamin B6 or methylcobalamin therapy is not better than placebo.

THE PEARLS

Carpal tunnel syndrome is a window in clinical medicine which helps the clinician to diagnose some subtle clinical diagnosis (e.g. myxedema). Medical intervention should be done early before the onset of wasting of abductor pollicis brevis.

It is worthwhile to remember that CTS may occur in conjunction with cervical nerve root compression, known as **double-crush syndrome**. So, a physician should be cautious in diagnosing these conditions when both are present.

Surgery is not recommended in pregnancy with CTS because of the likelihood of spontaneous recovery after delivery.

15

Claw Foot/Claw Hand

CLAW FOOT

Synonym

Pes cavus

Definition

A fixed deformity of foot where both feet are more or less symmetrically high-arched, i.e. there is gross exaggeration of the medial longitudinal arch of the feet (Fig. 15.1). It is just opposite to flat foot (pes planus) (Fig. 15.2) deformity.

Conditions Associated

- Familial
- Friedreich's ataxia
- Peroneal muscular atrophy

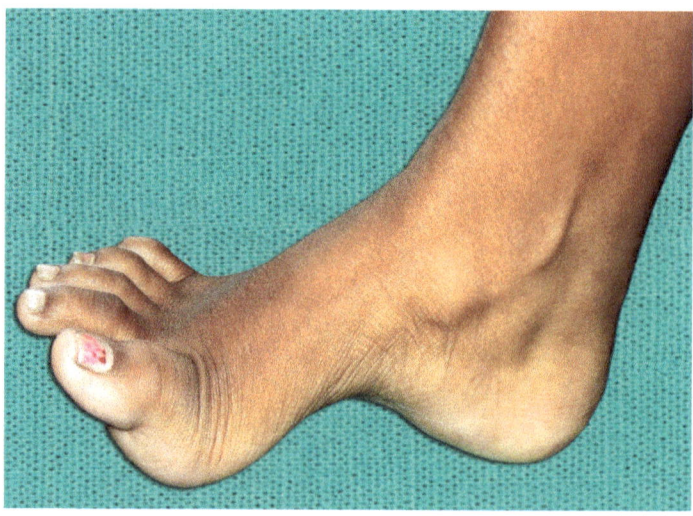

Fig. 15.1: Pes cavus (claw foot or high-arched foot) due to wasting of intrinsic muscles of foot in peroneal muscular atrophy

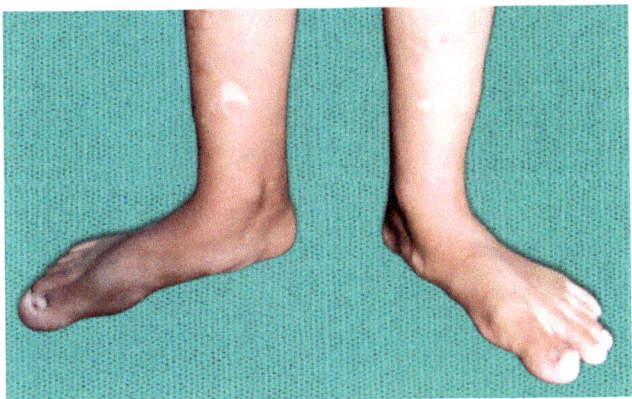

Fig. 15.2: Pes planus (flat foot)

- Spina bifida occulta
- Poliomyelitis
- Syringomyelia
- Cerebral palsy
- Refsum's disease
- Idiopathic.

Method of Demonstration

Take a foot-print on a white paper after painting the feet by lac-dye, or after immersing the feet in water, ask the patient to walk barefooted in the floor → observe the foot-prints.

GENU VARUM DEFORMITY

Bow legs are seen in:
- Rickets or osteomalacia
- Achondroplasia
- Paget's disease
- Severe osteoarthritis of knee joints.

GENU VALGUM DEFORMITY

Knock knees are seen in:
- Rickets
- Congenital deformity.

SKELETAL DEFORMITIES PRESENT WITH NEUROLOGICAL DISORDERS

- Kyphoscoliosis
- Pes cavus

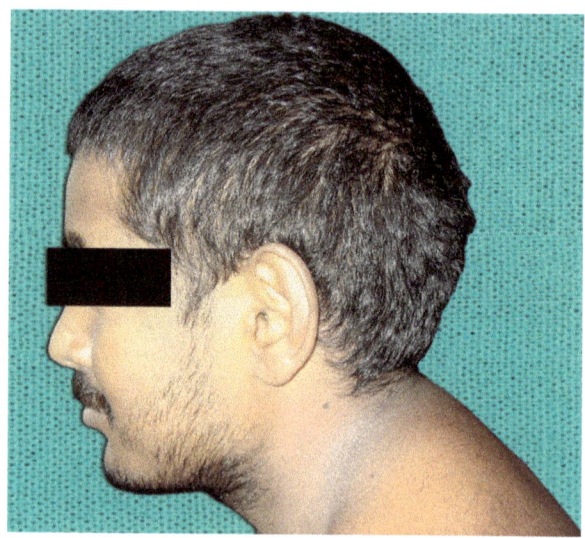

Fig. 15.3: Short neck and low hairline in craniovertebral anomaly (patient developed quadriplegia)

- High-arched palate
- Gibbus in spine
- Short neck (e.g. craniovertebral anomaly) (Fig. 15.3)
- Various skull deformities, e.g. craniostenosis.

HEEL PAD THICKNESS

A lateral view of patient's foot is taken by X-ray. The distance between the lower most point of calcaneum and the lower most point of the soft tissue shadow of heel is measured → **heel pad thickness**.

Increased Heel Pad Thickness

- More than 18 mm in women and more than 21 mm in men
- Conditions associated with heel pad thickness are as follows:
  - Acromegaly (most common cause)
  - Obesity
  - Edema-producing states.

DEFORMED OR MUTILATED FINGERS/TOES

- Leprosy
- Scleroderma (Fig. 15.4)
- Buerger's disease
- Congenital defects
- Diabetic foot
- Frost bite

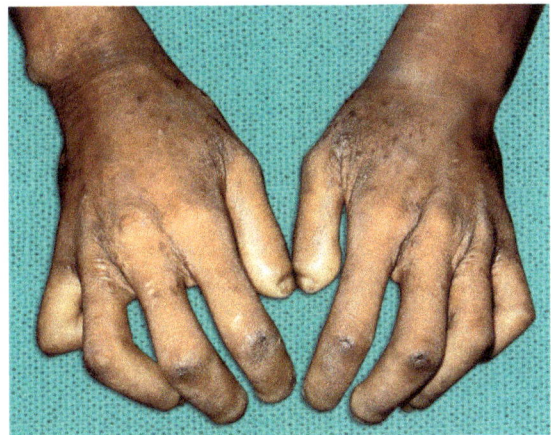

Fig. 15.4: Mutilated hands with pulp atrophy, sclerodactyly, limitation of full extension of fingers with dry, coarse skin in scleroderma

- Syringomyelia
- Vasculitis
- Antiphospholipid syndrome
- Atherothrombosis
- Arthritis mutilans (psoriasis)
- Trauma
- Atherothrombosis
- Porphyria
- Amyloid neuropathy
- Lesch-Nyhan syndrome.

SHORT NECK

When the ratio of length of the body to length of the neck is more than 13:1, it is called short neck. It is usually associated with low hair line (i.e. hairline below C4 vertebra) (Fig. 15.3). These are associated with craniovertebral anomaly. The common causes of short neck are:
- Craniovertebral anomaly
- Cretinism
- Down's syndrome
- Turner's syndrome
- Noonan's syndrome
- Hurler syndrome.

SHORT FOURTH METACARPALS (FIG. 15.5)

- Pseudohypoparathyroidism and pseudo-pseudohypoparathyroidism
- Down's syndrome
- Turner's syndrome
- Myositis ossificans progressiva.

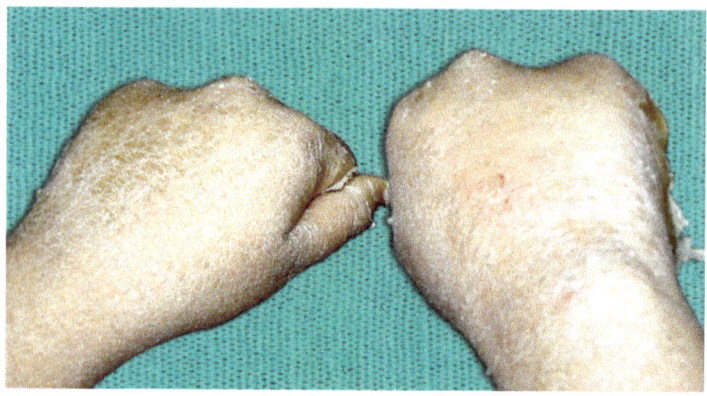

Fig. 15.5: Short fourth metacarpals in pseudohypoparathyroidism–'knuckle-knuckle dimple-dimple sign' (the patient shows peeling of skin of hands due to some drug reaction)

As the knuckles and dimples in closed fist of both hands are not symmetrical, presence of short fourth metacarpals is also known as ***knuckle-knuckle dimple-dimple sign*** (especially in pseudohypoparathyroidism).

CLAW HAND (FIG. 15.6)

Claw hand is a condition where the metacarpophalangeal (MCP) joints are hyperextended, and the proximal interphalangeal (PIP) and the distal interphalangeal (DIP) joints are flexed. Claw hand is produced as a result of paralysis of interossei and

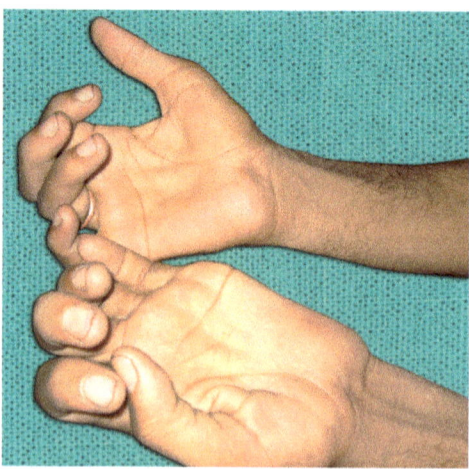

Fig. 15.6: Bilateral claw hand in motor neuron disease; wasting of small muscles of both hands are seen

lumbricals. Any lesion of T1 segment or the nerves will produce claw hand deformity. The common causes are:
- Combined lesion of ulnar and median nerve (e.g. leprosy)
- Motor neuron disease (Fig. 15.6), syringomyelia, intramedullary tumor
- Cervical rib
- Klumpke's paralysis
- Pseudo-claw hand—Dupuytren's contracture, Volkmann's ischemic contracture, post-burn.

THE PEARLS

These types of specific skeletal deformities, many a time, clinches the diagnosis of some hidden disease. These signs are equivalent to a positive serological test or radiological test in clinical medicine.

16

Coprolalia

DEFINITION

Offensive utterance of obscene words.

ASSOCIATIONS

- Psychosis (e.g. schizophrenia)
- Poisoning (e.g. organophosphorous)
- Atropinization or overdose of atropine
- Hepatic pre-coma
- Subdural hematoma
- Uremia
- Tourette syndrome
- Lesch-Nyhan syndrome
- Encephalitis or encephalopathy
- Habitual (personality disorder).

> Related to coprolalia there is coprographia i.e. making obscene writings or drawings, and copropraxia i.e. performing obscene gestures.

GILLES DE LA TOURETTE SYNDROME

Inherited neuropsychiatric disorder characterized by multiple motor (e.g. blinking, grimacing, head jerking) and vocal (e.g. clearing the throat or coprolalia) tics. Compulsive utterances of coprolalia is one of the most recognizable and distressing symptom, which appears a few years after disease onset. The disease starts in childhood or adolescence; hyperactive, non-specific ECG (electrocardiogram) abnormalities are seen in 50%; the cause is probably an inherited disorder of synaptic transmission.

Treatment is done by haloperidol (drug of choice), clonidine, clonazepam, pimozide or tetrabenazine.

SPEECH DISORDER

It is the symbolic expression of thought process in spoken or written words.

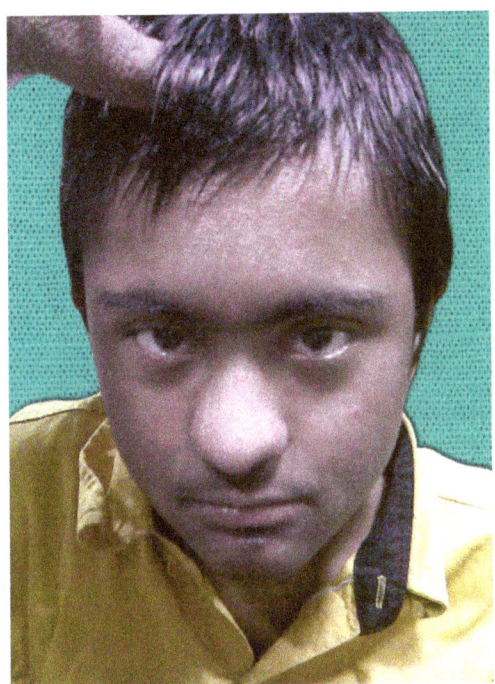

Fig. 16.1: Down's syndrome with lalling speech (baby speech)

- ***Aphasia or dysphasia:*** Unable to speak due to defect in higher center (e.g. Broca's or Wernicke's area in brain) with difficulty in language function.
- ***Dysarthria:*** Defect in articulation, commonly due to neuromuscular or muscular disorders resulting in impaired coordination of faciolingual muscles, e.g. slurring, stammering or mumbling.
- ***Dysphonia:*** Disorder of phonation where the defect lies in the vocal cord, e.g. hoarse voice, voice loss.
- ***Scanning or staccato speech:*** The patient speaks syllable by syllable with undue emphasis on a particular syllable. It is common in cerebellar dysfunction.
- ***Lalling speech (or baby speech):*** Common in children, mental retardation or Down's syndrome (Fig. 16.1).
- ***Slow, monotonous speech without any fluctuation:*** Seen in parkinsonism.
- ***Seventh nerve palsy:*** Labial dysarthria, and XIIth nerve palsy-lingual dysarthria.
- ***Echolalia:*** Repetition of examiner's word.
- ***Palilalia:*** Repetition of terminal words of own speech.
- ***Jargon aphasia:*** Neologisms (new words) making no sense at all.
- ***Perseveration:*** Repeated use of particular words or phrases.

THE PEARLS

Coprolalia is rarely seen but if present, may simplify the diagnosis for a clinician. It is mainly encountered by the psychiatrists.

17

Cough

DEFINITION

It is a reflex or voluntary expulsion of the inspired air by forced expiratory effort against a transitorily closed glottis. Cough is known to be one of the unique defensive reflex of human body designed to clear the tracheobronchial tree of secretion and foreign body. Though previously recognized as the 'watch-dog' (i.e. protective reflex) of the respiratory system, it may be regarded as a manifestation of diseases affecting many other systems including a major symptom of pulmonary diseases.

MECHANISM

It requires an intricate network of neurosensory-muscular coordination:
- *Afferent pathway:* It originates from the sensory receptors present in the epithelium of the airways (larynx, trachea and major bronchus), and the afferent nerves involved are trigeminal, glossopharyngeal, superior laryngeal and vagus.
- *Center:* Cough center is present in medulla oblongata.
- *Efferent pathway:* The efferent impulses reach the diaphragm, intercostal muscles, abdominal muscles, and to larynx through vagus, phrenic, recurrent laryngeal and spinal motor nerves which result in cough, while the laryngeal air velocities produced as a result of violent action of respiratory muscles make a sound.

Cough is usually associated with mucus secretion, bronchoconstriction and transient rise in systemic blood pressure.

THREE PHASES OF COUGH

1. Appropriate stimulus, i.e. mechanical (dust, mucus, foreign body), chemical (toxic gases, fumes, cigarette smoke), inflammatory (edema and hyperemia of respiratory mucus membrane) and thermal stimuli (inhalation of either very cold or hot air) initiate deep inspiration.
2. Glottic closure + contraction of muscles of expiration including accessory muscles + relaxation of diaphragm → resulting in maximum intrathoracic pressure → narrowing of trachea.
3. Opening of glottis → high flow rate generated as a result of pressure difference between the airways and the atmosphere associated with tracheal narrowing→ propels excessive mucus and foreign body outside.

ETIOLOGY

- ***Respiratory tract:*** Acute and chronic infection/neoplasm of larynx or pharynx, post-nasal drip, acute tracheobronchitis, cigarette smoking, pulmonary tuberculosis, bronchial asthma, chronic bronchitis, bronchiectasis, emphysema, interstitial pulmonary fibrosis, pneumonia, lung abscess, bronchogenic carcinoma, sarcoidosis, tropical eosinophilia, pneumoconiosis, cystic fibrosis, cough variant asthma, pleurisy, pleural effusion, mediastinal mass.
- ***System of ear, nose and throat:*** Inhalation of toxic gases, fumes, cooking fuels, dust or foreign body; otitis media, wax impacted in external ear, laryngitis, tracheitis, allergic rhinitis, sinusitis (maxillary) and post-nasal drip.
- ***Cardiovascular system:*** Pulmonary edema, pericardial effusion, aortic aneurysm, enlarged left atrium (from mitral stenosis commonly), left ventricular failure (LVF), or congestive cardiac failure (CCF).
- ***Gastrointestinal tract:*** Gastroesophageal reflux disease (GERD), hiatus hernia, achalasia cardia, esophageal diverticulum.
- ***Reflex:*** Happens to be due to irritation of vagus nerve and is commonly from wax impacted in external ear, otitis media, subdiaphragmatic abscess and acute distension of stomach.
- ***Drug-induced:*** Angiotensin converting enzyme (ACE) inhibitors (due to accumulation of bradykinin, substance P and prostaglandin E_2), β-blockers (indirect effect of bronchoconstriction).
- ***Psychogenic:*** Found in adolescents and self-conscious adults; usually smasmodic and explosive in nature; often it is barking (or 'honking') and loud in character → may be seen as a part of obsessional neurosis or coordinated tics.
- ***Idiopathic.***

CLASSIFICATION

- Acute (< 3 weeks), subacute (3–8 weeks) or chronic (> 8 weeks).
- Dry (upper respiratory tract infection, smoker's cough, early stage of pulmonary tuberculosis) or wet (e.g. bronchiectasis).
- Paroxysmal cough (usually lasts for 1–2 minutes): Whooping cough, tracheal obstruction, bronchial asthma, pulmonary edema, foreign body inhalation.

TYPES

Analysis of cough is a major task for clinicians.
- ***Dry or nonproductive:*** Acute laryngotracheobronchitis, acute dry pleurisy, smoker's cough, early stage of pulmonary tuberculosis, interstitial lung disease.
- ***Wet, productive or moist:*** Sputum production may be due to lung abscess, bronchiectasis, resolution stage of lobar pneumonia.
- ***Bovine (laryngeal cough):*** The explosive nature of cough is lost in recurrent laryngeal nerve palsy (commonly due to bronchogenic carcinoma).
- ***Brassy (or metallic):*** Dry cough with a metallic sound may be heard in carcinoma of larynx.

- **Whooping:** There is rapid succession of dry cough which gradually gathers speed and end in a deep inspiration when the characteristic 'whoop' (noise) is audible; found in pertussis.
- **Spluttering cough:** In tracheoesophageal fistula (cough during swallowing).
- **Hacking (pharyngeal cough):** Dry and irritable cough in heavy smokers.
- **Barking:** Harsh and loud cough; found in epiglottitis and hysteria.
- **Nocturnal:** Chronic bronchitis, LVF, tropical eosinophilia, post-nasal drip, aspiration (e.g. from GERD).
- **Nagging cough:** Commonly after use of ACE-inhibitors.
- **Croupy cough:** Laryngitis, especially in children.
- **Fetid cough:** In bronchiectasis and lung abscess, there is cough with foul smelling expectoration.
- **Suppressed cough:** Short spell of suppressed cough is found in pleurisy to avoid pain during coughing.
- **Paroxysmal cough:** Foreign body inhalation and aspiration, whooping cough.

FACTORS INFLUENCING COUGH

- Cough started acutely—foreign body aspiration, pulmonary thromboembolism (PTE), pulmonary edema, acute exacerbation of bronchial asthma, inhalation of fumes.
- Cough with wheeze—bronchial asthma, chronic bronchitis, PTE.
- Related to meals—hiatus hernia, esopheageal diverticulum, tracheoesophageal fistula, neurogenic dysphagia (e.g. bulbar palsy).
- Related to exertion—early left ventricular decompensation, mitral stenosis, bronchial asthma.
- Related to posture—bronchiectasis and lung abscess (cough evoked after change of posture in bed), GERD (cough evoked while lying horizontally).
- Related to seasonal variation—bronchial asthma and chronic bronchitis become worse in winter.
- Related to working hours—byssinosis (triggered by cotton dust).
- Induced after inhalation of cold air—bronchial asthma.
- Predominantly nocturnal cough—tropical eosinophilia, chronic bronchitis, bronchial asthma, LVF, esophageal disorders.
- Predominantly early morning cough—post-nasal drip, chronic bronchitis, sinusitis.
- Recurrent cough since childhood—cystic fibrosis, childhood asthma, congenital heart disease, cystic disease of lung, hypogammaglobulinemia.

HOW SPUTUM OR EXPECTORATION (PHLEGM) IS ANALYZED?

- Amount (profuse or not)
- Character (serous, mucoid, purulent, mucopurulent)
- Color (yellow, green, black, pinkish, rusty)
- Odor or taste (offensive or not)

- Mixed with blood (hemoptysis) or not
- Sputum production influenced by change of posture (bronchiectasis, lung abscess) or not.

Profuse sputum means approximately a 'teacupful' (> 100 mL) of sputum production per day. A 'teaspoonful' expectoration per day is known as small sputum.

PROFUSE AND FETID (FOUL-SMELLING) SPUTUM

- Bronchiectasis
- Lung abscess
- Pulmonary infection with anaerobic organism
- Infected cavity or neoplasm in the lung
- Empyema thoracis ruptured into bronchus.

DIFFERENT COLORS OF SPUTUM

- Red—hemoptysis (Fig. 17.1)
- Black—carbon particles from atmosphere, cough in coal-miners (benign in nature)
- Green—respiratory tract infection (verdoperoxidase from dead neutrophil turns yellow sputum to green), bronchial asthma (due to large number of eosinophils), pseudomonas infection
- Pink and frothy acute pulmonary edema
- Rusty or golden yellow—pneumonia (pneumococcal)
- Yellow—respiratory tract infection (creamy)
- Yellow (with sulphur granules)—actinomycosis of lung
- Brown to red + tenacious—*Klebsiella pneumoniae* infection

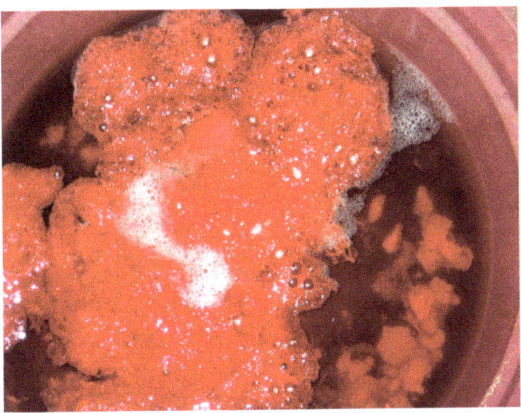

Fig. 17.1: Massive hemoptysis from bronchogenic carcinoma—air bubbles (froth) are mixed with blood

- Anchovy-sauce like—amebic liver abscess ruptured into lung
- Mucoid—chronic bronchitis, chronic obstructive pulmonary disease (COPD), chronic bronchial asthma
- Frothy—pulmonary edema, bronchoalveolar carcinoma (serous and frothy).

HOW COUGH IS ANALYZED AT THE BEDSIDE?

- Duration (days/months/years); acute < 3 weeks, subacute (3-8 weeks), chronic > 8 weeks
- Variability (daytime/nocturnal/morning)
- Precipitating factors (dust/fumes/pollen/cold air/lying down)
- Seasonal variation, pre-existing disease (allergic rhinitis, bronchial asthma), wheeze
- Types (dry/wet/bovine)
- Hemoptysis, present or not
- Change of character of cough in a chronic heavy smoker (e.g. development of COPD or bronchogenic carcinoma)
- Associated symptoms (port-nasal drip, GERD, occult asthma, fever, dyspnea)
- Chest pain (pleurisy) or breathlessness (COPD, pneumonia)
- History of drug intake—ACE-inhibitors or β-blockers.

EVALUATION OF CHRONIC COUGH

Common associations of chronic cough are:
- Viral infection
- GERD
- Post-nasal drip
- Cough variant asthma (present only with cough in the absence of wheezing or breathlessness)
- ACE-inhibitor induced.

POSSIBLE INVESTIGATIONS IN CHRONIC COUGH

- Chest X-ray (postero-anterior and oblique view)
- ENT (ear, nose and throat) check-up
- Paranasal sinus (PNS) X-ray and CT (computed tomography) scan of sinus for post-nasal drip
- Lung function tests and methacholine challenge testing for cough variant asthma
- CT scan of thorax (to exclude interstitial lung disease)
- Radionuclide ventilation/perfusion (V/Q) scan for recurrent PTE
- Fiberoptic bronchoscopy—to rule out inhaled foreign body or carcinoma of the bronchus
- Ambulatory esophageal pH monitoring for GERD
- ECG (echocardiography)—to exclude valvular lesion or left ventricular dysfunction (LVD).

A detailed history is very important in analyzing cough.

COMPLICATIONS

- Chest and abdominal wall soreness form harassing cough, exhaustion, headache and loss of sleep.
- Severe vomiting, rib fracture (especially in elderly with osteoporosis, multiple myeloma or osteolytic metastases), cough syncope (momentary unconsciousness due to raised intrathoracic pressure during coughing which impedes venous return to the heart and reduces cardiac output), spontaneous pneumothorax, subconjunctival hemorrhage, frenal ulcer (in tongue), urinary or fecal incontinence, prolapse of rectum/uterus/hernia.
- Postoperative wound dehiscence, rupture of rectus abdominis (rare), heart block (rare).

MANAGEMENT

Non-specific

- ***Antitussive agents***
  - Antihistamines—chlorpheniramine, clemastine, cetirizine
  - Sympathomimetic decongestants—pseudoephedrine, oxymetazoline, phenylephrine
  - Demulcents—menthol, tea with honey, and other household remedies (saline gurgle, putting ginger in mouth)
  - Others—narcotic and non-narcotic analgesics, bronchodilators in asthma.
- ***Protussive agents*** (or cough enhancing agent)
  - Expectorants—guaifenesin
  - Mucolytics—bromhexine, carbocisteine, acetylcysteine, dornase alpha, ambroxol (a metabolite of bromhexine)
  - Hypertonic saline aerosol (for chronic bronchitis).

Specific

Cessation of smoking, administration of antibiotics, stoppage of ACE-inhibitors, treatment of LVF.

🕮 THE PEARLS

Cough is one of the cardinal symptom in respiratory system. Analysis of cough and expectoration, many a time, clinches the etiological diagnosis. A simple cough may herald the onset of a serious underlying disease.

A bedside clinician often asks his patient to cough while auscultating the respiratory system in a target to (a) clear the throat (if throat sound appears), (b) note the changes in crepitations (many a time helps to differentiate crepitations and pleural rub, where plural rub does not alter with cough), and (c) auscultating for post-tussive crepitations (especially in tuberculous cavity where crepitations evoke after coughing).

18

Cramps

DEFINITION

It is the painful, involuntary contractions of a single or a group of muscles. Cramps are seen in normal healthy persons or may be precipitated by voluntary movements. Cramps in the calf muscles are so common as to be regarded normal, but a more generalized cramps may be a sign of chronic disease of motor neuron.

ETIOPATHOGENESIS

Not truely known but may be due to:
- Overactivity of muscle/nerve membranes
- Electrolyte imbalance.

Pain associated with cramp is possibly due to:
- Focal ischemia
- Accumulation of metabolites within the muscles.

> Pathological cramps may be due to an abnormality anywhere in the pathway including anterior horn cells, peripheral nerve, neuromuscular junction and muscle membrane.

POSSIBLE CAUSES (LEG CRAMP)

- Normally occurs in healthy individual at night.
- Electrolyte imbalance ($\downarrow$Ca, $\downarrow$Mg, $\downarrow$Na, $\downarrow$K, $\downarrow$PO$_4$).
- Overexertion (producing dehydration by profuse sweating, heat cramps, miner's cramp, heat cramp, swimmer's cramps, leg cramps in long distance bus drivers).
- Motor neuron disease, e.g. amyotrophic lateral sclerosis.
- *Metabolic:* Chronic renal failure, hypothyroidism, McArdle's disease, phosphofructokinase deficiency, hemodialysis.
- *Peripheral neuropathy:* Diabetes mellitus, alcohol or vincristine-induced.
- *Cramps in professionals:* Writers, tailors, typists.
- *Muscular dystrophies:* X-linked variety, myotonia.
- *Others:* Chronic wasting disease (e.g. tuberculosis), pregnancy, dehydration due to any cause, tetany, peripheral arterial disease, deep vein thrombosis.

Muscle spasm may occur in tetanus, tetany, epilepsy, myoclonus, etc.

NOCTURNAL LEG CRAMPS

Majority of healthy persons at sometime or other had experienced muscle cramp. Usually it occurs at night, especially when the feet are cold, after a day of unusually strenous activity. Muscles of calf and foot are commonly affected. The onset is sudden and may awake the person. The muscle is visibly and palpably taut, as well as painful. Massage and vigorous stretch of the cramped muscle may give relief. Visible fasciculations may precede and follow muscle cramp. This type of nocturnal cramps are nortorious for recurrence.

All causes mentioned above are responsible for nocturnal cramps with a special reference to:
- Idiopathic
- Electrolyte abnormalities (especially by diuretics)
- Deep vein thrombosis
- Hypoglycemia
- Diabetic neuropathy
- Chronic renal failure or patient on hemodialysis
- Peripheral vascular insufficiency
- Alcohol use, statins.

DIFFERENTIAL DIAGNOSIS (CRAMP)

The single most important condition to be differentiated is intermittent claudication.

POST-EXERCISE LEG PAIN

Think of:
- Arteriosclerosis obliterans
- Buerger's disease
- Deep vein thrombosis
- Lumbar canal stenosis (i.e. neurogenic)
- Venous claudication
- Popliteal cyst
- McArdle's disease (muscle phosphorylase deficiency)
- Popliteal artery entrapment syndrome
- Tetany (↓Ca, ↓Mg or alkalosis).

CALF PAIN (COMMON CAUSES)

- Intermittent claudication (needs meticulous clinical examination, e.g. examination of pedal pulses)

- Deep vein thrombosis (perform Doppler studies)
- Rupture of Baker's cyst (perform arthrography of knee joint)
- Referred pain from lumbar spine [magnetic resonance imaging (MRI) scan of lumbar cord to demonstrate compression]
- Spastic calf muscle (diagnosed by clinical examination)

CALF SWELLING (UNILATERAL)

This may be due to local inflammation, or obstruction/damage to a vein or lymph channel. The possibilities are:
- Deep vein thrombosis (↓ flow on Doppler ultrasound scan, filling defect in venogram)
- Cellulitis (↑ leukocytes, response to antibiotics)
- Ruptured Baker's cyst (usually suffering from rheumatoid arthritis. Arthrogram reveals leakage of contrast from joint capsule)
- Traumatic (may have tender hematoma formation)
- Filariasis or abnormal lymphatic drainage (e.g. trypanosomiasis in tropics, or pelvic malignancy)—obstruction revealed in lymphangiogram.

CALF SWELLING (BILATERAL)

- True hypertrophy (elastic in feel)
  - Manual labourers
  - Athletes
  - Myotonia (Fig. 18.1)
  - Sometimes, in cysticercosis in muscles
  - Acromegaly
  - Hemangioma or arteriovenous malformations in muscle (may be unilateral).
- Pseudohypertrophy (doughy in feel)
  - Myopathy (e.g. Duchenne type) (Fig. 18.2)
  - Hypothyroidism
  - Glycogen storage disease
  - Rarely in trichinosis.

TETANY

It is increased neuromuscular irritability due to decrease in the concentration of free calcium ion in the plasma. This special variety of paroxysmal cramps occur mainly in the extremities. Normally the serum calcium level is 9–11 mg/dL and the ionic fraction is 4.5–5.6 mg/dL.

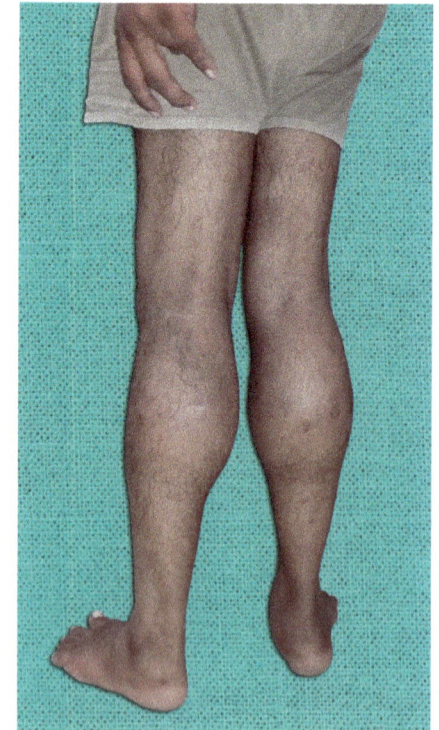

Fig. 18.1: Calf muscles hypertrophy (true) in myotonia dystrophica

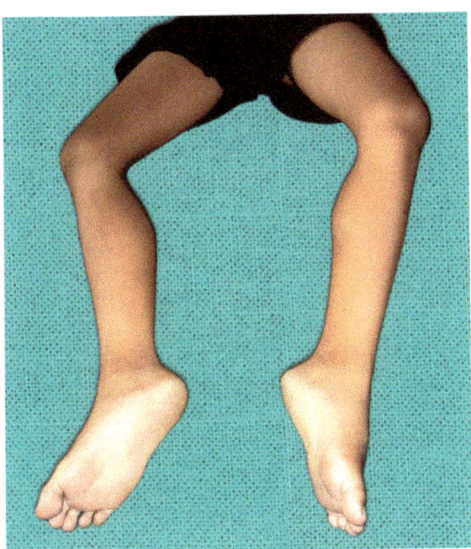

Fig. 18.2: Duchenne muscular dystrophy with calf muscles hypertrophy (pseudo)

The common symptoms are:
- Irritability
- Muscle cramp (carpopedal spasm)
- Peripheral paresthesia
- Triad of symptoms in children, i.e. carpopedal spasm, laryngismus stridulus (stridor, respiratory distress, cyanosis) and convulsions
- Dysphagia, dyspnea, dysuria, abdominal colic.

Physical Signs

- ***Trousseau's sign:*** When the pressure is raised above the systolic blood pressure (BP) for 2–3 minutes, typical carpal spasm occurs in hands within 3 minutes. There is flexion of metacarpophalangeal (MCP) joints with extension of interphalangeal joints, and the flexed thumb takes its position in between the index and the middle finger (opposition of thumb). This is known as **main d'accoucheur** or obstetrician's hand. Pedal spasm is less frequently demonstrated. Latent tetany is best demonstrated by this sign (Fig. 18.3).
- ***Chvostek's sign:*** Tapping of the facial nerve (by finger or hammer) in front of the ear will produce twitching of facial muscles.
- ***Erb's sign:*** Muscular contractions can be produced by application of subthreshold electrical stimulation (0.5–2.0 mAmp).
- ***Peroneal sign:*** Tapping of peroneal nerve at the neck of fibula will produce pedal spasm, i.e. plantar flexion and adduction of the foot, while the knee is extended.
- *[**Electrocardiography (ECG):** Prolonged Q-T interval].*

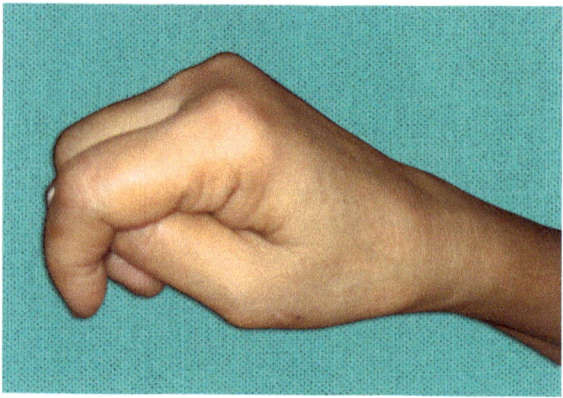

Fig. 18.3: Carpal spasm in tetany (hypocalcemia resulting from hypoparathyroidism)

All are the features of increased neuromuscular irritability. Tetany is due to **unstable depolarization** of the distal segments of the motor nerves. Carpopedal spasm may uncommonly spread over face, neck and trunk muscles (except the eye muscles). Psychoneurotic patients may have tetany during hyperventilation. Hyperventilation and ischemia of muscles increase the tendency of carpopedal spasm.

TREATMENT OF CRAMPS

- Massaging, and passive and vigrous stretching of the affected muscles.
- **Tetany:** Injection of calcium gluconate (10% solution) 10 mL by intravenous route, slowly (injection calcium chloride may be given). If tetany is not controlled by calcium, administration of magnesium may be necessary.
- Tab quinine sulfate—300–600 mg three times daily.
- Tab procainamide—250–500 mg three times daily.
- Tab diphenhydramine hydrochloride—50 mg at bedtime.
- Carbamazepine, clonazepam, muscles relaxants (e.g. tizanidine) may be of some help.
- Idiopathic nocturnal cramp may be alleviated by tocopherol, 400 mg twice daily; carnitine may be of some help.

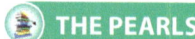 **THE PEARLS**

Cramps are usually temporary and non-damaging but may cause mild-to-excruciating pain. They may be recurrent. Proper history-taking (occupation, drug intake) and judicious investigations—nerve conduction velocity (NCV), electromyography (EMG), Doppler studies, electrolyte analysis, serum creative kinase (CK) and aldolase often solve this nagging problem.

Depressed Bridge of the Nose

POSSIBILITIES

1. *Lepromatous leprosy (Fig. 19.1)* (thick and coarse skin of face, especially the infiltrated earlobes, madarosis, occasional perforated nasal septum, deeper lines of face, bronzed hyperpigmentation, leonine face).
2. *Thalassemia major* (frontal bossing, hypertelorism, mongoloid slant of eyes, malar prominence, dental malocclusion, icterus and pallor → the 'chipmunk' facies).

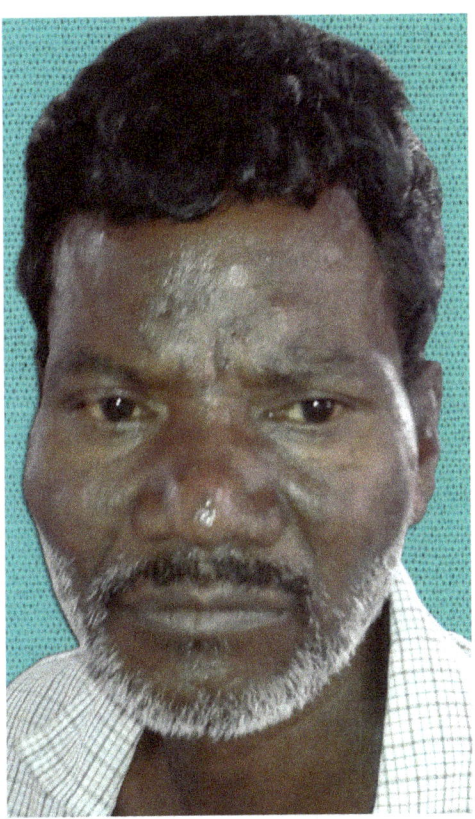

Fig. 19.1: Depressed bridge of the nose in lepromatous leprosy

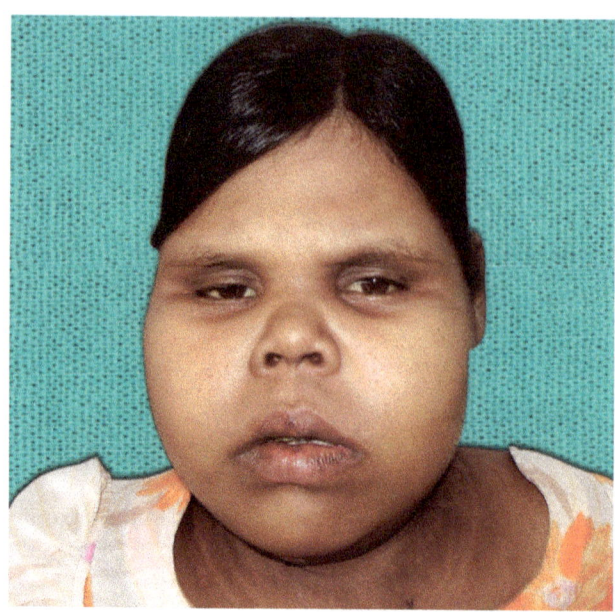

Fig. 19.2: A rare patient of congenital syphilis having saddle-nose deformity with depressed bridge of the nose and peg-shaped upper central incisors (part of Hutchinson's triad)

3. ***Down's syndrome (see Fig. 16.1)*** (microcephaly, upwards slanting of eyes with epicanthic folds, low set ears, hypertelorism, high-arched palate, large and fissured tongue with an idiotic look → mongol facies).
4. ***Cretinism*** (broad-flat nose with big nostrils, hypertelorism, thick-everted lower lip with macroglossia, sparse and dry skin, dull and idiotic look).
5. ***Congenital syphilis (Fig. 19.2)*** [frontal bossing, small and broad nose, poorly developed maxilla, ground-glass cornea, Hutchinson's teeth, 'Mulberry' molars (sixth years molars have multiple poorly developed cusps instead of four) and rhagades at the angle of mouth].
6. ***Ectodermal dysplasia (Fig. 19.3)*** (frontal bossing, small and broad nose, fine wrinkling in skin of face, sparse and dry hair, poor dentition with conical and pointed tip of teeth, poorly developed maxilla and often there is absence of sweating).
7. ***Wegener's granulomatosis*** (purulent or bloody nasal discharge, small and broad nose may result from nasal septal perforation).
8. ***Midline granuloma*** (small and broad nose, nasal discharge with septal perforation, perforation of soft and hard palate, conjunctival inflammation or ulceration, and loosening of teeth).
9. ***Sarcoidosis*** [lupus pernio in the skin of face (deeper nodules and plaques), conjunctival nodules, uveitis, dry eye with destruction of nasal bone may be present].
10. ***Others:*** Racial, achondroplasia, osteopetrosis, Hurler syndrome, blastomycosis, yaws, carcinoma of the nose or nasopharynx, vasculitis.

Chapter 19 Depressed Bridge of the Nose

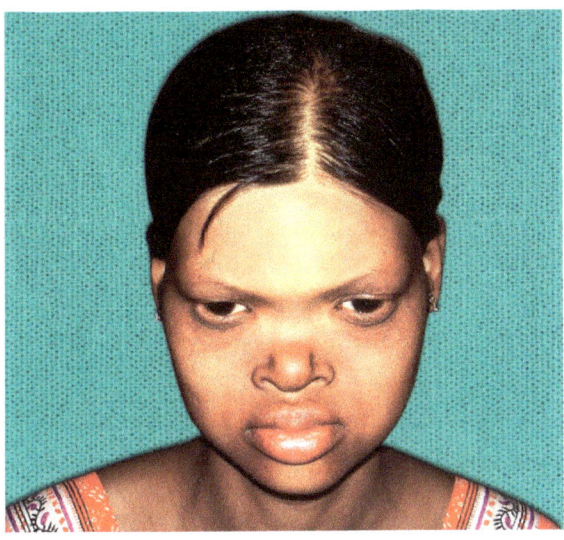

Fig. 19.3: Typical saddle-nose deformity in a patient with ectodermal dysplasia

- Saddle-nose deformity is classically found in 1, 5, 6, 7, 8 of above mentioned possibilities; also seen after overzealous septal excision operation or in polychondritis.
- 'Destruction of nasal structures' are seen in 1, 7, 8 and lupus vulgaris.

MECHANISMS RESPONSIBLE

- Due to hyperplasia of lesser wing of sphenoid bone in thalassemia.
- In others, it is due to chronic granulomatous destruction of anterior nasal septum.

SADDLE-NOSE DEFORMITY (FIG. 19.3)

- Small and broad nose
- Big nostrils
- Depressed bridge of the nose.

FRONTAL BOSSING OF SKULL (PROMINENT FOREHEAD)

- Thalassemia major
- Rickets
- Hydrocephalus
- Congenital syphilis
- Ectodermal dysplasia
- Acromegaly

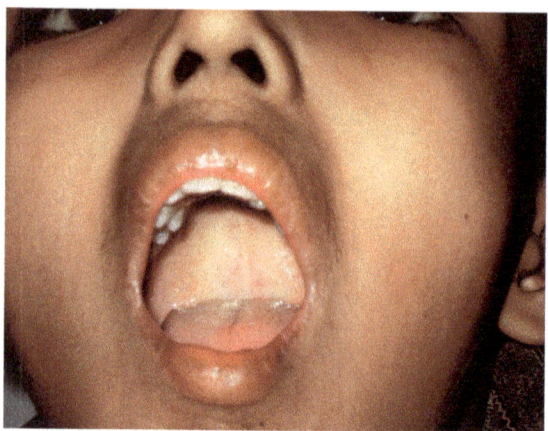

Fig. 19.4: High-arched palate in a suspected case of Marfan's syndrome

- Achondroplasia
- Ehlers-Danlos syndrome.

HIGH-ARCHED PALATE (FIG. 19.4)

Arbitrarily diagnosed if the roof of the palate is not visible when the examiner's eyes are kept at the level of the patient's upper incisor teeth—
- Down's syndrome
- Marfan's syndrome
- Thalassemia
- Cyanotic congenital heart diseases
- Turner's syndrome.

SABRE TIBIA (ANTERIOR TIBIAL BOWING)

- Rickets
- Congenital syphilis
- Paget's disease
- Osteogenesis imperfecta.

'Sabre' literally means cavalry sword with curved blade. In sabre tibia, the anterior border of tibia mimics the sword.

HUTCHINSON'S TRIAD (FIG. 19.2)

- Hutchinson's teeth (centrally notched, widely spaced, peg-shaped upper central incisor)
- Interstitial keratitis
- Nerve deafness.

Hutchinson's triad is a stigma of congenital syphilis.

SLANTING OF EYES

- ***Mongoloid:*** Racial, Down's syndrome, ectodermal dysplasia, Prader-Willi syndrome.
- ***Anti-mongoloid:*** Noonan's syndrome, Turner's syndrome, Apert's syndrome, Alport syndrome.

SMALL CHINS (MICROGNATHIA)

- Treacher collins syndrome
- Turner's syndrome
- Pierre-Robin syndrome
- Fetal alcohol syndrome.

PROMINENT SUPRAORBITAL RIDGES

- Racial
- Acromegaly
- Achondroplasia
- Hydrocephalus
- Thalassemia
- Paget's disease.

BIG LIPS

- Acromegaly
- Cretinism
- Hemangioma or lymphangioma of lip.

THE PEARLS

Depressed bridge of the nose, saddle-nose, high-arched palate, etc. are different windows in clinical medicine and are regarded as clinician's paradise to diagnose a common disease or to have a difficult syndromic analysis.

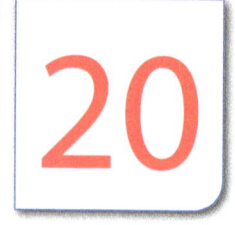

Dextrocardia

PROLOGUE

Dextrocardia is a rare congenital defect where the apex of the heart is situated on the right side of the chest rather than the left chest, as is the usual case (dextro means *right* in Latin).

There are two main types of dextrocardia:
1. **Isolated dextrocardia** (almost always have cardiac malformations; 5% normal heart).
2. **Dextrocardia with situs inversus** (heart per se does not show any abnormality; 95% normal heart).

SITUS INVERSUS

It is the rotation of abdominal/thoracic organs to opposite side, either totally (situs inversus totalis) or partially (situs inversus partialis).

In situs inversus, there is right-sided apex beat, right-sided stomach, right-sided descending aorta, left-sided liver. The right atrium is present on the left side as evidenced by inverted P wave in lead I in electrocardiography (ECG). The right lung has two lobes and left lung has three lobes (pulmonary isomerism) (Fig. 20.1).

> Heterotaxy is defined as an abnormality where the thoraco-abdominal organs demonstrate arrangement across the left-right axis of the body. Situs solitus is the normal position of thoracic and abdominal organs. When components of situs solitus and situs inversus are present in the same person, it is known as situs ambiguous.

COMMON PRESENTATIONS

The patients are usually asymptomatic (detected accidentally on chest X-ray done as a part of routine investigation).

There may be history of recurrent sinusitis (fever, cough, sneezing) and bronchiectasis (cough with profuse and fetid sputum); infertility in males may be noted—*vide* Kartagener's syndrome (*see* page 78).

On examination—there may be tender frontal sinuses, pyrexia and clubbing. Apex beat is present on the right side of the chest and the heart sounds are heard

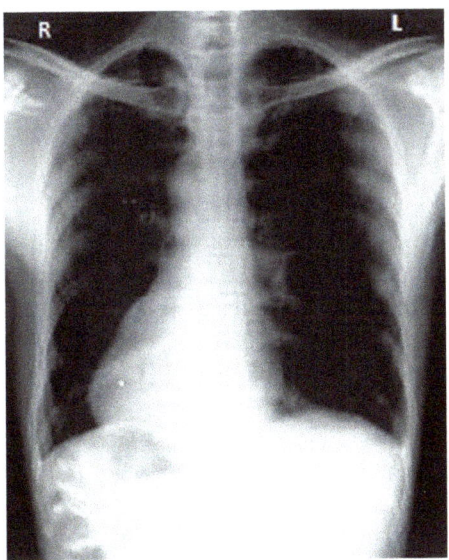

Fig. 20.1: Dextrocardia with situs inversus—cardiac apex is in right hemithorax; the left diaphragm is slightly higher than the right one. Fundal gas shadow seems to be on the right side

better on the right side than on the left side of the chest. Traube's space tympanicity is noted on the right side (as stomach is present on right side). The upper border of liver dullness is elicited on the left 5th intercostal space. Heart may reveal murmur, if associated with any cardiac abnormality (not common). Auscultation of lungs may reveal bilateral and basal crepitations (crackles) and rhonchi (wheezes), if associated with bronchiectasis.

DIFFERENT POSITIONS OF HEART

- Levocardia (situs solitus, i.e. normal position of heart)—cardiac apex on the left side of the chest
- Dextrocardia—cardiac apex on the right side of the chest
- Dextrocardia with situs inversus
- Isolated dextrocardia—dextrocardia without situs inversus
- Mesocardia—cardiac apex over the center of the chest
- Isolated levocardia—cardiac apex on the left side with viscera rotated (partially or totally) to the opposite side.

DEXTROVERSION

The cardiac apex is always on the right side due to extracardiac causes like right-sided collapse/fibrosis of the lung or left-sided pleural effusion/pneumothorax (i.e. shifting of the mediastinum to right side by push-pull effects). The trachea is moved to the right side too.

To differentiate dextrocardia from dextroversion, **always palpate the trachea**. In dextrocardia, trachea remains central in position, while in dextroversion trachea shifts to the right side.

CONGENITAL ANOMALIES ASSOCIATED WITH DEXTROCARDIA

- *Cardiac:*
  - Ventricular septal defect (VSD)/double-outlet right ventricle (DORV)
  - Single ventricle/single atrium
  - Pulmonary stenosis/pulmonary atresia
  - Right-sided aortic arch/aortic atresia
  - 'Corrected' transposition of great arteries (TGA)
  - Endocardial cushion defects.
- *Extracardiac:* Asplenia [evidenced by **Howell-Jolly bodies**—remnants of nuclear material in red blood cell (RBC), and **Heinz bodies**—formed from denatured aggregated hemoglobin, in peripheral blood smear] and polysplenia syndrome (manifested by multiple small accessory spleens).

KARTAGENER'S SYNDROME

This is also known as *immotile cilia syndrome*, which results in male infertility. This syndrome is the triad of:
- Bronchiectasis
- Dextrocardia/situs inversus
- Recurrent sinusitis.

Kartagener's syndrome is a variety of **primary ciliary dyskinsia** where there is immotility of cilia present in respiratory tract epithelium and sperm.

CHEST X-RAY AND ECG FINDINGS OF DEXTROCARDIA

- *Chest X-ray (postero-anterior view):* See the radiographer's labelling of "R" in the X-ray plate. The cardiac apex is in the right hemithorax with major portions of heart on the right side. The left dome of the diaphragm is elevated with fundal gas shadow seen below the left dome. Trachea remains central.
  In situs inversus, fundal gas shadow will be on the right side. Some cases may have associated bronchiectasis.
- *Electrocardiography:* P wave is inverted (negative) in lead I. QRS complex and T wave are also inverted in lead I. Upright (positive) P wave is seen in lead aVR. Tallest QRS complexes are seen in the precordial leads, i.e. in V_1 and V_2, which progressively diminishes to the left. That is to say, there is gradual diminution of height of R wave from V_1 to V_6.

Confirmation of diagnosis is done by chest X-ray, ECG and echocardiography.

TECHNICAL DEXTROCARDIA

It is the faulty interchange of right and left arm electrodes in ECG by a technician. Here, lead I, II, III, aVR, aVL, aVF will have similar changes like true dextrocardia but there will be no alteration of normal ECG pattern in precordial leads (precordial leads, i.e. lead V_1 to V_6 will be normal as is seen in healthy normal people).

THE PEARLS

Diagnosis of dextrocardia evokes much interest in the medical fraternity. Many detective stories and novels are based on person who has dextrocardia. It is the duty of the physician to disclose the diagnosis to the patient that he/she has a heart which is right-sided. The physician should search for associated anomalies, which may or may not be present. The patient should always be reassured.

Dextrocardia is believed to occur in 1 in 12,000 people approximately. When defibrillating a person with dextrocardia (for cardioversion), the pads should be placed in reverse position, i.e. instead of upper right and lower left, pads should be placed upper left and lower right.

21 Diffuse Aches and Pains

POSSIBLE ETIOLOGY

Diffuse aches and pains all over the body are due to:
- Soft-tissue rheumatism
- Fibromyalgia
- Post-viral myalgia
- Myxedema
- Polymyalgia rheumatica
- Hypermobility
- Chronic fatigue syndrome
- Hypophosphatemia
- Polymyositis/dermatomyositis
- Myopathy
- Metabolic bone disease
- Paraneoplastic syndrome.

> One should never forget osteomalacia and multiple myeloma as causes of diffuse pain in the body.

COMMON REGIONAL MUSCULOSKELETAL PROBLEMS

Neck and Shoulder Pain

- Cervical spondylosis
- Musculoskeletal (MSK) strain (mechanical or muscular neck pain)
- Trauma
- Cervical disc prolapse (nerve root entrapment)
- Rotator cuff syndrome
- Bicipital tendonitis
- Adhesive capsulitis (true *frozen shoulder*)
- Ankylosing spondylitis
- Polymyalgia rheumatica
- Glenohumeral or acromioclavicular arthritis

- Pancoast tumor or thoracic inlet syndrome
- Ischemic heart disease
- Chronic burning neck pain (muscle tension from anxiety and stress).

Hand and Wrist Pain

- Tenosynovitis (e.g. De Quervain's)
- Carpal tunnel syndrome
- Inflammatory arthritis (e.g. rheumatoid arthritis)
- Gout and pseudogout
- Nodal osteoarthritis
- Cellulitis, lymphangitis, thrombophlebitis
- Trauma (e.g. scaphoid fracture)
- Raynaud's phenomenon
- Leprosy, sickle cell anemia
- Chronic regional pain syndrome.

Low Back Pain

- Trauma
- Lumbar spondylosis
- Lumbar disc prolapse
- Facet joint syndrome
- Spondylolisthesis
- Ankylosing spondylitis
- Multiple myeloma, metastases
- Osteomalacia
- Osteoporosis with spinal fracture
- Miscellanous—pregnancy, dysmenorrhea, psoriatic or reactive arthritis, subarachnoid hemorrhage, fibromyalgia, osteomyelitis, muscular or ligamentous strain, anxiety, malingering.

Hip Pain

- Sacroiliitis (e.g. ankylosing spondylitis)
- Trochanteric bursitis
- Neck femur fracture or trochanteric fracture
- Avascular necrosis or osteonecrosis
- Inflammatory arthritis (e.g. ankylosing spondylitis)
- Tuberculosis of the hip joint
- Meralgia paraesthetica
- Lumbar radiculopathy
- Osteoarthritis of hip joint
- Osteomalacia (with 'pseudofractures').

Knee Pain

- Osteoarthritis
- Spondyloarthropathy, rheumatoid arthritis
- Gout, pseudogout
- Septic arthritis
- Meniscal tears or cruciate ligament tears
- Baker's cyst
- Hypermobility syndrome
- Chondromalacia patellae.

Foot and Heel Pain

- ***Foot pain***
    - High-arched or flat foot
    - Gout
    - Buerger's disease
    - Inflammatory arthritis (e.g. rheumatoid arthritis)
    - Stress fracture
    - Metatarsalgia
    - Tarsal tunnel syndrome
    - Plantar fasciitis
    - Calcaneal spur
    - Hallux rigidus
- ***Heel pain***
    - Ulcer, fissure, keratoses, panniculitis, verruca
    - Plantar fasciitis
    - Achilles tendinosis
    - Calcanean spur
    - Sever's disease (i.e. traction apophysitis of Achilles tendon).

CHRONIC FATIGUE SYNDROME

Controversial topic; previously known as **neurasthenia** or myalgic encephalomyelitis. Commonly seen in females in between ages 20 and 50 years. The chief complaint is chronic fatigue which is made worse by minimal exertion. It is a combined physical and mental (e.g. poor concentration, irritability) fatiguability. Etiological factors are post-viral (e.g. viral hepatitis, influenza, infectious mononucleosis), physical inactivity and sleep difficulties. Though the role of stress is uncertain, there is presence of mood disorder in many patients. The onset may be sudden (fibromyalgia is insidious in onset) and tender trigger points are not associated with chronic fatigue syndrome (CFS). Psychotherepy is essential; antidepressants work better in the presence of mood disorder or insomnia. Graded exercise therapy and cognitive behavioural therapy work better.

FIBROMYALGIA (FIBROSITIS SYNDROME)

It is a chronic multisystem illness characterized by widespread pain (present for more than 3 months both above and below the waist) and associated with neuropsychological symptoms including fatigue, anxiety, depression and many medically unexplained symptoms in other systems. Objective signs of inflammation are absent with normal laboratory studies including erythrocyte sedimentation rate (ESR). It is very often a diagnosis of exclusion; the cardinal feature is specific tender trigger points (Note: in anxiety, tender points are present 'all over' the body). Women are the worst sufferer (female: male; F:M=10:1) who struggles much in family/day to day life. History of (H/O) familial disharmony is present in some patients; many have sleep disturbances who awake unrefreshed with poor mental concentration. There is widespread, unremitting pain. The patient may also suffer from irritable bowel syndrome, CFS, tension headache or premenstrual syndrome. There is associated subjective feeling of muscle swelling. Available evidence implicates the central nervous system as key in maintaining pain and other core symptoms of fibromyalgia. It is a ***pain amplification syndrome*** due to abnormalities in serotonin, substance P and cortisol levels. Reassurance, sympathetic attitude, aerobic exercise, nonsteroidal anti-inflammatory drugs (NSAIDs), antidepressants (amitriptyline, dothiepin), trigger point injections (local anesthetics/corticosteroid), cognitive behavioural therapy or acupuncture may be of some help. Many patients do not respond to therapy.

SOFT-TISSUE RHEUMATISM

Soft-tissue rheumatism (STR) forms the major chunk of MSK disorders in any outpatient clinic. This refers to aches and pains which arise from structures surrounding the joint (i.e. non-articular) such as tendons, muscles, bursae and ligaments.

Differential diagnosis with arthritis is done by:
- Tenderness away from the joint-line margin
- Pain aggravated more with active movements than on passive movements
- Swelling usually away from the joint-line
- Dramatic relief with local injections of corticosteroid.

ANATOMICAL BASIS OF PAIN ARISING IN MUSCULOSKELETAL SYSTEM

- ***Joint***
  - Synovium—synovitis
  - Joint capsule—capsulitis
- ***Periarticular (soft tissue) rheumatism***
  - Bursa—bursitis
  - Tendon—tendonitis
  - Tendon sheath—tenosynovitis
  - Insertion of tendon, ligaments—enthesitis
- ***Bone:*** Osteoporosis, ostemalacia, osteonecrosis, multiple myeloma.

FUNCTIONAL SOMATIC SYNDROMES

The functional somatoform disorders are probably stress-induced psychosomatic disorders. Often they are not explanable to the physician himself and thus they are called **all in the mind** of the patient. They are as follows:
- Tension headache
- Atypical facial or chest pain
- Fibromyalgia
- Chronic fatigue syndrome
- Chemical sensitivity
- Irritable bowel syndrome
- Premenstrual syndrome
- Irritable bladder.

TINGLING AND NUMBNESS

This is the most common paresthesia in clinical practice → may occur in health due to sitting or sleeping in abnormal awkward position (e.g. sitting in the front rod of a bicycle) for some time (as a result of neuropraxia). Usually these are features of lesion in nerves (peripheral neuropathy), spinal roots (radiculopathy) or spinal tracts. Tingling sensation usually leads to numbness when there is total loss of function of touch as well as pain fibers. Common causes encountered in clinical practice are:
- Peripheral neuropathy
- Carpal tunnel syndrome
- Cervical spondylitis
- Prolapsed intervertebral disc
- Lumbar canal stenosis
- Radiculopathy (e.g. from diabetes mellitus)
- Hyperventilation (hysterical, salicylate overdose).

THE PEARLS

The major manifestations of MSK disorders are pain and impairment of locomotor functions. Non-inflammatory conditions are for more prevalent than the inflammatory disorders. Most of the MSK disorders are common in women. Early recognition and subsequent treatment by rheumatologists lead to better symptom control.

22

Diplopia

DEFINITION

It is the perception of **double vision** of a single object.

MECHANISM OF PRODUCTION

In health, coordination of ocular muscles gives rise to conjugate movements of the eyes, and as a result binocular vision is achieved. Thus, the visual stimulus falls exactly on the similar parts of two retinae (macula), and an object is perceived as a single unit. Conjugate movements of the eyes are maintained by cortex, brainstem, and via the IIIrd, IVth and VIth cranial nerves. Defective movement of one eye may result in images (from the two eyes) arising from different points on the two retinae → as a result binocular fusion cannot occur in visual cortex → two separate or overlapping images are formed. In paralytic squint, the image from the healthy eye (true image) is clear and distinct, but the image produced on the affected eye is indistinct and blurred (false image; image derived from the retina outside macula) → false image is perceived in the true direction of action of the weak extraocular muscle.

Many a time, the head may be involuntarily turned in the direction of action of paralyzed or weak muscles (head tilt to avoid diplopia in IVth cranial nerve palsy). True diplopia becomes single, if one eye is covered by hollow of the palm. Sudden appearance of diplopia usually points towards a neurological lesion.

Diplopia results from loss of parallel visual axes, and is commonly due to IIIrd, IVth and VIth nerve palsy, myasthenia gravis and myopathy (e.g. thyrotoxicosis). Diplopia should be clinically assessed in nine cardinal direction of gaze (i.e. as done in the test of voluntary movements of extraocular muscles) by asking the patient to follow the examiner's finger.

Cover one eye with a red glass, and ask the patient whether the red or the normally colored image is the true imge → this **red glass test** often indicates the affected eye.

WHY THERE IS NO DIPLOPIA IN CONCOMITANT (NON-PARALYTIC) SQUINT?

Squint is of two types—paralytic and concomitant (non-paralytic).

In case of paralytic squint, the image on the paralyzed side does not fall on the macula and thus diplopia occurs. Diplopia is maximum if the eye is moved in the direction of weak muscle. Whereas in concomitant squint, the image formed by the defective eye is either rejected or suppressed by the occipital (visual) cortex and thus, there is no diplopia.

TYPES

There are two types of diplopia:
1. **Binocular:** Diplopia perceived when both eyes remain open
2. **Uniocular:** Diplopia perceived when one eye remains open.

Possible Associations of Binocular Diplopia

- **Loss of parallel visual axes:** Displacement of eyeball by intraocular space occupying lesion (SOL), orbital pseudotumor
- **IIIrd, IVth, VIth cranial nerve palsy:** Intracranial SOL, demyelinating disease, brainstem infarction or hemorrhage, cavernous sinus thrombosis, raised intracranial tension, meningitis, diabetes mellitus, vasculitis, vertebrobasilar insufficiency
- **Muscle disorders:** Congenital weakness of extraocular muscles, myasthenia gravis, muscular dystrophy, severe exophthalmos from thyrotoxicosis, botulism.
- **Miscellaneous:** Ophthalmoplegic migraine, temporal arteritis, syphilis, restriction of eye movement (e.g. in pterygium, symblepharon).

Possible Associations of Monocular Diplopia

Rare and due to eye disorders like:
- Incipient stage of cataract (water molecule within lens)
- Subluxation of the lens
- Peripheral iridectomy (large)
- Astigmatism
- Keratoconus
- Iridolysis as a result of injury
- Defective contact lens or poorly-fitting bifocals
- Hysteria.

THE PEARLS

- Unilateral IIIrd nerve palsy does not produce diplopia because of the presence of complete ptosis. Diplopia is complained by the patient as soon as the affected drooped upper eyelid is elevated by fingers
- In IIIrd, IVth and VIth nerve palsy, there is paralytic squint over and above diplopia
- In myasthenia gravis, diplopia is associated with diurnal variation of ptosis
- In concomitant squint, diplopia is absent

Contd...

Contd…

- In IVth nerve palsy, double vision is present for reading and walking downstairs. In IIIrd nerve palsy, diplopia and squint are maximum on looking up and in, while in VIth nerve palsy diplopia occurs in looking in the direction of affected muscle. In myesthenia gravis and Graves' disease, diplopia occurs in all directions of gaze
- Common investigations done for diplopia are blood for total leukocyte count (TLC), differential leukocyte count (DLC), erythrocyte sedimentation rate (ESR) and computed tomography (CT) or magnetic resonance imaging (MRI) of brain and Tensilon test (to diagnose myasthenia gravis) over and above meticulous clinical examination.
- Treatment is aimed at correction of the primary defect. In incapacitating diplopia, shielding of the affected eye is advised. Exercise of the external ocular muscles with the help of optometrist and electrophysiotherapy of the paralyzed eye muscles are advised; surgical correction is needed in selective patients (e.g. lesion persisting >6 months).

23

Discolored Teeth

POSSIBILITIES OF STAINED TEETH

- Chronic betel-leaf chewer, tobacco staining by smokers; coffee, tea, cola and wines can stain the teeth
- Unhealthy oral hygiene (the yellowish-brown discoloration may be eradicated after repeated mouth wash/brushing)
- Tetracycline therapy (if given during second half of pregnancy, in infancy or in childhood < 8 years of age → permanent discoloration of teeth by greyish-blue to brownish-yellow color as well as enamel hypoplasia)—irregularly stained appearance
- Minocycline therapy (affects middle part of teeth with a greyish pigmentation; involves permanent teeth in comparison to tetracycline which affects temporary teeth. The drug is used in leprosy and nocardiosis)
- Fluorosis (produces chalky-while patches, yellowish-brown discoloration)
- Congenital erythropoietic porphyria (teeth are brownish-pink) → erythrodonita, as a result of high porphyrin content → orange-red fluorescence under Wood's lamp
- Kernicterus, caries tooth and osteogenesis imperfecta may develop into brownish discoloration of teeth. Trauma can discolor the adult teeth.

GRADES OF DENTAL FLUOROSIS

Three grades of dental fluorosis are as follows:
1. White chalky opacities of patches on enamel with or without faint yellow lines.
2. Distinct brownish discolouration.
3. Pitting of enamel surface, sometimes with chipping of edges.

Dental fluorosis, classically known as ***mottled enamel***, is essentially a dental hypoplasia with areas of decreased calcification and mineralization.

In Punjab (India), fluorosis manifests in one of the severest forms leading to advanced invalidism. In fluorosis, considerable disability is associated with spinal rigidity, restricted movements of the joints, and flexion deformity of the hips and knees. There is increased bone density; tendons, ligaments and even muscles may be mineralized. Ultimately, compressive myelopathy leads to progressive neurological disability.

OSTEOSCLEROSIS (BONE TURNS ABSOLUTELY WHITISH IN X-RAY)

- Fluorosis
- Metastatic deposits from carcinoma of prostate (commonly), and rarely from breast, intestine or bronchus
- Hodgkin's disease (ivory vertebra)
- Marble bone disease (osteopetrosis)
- Osteopoikilosis
- Vitamin A or D toxicity
- Jaw in Paget's disease
- Diffuse idiopathic skeletal hyperostosis (DISH)
- Renal osteodystrophy (Rugger-jersey spine).

THE PEARLS

Discolored teeth is also a window in clinical medicine with special reference to fluorosis. The patient should be immediately referred to a dentist with a goal to prevent the systemic manifestations of the disease.

Unhealthy oral hygiene and tobacco staining are probably the most common causes.

24

Drop Attacks

DEFINITION

A fall occurring without warning (instant), giddiness, tripping, apparent paralysis or loss of consciousness due to unexpected episodes of lower limb weakness.

THE FALL

The victims are usually middle-aged or elderly women. They suddenly drop (i.e. fall) to the floor while standing or walking. She/he feels her/himself falling (intense leg weakness), then crashes the ground (knees buckle, striking the knees/nose upon the ground) and picks her/himself up almost immediately. Some patients describe sudden and momentary loss of power in the legs, who are unable to prevent the fall by raising their hands. Drop attacks are presumably of brainstem origin, rather than thromboembolism and consciousness is preserved throughout. No post-incidence confusion is there but considerable embarrassment persists.

COMMON ASSOCIATIONS

- No obvious cause
- Vertebrobasilar insufficiency (may complain diplopia)–one of the very common cause of drop attack
- Epilepsy
- Hydrocephalus, third ventricular tumor (both the patients are young)
- Parkinson's disease
- Quadriceps weakness (they fall simply due to knees flexing; may be able to protect the face by raising the arms)
- Causes of *falls in the elderly* (see below).

INVESTIGATIONS

- Blood sugar (fasting)
- X-ray of neck to rule out cervical spondylosis (as a cause of vertebrobasilar insufficiency)
- Electroencephalogram (EEG)
- Computed tomography (CT) or magnetic resonance imaging (MRI) scan to rule out any organic lesion in brain
- Doppler studies of carotid/vertebral arteries.

CAUSES OF FALLS WITH DISTURBED CONSCIOUSNESS

1. Epilepsy
2. Syncope (simple faints, cough/micturition/carotid sinus)
3. Transient ischemic attack (TIA)
4. Cardiac dysrhythmias
5. Pseudoseizures (non-epileptic attacks)
6. Panic attacks
7. Vertigo
8. Hyperventilation
9. Breath-holding (children)
10. Pheochromocytoma, carcinoid syndrome, drug reactions
11. Hypoglycemia, hypocalcemia.

One should do electrocardiography (ECG) and Holter monitoring (24-hours ambulatory ECG), if necessary.

MAJOR CAUSES OF FALLS IN THE ELDERLY

Falls are the leading cause of accidental death among older adults and thus every effort should be made to prevent them. Major causes of falls in the elderly are as follows:
- Visual impairment (e.g. cataract)
- Reduced hearing
- Muscle weakness
- Postural hypotension (e.g. use of antihypertensives or diuretics)
- Lack of concentration
- Musculoskeletal disorder (e.g. rheumatoid arthritis)
- Use of medications (sedatives, antidepressants, diuretics)
- Foot disorders (deformities/edema)
- Postural instability/vestibular dysfunction
- Gait or balance abnormalities (e.g. acute labyrinthitis)
- Depression
- Cognitive impairment
- Environmental—insufficient light, high-stepping stairs, waxed slippery mozaic floor, uneven carpet edge, raised toilet seat in bathroom, uneven/high heel shoes.

DIFFERENTIAL DIAGNOSIS OF FITS IN CLINICAL PRACTICE

- ***Idiopathic epilepsy:*** History of (H/O) previous fits; perform EEG (abnormal) and CT scan (normal)
- ***Febrile convulsions:*** Age ranges 6 months to 5 years, often with a positive family history; normal EEG and CT scan. Always associated with febrile illness

- ***Intracranial space occupying lesion (ICSOL):*** Any age, headache, papilloedema; confirmed by CT or MRI scan
- ***Convulsions due to meningitis or meningoencephalitis:*** Pyrexia, altered consciousness, positive neck rigidity; confirmed by lumbar puncture and CT scan
- ***Hypoglycemia:*** Perspiration, increase hunger, a diabetic on insulin or oral hypoglycemic agents; confirmed by blood sugar level during the attack (hypoglycaemic symptoms occur when blood sugar is less than 50 mg/dL and convulsions occur when it is less than 36 mg/dL).
- ***Alcohol withdrawal:*** History from relatives is diagnostic and is often suggested by recent heavy intake of alcohol; confirmed by recurrent episodes in similar circumstances
- ***Severe dyselectrolytemia (↓Na, ↑Na, ↓Ca, ↓Mg):*** Confirmed by serum biochemistry. No recurrence after correction of metabolic abnormality
- ***Severe hypotension (sudden):*** Pulse not palpable, blood pressure (BP) not recordable, central and peripheral cyanosis; ECG shows asystole or electromechanical dissociation
- ***Pseudoseizures (functional):*** Always happens to occur in front of people/relatives and eyes closed during seizure; normal EEG and CT scan.

SOME DEFINITIONS

- ***Syncope:*** Sudden and transient loss of consciousness with inability to stand upright as a result of impairment of cerebral blood flow (i.e. postural collapse)
- ***Vertigo:*** A sense of loss of balance and unsteadiness with a feeling of rotation of environment or body
- ***Dizziness:*** A sensation of light headedness or faintness
- ***Convulsions/fits/seizures:*** It is a paroxysmal event of violent and irregular movement of body due to abnormal excessive or synchronous neuronal activity (discharge) in the brain
- ***Conversion disorder (previous hysteria):*** It is a loss or distorsion of neurological function not fully explained by organic disease, e.g. aphonia, paralysis of limb, blindness, etc.

🐚 THE PEARLS

Drop attacks, fits or syncope should never be ignored whatever the age of the patient is. It should always be investigated as an emergency basis. Remember, in drop attacks the patient remains conscious in contrast to syncope or fits, where transient loss of consciousness is the rule.

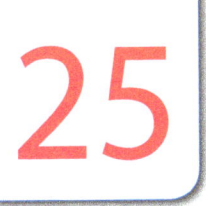

25 Erectile Dysfunction (Impotence)

DEFINITION

Inability of the male to achieve an erection of penis during sexual activity is impotence (a better terminology is erectile dysfunction, ED). Male erection is a neurovascular reflex, which depends on a healthy anatomy of penis with an ideal hormonal environment. Impotence is of two types—primary (ED from the beginning) and secondary (initiates after a period of normal penile erection).

BASICS

Three basic mechanisms needed to develop ED are as follows:
1. Failure to initiate (psychogenic, endrocrinologic or neurogenic)
2. Failure to fill (arteriogenic)
3. Failure to store (veno-occlusive dysfunction) sufficient volume of blood within the lacunar network of penis.

Multiple factors contribute to ED in many patients. Diabetes mellitus, atherosclerosis, and drug-related etiologies are responsible for major causes of ED in older people.

POSSIBLE ASSOCIATIONS

Psychological (Situational)

Variety of psychogenic inputs like anxiety, depression, sexual inhibition, sexual abuse in childhood, fear of pregnancy, sexually transmitted diseases (STDs), sense of guilt, ignorance of sex act, marital conflict, conflicted parent-child relationship or religious orthodoxy.

Organic (Constitutional)

- **Endocrine disorders:** Kallmann syndrome, hypopituitarism, hyperprolactinemia, pituitary tumor, Klinefelter's syndrome, testicular tumor/trauma/orchitis, alcoholic liver disease-induced testicular atrophy, hypogonadism, andropause, Addison's disease, hypo- or hyperthyroidism
- **Diabetes mellitus (DM):** DM-associated neurologic as well as vascular complications are responsible for ED in 35–75% patients

- ***Vascular:*** Atherosclerosis (e.g. Leriche's syndrome) or traumatic arterial disease
- ***Neurogenic:*** Autonomic neuropathy (e.g. from DM), cauda equina lesion, multiple sclerosis, peripheral neuropathy (e.g. alcoholism), following pelvic surgery, spinal cord injury, alcohol excess
- ***Drug-induced:*** Antihypertensives, antidepressants, tranquilizers, psychotropics, anticholinergics, cytotoxic drugs, hormones (e.g. oestrogens), β-blockers
- ***Miscellaneous:*** Recreational drugs or addictions (alcohol, cocaine, marijuana), chronic debilitating diseases (chronic renal failure, motor neuron disease), pelvic fracture, mechanical interference from morbid obesity, prostatectomy, penile trauma, Peyronie's disease.

CLINICAL EVALUATION

A close-door sympathetic interview with the patient is the first task of the physician. Differentiate organic from psychological causes; ED with only one partner, of sudden onset, intermittent (i.e. not permanent), with ability to masturbate, having nocturnal and early morning erections, and with normal nocturnal penile tumescence (NPT) test (a plethysmograph placed around the penis overnight to determine the neurovascular action sufficient to produce erection during sleep) suggest psychogenic ED. Organic ED is characterized by impotence of gradual onset, with all partners, permanent with total decline of erectile ability (diurnal as well as nocturnal), and with abnormal NPT test. Other aspect of history should focus on duration and persistence of ED, symptoms suggestive of endocrine disorders, neuropathy, vascular disease or diabetes.

Normal level of testosterone, gonadotrophin and prolactin with history of nocturnal emissions and frequent satisfactory morning erections make endocrine disorders unlikely. A careful history of stress, alcohol abuse, drugs (mentioned above) should be taken.

Detail physical examination of blood pressure (BP), thyroid, liver, cardiovascular system (CVS), renal system should be sought for. Size of testicles and penis, secondary sexual characters, and testing of peripheral neuropathy must be done.

In selected patients, specialized testing may give clue to diagnosis:
- Studies of NPT and rigidity
- Vascular testing [penile Doppler ultrasonography (USG), penile angiography, dynamic infusion cavernosometry]
- Neurologic testings (vibratory perception; so called somatosensory evoked potentials)
- Psychological diagnostic tests.

It is important to remember that, psychogenic ED is frequently a diagnosis of exclusion.

- *Impotence with reduced libido (sexual desire):* hypogonadism and depression
  Impotence with intact libido: Others including psychological problems
- NPT test is normal in psychogenic ED and abnormal in organic ED.

DRUGS ASSOCIATED WITH ERECTILE DYSFUNCTION

- Antidepressants [selective serotonin reuptake inhibitor (SSRI), tricyclic antidepressant]
- Tranquilizers (phenothiazines)
- Cardiac drugs (digoxin, gemfibrozil)
- Antihypertensives [β-blockers, calcium channel blockers (CCB), clonidine]
- Diuretics (thiazides, spironolactone)
- Hormones [corticosteroids, gonadotropin-releasing hormone agonist (GnRHa)]
- Anticholinergics (anticonvulsants)
- Cytotoxics (cyclophosphamide)
- Recreational (ethanol, cocaine).

MANAGEMENT

- Patient education is started with gynecological examination of the female partner to rule out any obstructive pathology in female genital tract. Psychiatric examination of both the partners is mandatory. It is important to discuss the matter frankly with the patient
- **Drugs:** Phosphodiesterase type-5 (PDE5) inhibitors (sildenafil, tadalafil, vardenafil, avanafil) increase penile blood flow and remain the first line of drug therapy in ED (by enhancing the effects of nitric oxide on smooth muscles); apomorphine, intraurethral or intracavernosal self-injections of alprostadil, papaverine or phentolamine
- **Androgen therapy:** Androgen replacement treatment is used in primary and secondary causes of hypogonadism. Loss of libido is corrected by androgen therapy
- **Devices:** Vacuum constriction devices, insertion of inflatable penile prosthesis or revascularization surgery may be done in selected cases
- **Sex therapy:** It addresses specific interpersonal factors; and consists of in-session discussion and at-home exercises specific to the person and the relationship. Both the partners should be involved in sex therapy to have a favorable outcome.

PREMATURE EJACULATION

It is the discharge of the semen before the orgasm is attained, i.e. it is an early orgasmic response. If it is persistently or recurrently experienced, one seeks advice of a doctor. The main causes in clinical practice are as follows:

- Psychological (no sexual experience, anxiety)
- Injury to genitourinary tract, genital anomalies or urinary infection (e.g. burning micturition)
- Diabetic autonomic neuropathy (affects parasympathetic control)
- Spinal cord injury.

While treating the patient, the physician should consider duration of excitement phase, age of the patient, frequency and duration of coitus; in day to day practice, it is seen in young patients with lack of sex knowledge. Usually, it requires no treatment but psychiatric counselling with clearing of myths/misconceptions, empathic attitude, or application of anti-anxiety drugs (sertraline, fluoxetine) may be of some help.

CARDINAL ELEMENTS OF NORMAL SEXUAL FUNCTION

Libido (sexual desire)
↓
Erection (lubrication in female)
↓
Intromission (inserting penis into the vagina)
↓
Ejaculation and orgasm (only orgasm in female).

PRIAPISM

It is the unwanted, painful and persistent erection of penis, and is commonly due to:
- Sickle cell anemia
- Hypercoagulable states
- Chronic myeloid leukemia
- Spinal cord injury
- Injection of vasodilators (e.g. papavarine) into penis
- Pelvic vascular thrombosis (e.g. idiopathic thrombosis of prostatic venous plexus)
- Secondary malignant deposits in the corpora cavernosa
- Megapenis.

It is a very embarrassing situation for the patient. Local applications are useless. Anastomosis of saphenous vein to one corpus cavernosum is effective, if done within 48 hours; a trial of anticoagulant therapy for 14 days can be given. To treat the first 3 causes, analgesics, hydration and α-adrenergic blockers are used. In others, treatment of the etiology is solicited.

RETROGRADE EJACULATION

The process of ejaculation starts by → stimulation of sympathetic nervous system → contraction of vas deferens + seminal vesicles + prostate → seminal fluid entering into urethra, associated with rhythmic contractions of bulbocavernosus and ischiocavernosus muscles → ejaculation follows. When the internal urethral sphincter remains open during the process of ejaculation, semen enters into urinary bladder, and is known as *retrograde ejaculation*. It is commonly seen in diabetic patients with autonomic neuropathy, multiple sclerosis, spinal cord injury or after surgery involving the bladder neck. A dry climax (orgasm without semen) is the primary sign of retrograde ejaculation.

FECAL AND URINARY INCONTINENCE

- Neurogenic bladder (patient having paraplegia)
- Dementia (e.g. Alzheimer's disease)

- Epileptic convulsions [history of tongue bite, positive electroencephalogram (EEG)]
- Severe depression (low mood, lack of motivation)
- Impacted feces with overflow (very hard, rock-like feces in rectum).

THE PEARLS

The prevalence of ED is like this: 7% men between 18 and 29 years, 18% in their 50s, 25% in their 60s and 80% in their 80s.

First try to rule out diabetes, ↑ lipids, ↑ prolactin, ↓ androgen, hypo- or hyperthyroidism. In neurological examination, penile and perianal sensations are carefully examined. PDE5 inhibitors are treatment of choice keeping in mind its contraindications like hypotension, nitrate use, decompensated cardiac disease and concomitant use of α-adrenergic blockers.

26 Eyes: A Clue to Diagnosis

Very often the face, especially the eyes speak for a diagnosis of medical illness as many diseases may have manifestations in and around the eyes:
- Ptosis (pseudoptosis too) → oculomotor (or cervical sympathetic) nerve palsy (Fig. 26.1)
- Exophthalmos (proptosis), e.g. thyrotoxicosis, retro-orbital tumor (Fig. 26.2)
- Retraction of upper eyelids → hyperthyroidism
- Photophobia (↑ sensitivity to light) → meningitis, painful diseases of the eye (or 'red eyes'), migraine, tetanus, albinism
- Voluntary closure of eyes with occasional blinking → hysteria

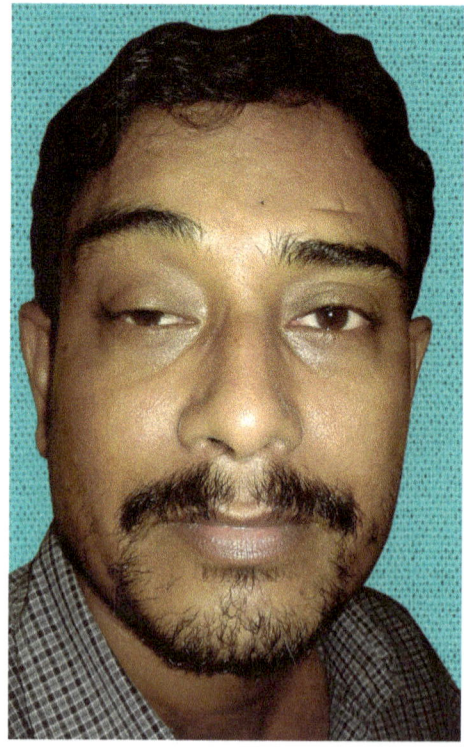

Fig. 26.1: Congenital ptosis of right eye (right upper eyelid is smooth and devoid of any cutaneous fold)

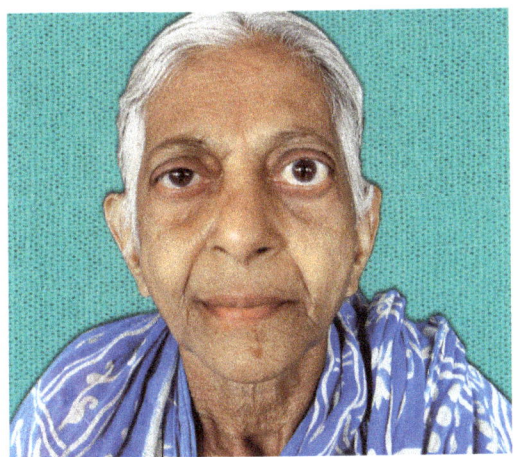

Fig. 26.2: Proptosis (exophthalmos) in left eye due to retro-orbital tumor

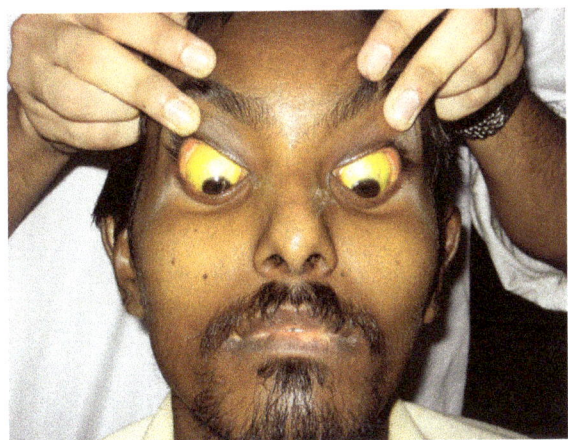

Fig. 26.3: Jaundice demonstrated in yellowish upper bulbar conjunctiva

- Periorbital edema → nephrotic syndrome, angioedema, drug hypersensitivity, acute glomerulonephritis, hypothyroidism, infection with *Trichinella spiralis* (trichinosis), congestive cardiac failure, dermatomyositis, excessive crying
- Xanthelasma around the eyes (often indicates hypercholesterolemia)
- Pallor or polycythemia → the lower palpebral conjunctiva
- Jaundice → the upper bulbar conjunctiva (Fig. 26.3)
- Cyanosis → the lower palpebral conjunctiva
- Chemosis (edema) of conjunctiva → type II respiratory failure (hypercapnia), superior vena caval (SVC) syndrome, severe exophthalmos, alcoholism, Weil's disease, hypoalbuminaemia
- Subconjunctival hemorrhage → severe cough (e.g. whooping cough), bleeding disorder, fracture of skull (Fig. 26.4), snake bite (Fig. 26.5), SVC syndrome, anticoagulant therapy or without any obvious cause

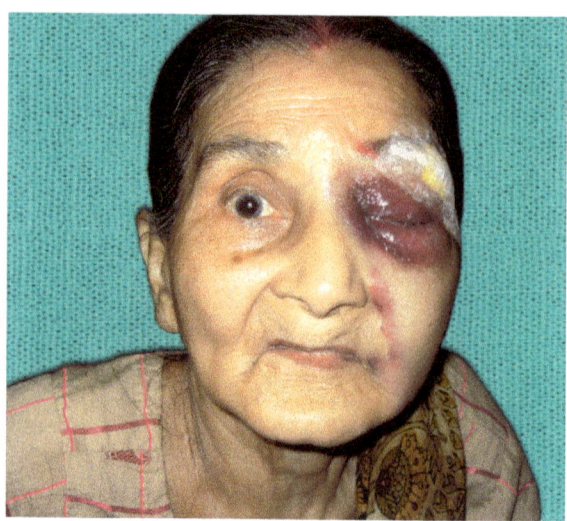

Fig. 26.4: Periorbital hematoma from head injury

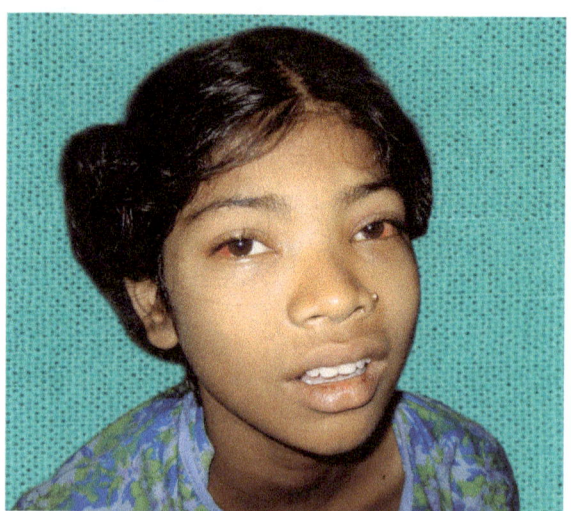

Fig. 26.5: Bilateral subconjunctival hemorrhage in the second day of viperidae snake bite

- Blue sclera → osteogenesis imperfecta (see Chapter 10)
- Scleromalacia perforans (choroidal pigments are seen as small brown patches on either side of the iris) → rheumatoid arthritis
- Corneal damage or opacities → trauma, infection, malignant exophthalmos, xerophthalmia from Sjögren's syndrome, Bell's palsy, Vth cranial nerve palsy
- Arcus senilis→ indirect clue to atherosclerosis
- Kayser-Fleischer (K-F) ring → Wilson's disease (see Chapter 66), prolonged cholestasis
- Phlyctenular conjunctivitis→allergic reaction to primary tuberculosis

- Iridocyclitis → tuberculosis, sarcoidosis, seronegative arthritis
- Cataract → hypoparathyroidism, diabetes mellitus, galactosemia, prolonged steroid therapy, Down's syndrome, Wilson's disease, myotonia dystrophica, atopic dermatitis.
- Enlarged lacrimal glands → Sjögren's syndrome, sarcoidosis
- Ectopia lentis → look for iridodonesis
  Upward subluxation: Marfan's syndrome
  Downward subluxation: Homocystinuria
- Bitot's spot → vitamin A deficiency (whitish, foamy, raised and triangular spot with its base towards limbus; present on the bulbar conjunctiva, a little away from limbus)
- Brushfield's spot → Down's syndrome (radially arranged small whitish inclusions having the appearance of grains of salt, present in between middle and outer third of iris)
- Squint (concomitant or paralytic) → in paralytic squint, it indicates external ophthalmoplegia (IIIrd, IVth, or VIth cranial nerve palsy)
- Epicanthic folds at inner angle of eyes → Down's syndrome, Treacher Collins syndrome
- Hypertelorism (widely set eyes) → Down's syndrome, associated with congenital supravalvular aortic stenosis (elfin facies) or pulmonary stenosis, mental retardation, thalassemia, craniofacial dysostosis and carpenter syndrome
- Pupil → miosis, mydriasis or anisocoria (unequal pupils)
- Nystagmus → Pendular nystagmus when the patient looks forward; jerky nystagmus on fixation of gaze laterally
- Myokymia → benign phenomenon in fatigued or anxious person (persistent twitching and occasionally rhythmical movement, especially of periorbital muscles)
- Corneal opacities → 'band keratopathy' (i.e. corneal calcification) due to hypercalcemia; cholesterol deposition (arcus senilis) due to hypercholesterolemia; chloroquine crystals as a result of treatment in systemic lupus erythematosus (SLE) and discoid lupus erythematosus (DLE); copper deposition Kayser-Fleischer (KF) ring in Wilson's disease; cystine crystals in cystinosis; deposition of amiodarone used in the treatment of cardiac dysrhythmias; keratitis with corneal opacities in herpes zoster or simplex infection, congenital syphilis, Reiter's syndrome (Fig. 26.6)
- Grey-brown sclera → alkaptonuria
- Madarosis (loss of hair in lateral one-third of eyebrows) → myxedema, lepromatous leprosy, amyloidosis and neurodermatitis
- Palpebral fissure:
  Wide → exophthalmos
  Narrow → partial ptosis, photophobia and blepharospasm
  Oblique → Down's syndrome
  Absent → Evisceration or enucleation of eyeball.
- Red eyes → trauma, conjunctivitis, keratitis, scleritis, episcleritis, uveitis, subconjunctival hemorrhage, acute congestive glaucoma
- 'Bags under the eyes' → may not have any clinical value but often associated with insomnia, senility, chronic alcoholism and myxedema

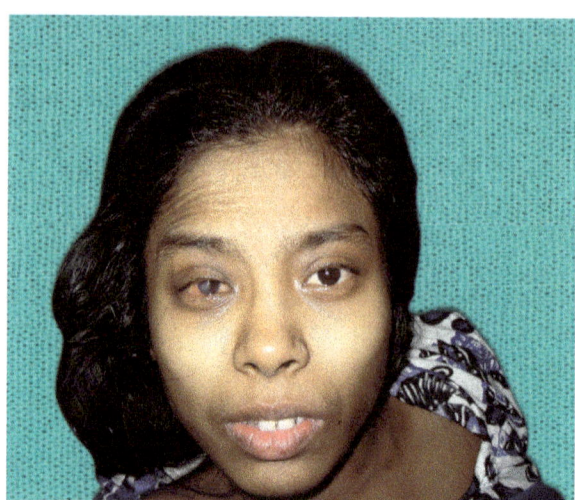

Fig. 26.6: Keratitis as well as conjunctivitis in reactive arthritis (Reiter's syndrome)

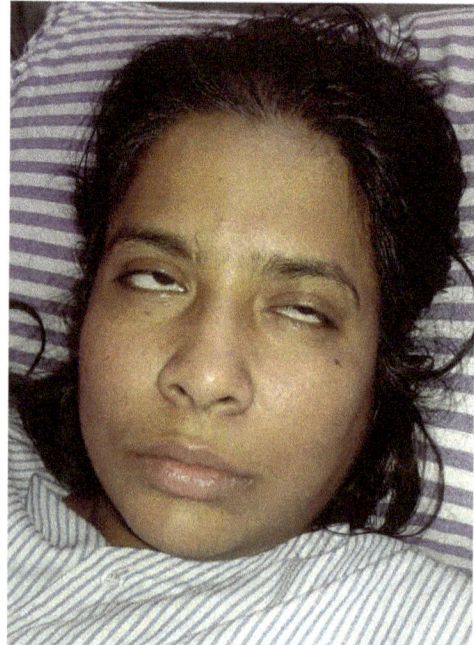

Fig. 26.7: Lagophthalmos due to bilateral Bell's palsy in Guillain-Barré syndrome

- Blepharospasm → involuntary spasmodic closure of eyelids (a form of dystonia)
- Enophthalmos → senility, phthisis bulbi, microphthalmos, Horner's syndrome, severe dehydration, as a consequence of resolved orbital cellulitis
- Lagophthalmos → physiological, extreme degree of proptosis, Bell's palsy (Fig. 26.7), eyelid scarring

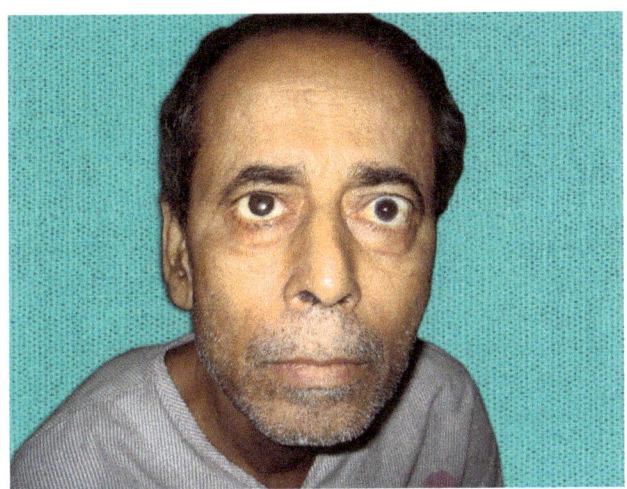

Fig. 26.8: Dry and lustreless artificial right eye (glass eye), which is devoid of blood vessels and pupillary reactions

- Dry eyes (xerophthalmia) → Sjögren's syndrome, vitamin A deficiency, Stevens-Johnson syndrome, burns, pemphigoid and medications (e.g. antihistamines, scopolamine)
- Shrunken eyes → malnutrition, dehydration, poverty.

FIVE COMMON CAUSES OF PAINFUL EYE

1. Conjunctivitis
2. Iritis
3. Corneal ulcer
4. Acute glaucoma
5. Retrobulbar neuritis.

- **Aching pain** indicates internal cause while **gritty pain** points towards external cause. Increased sensitivity to light is always associated with inflammation of eyes.
- Other important causes are foreign body, trauma, Herpes zoster, uveitis and dry eyes.

COMMON CAUSES OF TUBULAR VISION

- Hysteria (tunnel vision)
- Glaucoma (terminal)
- Retinitis pigmentosa (advanced)
- Papilledema
- Migraine
- Posterior cerebral artery occlusion.

Tubular vision is the result of peripheral constriction of visual field.

PUPIL

Normally pupils are **round and regular** in outline, centered in the iris, and equal in size. The size of pupil varies in between 3 and 5 mm. If it is less than 3 mm, it is known as **miosis**; if more than 5 mm, it is called **mydriasis**.

Constrictors of the pupil are supplied by parasympathetics (via oculomotor nerve), while the dilator fibers are controlled by sympathetic nervous system. Changes in the size of the pupil do not affect vision.

Miosis (Constriction) of the Pupil

- Unilateral
  - Horner's syndrome
- Bilateral
  - Old age (senile miosis)
  - Pontine hemorrhage
  - Organophosphorus poisoning
  - Argyll Robertson pupil
  - Application of pilocarpine drops
  - Overdose of neostigmine
  - Iritis.

Mydriasis (Dilatation) of the Pupil

- Unilateral
  - IIIrd cranial nerve palsy
  - Optic atrophy
  - Acute congestive glaucoma
  - Head injury
  - Adie's pupil
  - Tentorial herniation (same side)
- Bilateral
  - Childhood, anxiety, fear
  - Application of mydriatic (atropine)
  - Datura poisoning
  - Deep coma
  - Severe raised intracranial tension
  - Cerebral anoxia, death.

- Pin-point pupil (pupil 1 mm or less) is common in pontine hemorrhage, organophosphorus/morphine/barbiturate poisoning, heat stroke and after application of pilocarpine drops.
- Anisocoria (unequal pupils) is due to application of mydriatic in one eye; other causes are idiopathic, unilateral IIIrd nerve or sympathetic palsy, head injury, encephalitis or iritis.

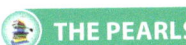 THE PEARLS

Eyes are the two pearls in the face which are clinician's paradise to target a diagnosis. Other than the manifestations of emotion, eyes display many diseases. Examine all the sectors of both the eyes. Ophthalmoscopy gives clue to diabetes mellitus, hypertension and many of the ophthalmic disorders.

27

Face Reading

PROLOGUE

Reading the *facial expression* of the patients or *facies* many a time suggests an instant or 'spot' diagnosis. Experience teaches a doctor to read the face vividly. One may prove to be wrong in face reading but every doctor should learn how to read the emotional play, response to questioning and intellectual shadows in the patient's face. The vacant stare of a mentally retarded child, sad appearance of depression or anxious facies of thyrotoxicosis (Fig. 27.1) can never be overlooked. Though the *facies* may be deceptive, one should meticulously examine for complexion, eyes, eyebrows (Fig. 27.2), skin of cheeks (Fig. 27.3), mouth, nose, nasolabial folds, head, hairs or any sign of wasting present or not.

Few *facies* are described below where the patient carry their diagnosis in the face.

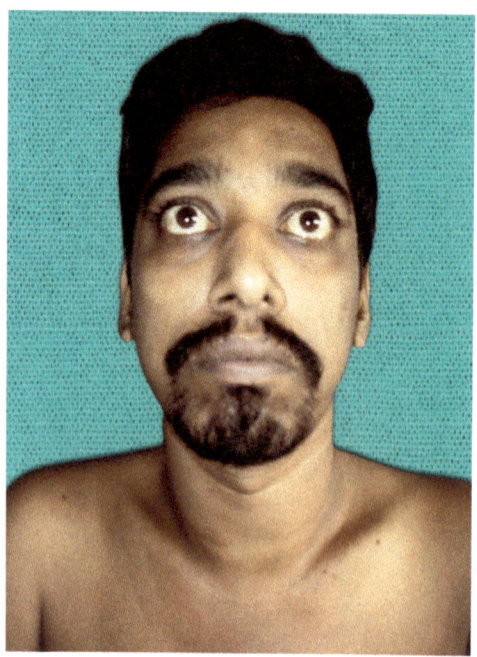

Fig. 27.1: Exophthalmos in a patient with thyrotoxicosis

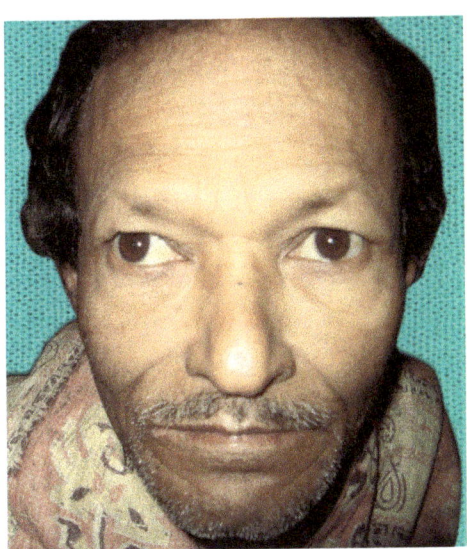

Fig. 27.2: Madarosis (loss of hair in lateral third of eyebrows) with concomitant squint in a male hypothyroid

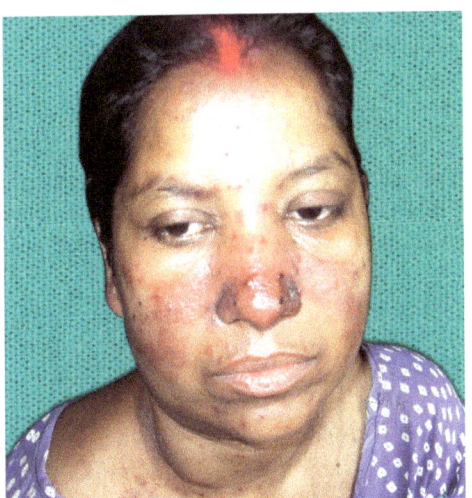

Fig. 27.3: Classical photosensitive butterfly rash over face with erythema, edema and telangiectasia in a patient of systemic lupus erythematosus (SLE)

DIFFERENT FACIES IN CLINICAL MEDICINE

ACROMEGALY (FIG. 27.4)

- Prognathism (lantern or bull-dog jaw) where the lower incisors (mandible) protrude in front of the upper jaw (maxilla), and widened spaces between upper and lower teeth; heavy chin.

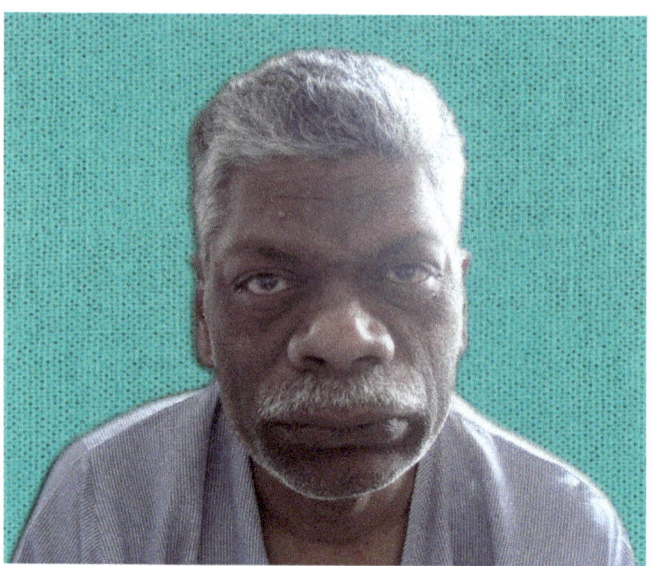

Fig. 27.4: A case of acromegaly with facial enlargement

- Facial enlargement (large wide face) with prominent supraorbital ridges as a result of enlargement of maxillary, frontal and ethmoid sinuses. Frontal bossing may be associated with
- Macroglossia with thick lips, and large ears and nose; wide spacing of teeth may be present
- Thick skin with hypertrichosis (e.g. bushy eyebrows), hyperhidrosis and increased sebum production (skin becomes greasy); exaggerated nasolabial folds
- Deep, husky and resonant voice due to increased thickness of vocal cord.

THYROTOXICOSIS (FIG. 27.1)

- Staring as well as anxious look
- Exophthalmos
- Lid retraction reading to an anxious startled look
- Infrequent blinking
- Lack of harmonious movement between the eyeball and the eyelid
- Moist skin of face with a malar flush.

A goiter may be noticed in the front of the neck in thyrotoxicosis.

BELL'S PALSY (SEE FIGS 3.1 AND 26.8)

1. Facial asymmetry
2. Asymmetry of blinking and eye closure

3. Lack of spontaneous movements of face
4. Wide palpebral fissure with epiphora
5. Bell's phenomenon (the eyeball rolls upwards and inwards during attempted forced eye closure)
6. Loss of nasolabial fold
7. Angle of the mouth is drawn to the healthy side when asked to show the upper teeth
8. Inability to blow or whistle properly.

2 to 6 are noticed on the affected side of facial paralysis.

THALASSAEMIA (MONGOLOID)

- Frontal bossing (prominent forehead as a result of marrow hyperplasia)
- Depressed bridge of the nose (due to hyperplasia of lesser wing of sphenoid)
- Hypertelorism (widely set eyes)
- Apparent mongoloid slant of the eyes
- Malar prominence (due to marrow hyperplasia)—*Chipmunk facies*
- Dental malocclusion with prominent upper incisors
- Associated with mild icteric tinge of the conjunctiva, and pallor.

DOWN'S SYNDROME (MONGOL) (SEE FIG. 16.1)

- Small, round and flat face, brachycephaly; downy forehead; short fleshy neck
- Upwards—slanting eyes (oblique orbital fissure) with epicanthic folds at inner angles
- Low set ears; ears are small and dysplastic
- Small nose with depressed bridge of the nose
- Hypertelorism
- High arched palate with small teeth
- Open mouth with protruded and furrowed tongue (macroglossia), with an idiotic look (often called as *cheerful idiot*).

CRETINISM (FIG. 27.5)

- Dull, expressionless and idiotic look; large head with scanty scalp hair
- Depressed bridge of the nose, blood flat nose with big nostrils
- Hypertelorism with wrinkling of eyebrows; narrow palpebral fissures
- Sparse, coarse and brittle hair with dry skin
- Thick and everted lips with big, fissured, protruded tongue (macroglossia)
- Delayed dentition with hoarse voice.

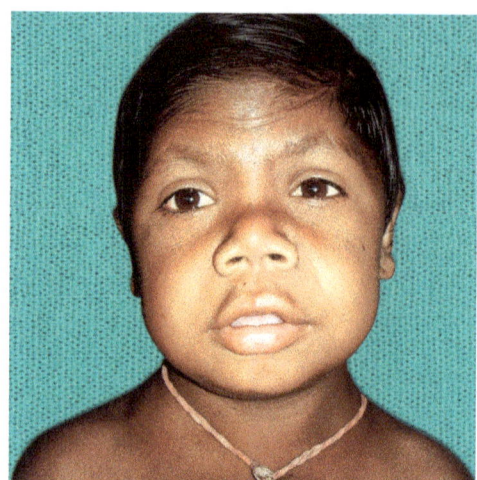

Fig. 27.5: Classical facies of cretinism: a dull and idiotic look associated with depressed bridge of the nose, wrinkled eyebrows, broad flat nose with big nostrils, narrow palpebral fissures, thick and everted lips

TABETIC

This is the classical facies of tabes dorsalis and is rarely seen nowadays.
- Bilateral partial ptosis
- Compensatory wrinkling in the forehead
- Elevated eyebrows
- Very little subcutaneous fat with loss of emotional reflexes
- Accompanied by Argyll Robertson pupil.

DEHYDRATION (FACIES HIPPOCRATICUS)

- Face is drawn
- Shrunken eyes; the eyeballs are soft as a result of lowering of intraocular tension
- Pinched-up nose
- Parched lips
- Hollowed temporal fossa; depressed anterior fontanelle (infants)
- Tongue is dry and coated
- Skin is dry and wrinkled.

HEPATIC (SEE FIG. 31.1)

- Shrunken eyes
- Hollowed temporal fossa
- Pinched-up nose associated with malar prominence
- Parched lips
- Muddy complexion of skin (blending of pallor, jaundice and melanosis)
- Shallow and dry face
- Icteric tinge of conjunctiva.

Hepatic facies is characteristic of chronic liver disease (e.g. cirrhosis of liver)

MOON FACE (FIGS 27.6, 27.7, 40.1 AND 41.1)

The face looks bloated and rounded (like the full moon). Moon face is commonly associated with:
- Cushing's syndrome (facial plethora + hirsutism)

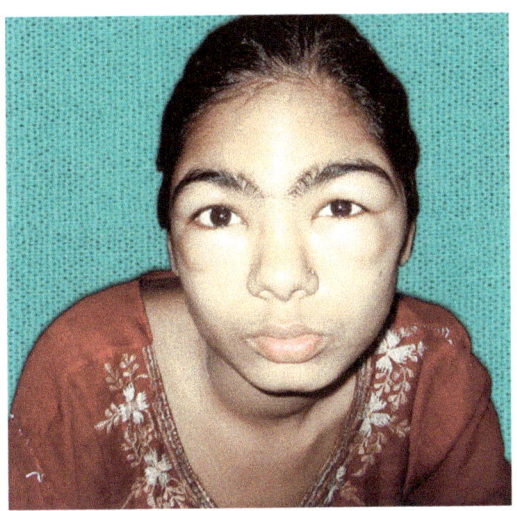

Fig. 27.6: Periorbital edema in nephrotic syndrome

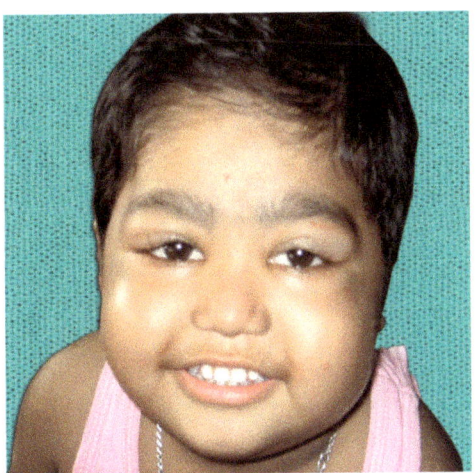

Fig. 27.7: Cushingoid facies in a child suffering from steroid-dependent minimal lesion nephropathy (nephrotic syndrome)

- Nephrotic syndrome (periorbital edema)
- Acute glomerulonephritis (periorbital edema)
- Myxedema (baggy lower eyelids)
- Prolonged corticosteroid therapy (facial plethora + hirsutism)
- Superior mediastinal syndrome (prominent veins in forehead and temple)
- Angioneurotic edema of face (patchy involvement; lips are swollen ++)
- Subcutaneous emphysema of face, extending from chest (asymmetrical).
- Rarely advanced congentive cardiac failure (CCF), severe hypoproteinemia and alcoholism (puffy face).

NEPHRITIC (ACUTE GLOMERULONEPHRITIS/AGN) SYNDROME

- The face is pale and puffy
- Pronounced periorbital edema with narrowing of the parpebral fissure.

NEPHROTIC SYNDROME (FIGS 27.6 AND 27.8)

The face looks like nephritic one but the features of moon face is more pronounced in nephrotic syndrome, especially the periorbital edema.

SYSTEMIC LUPUS ERYTHEMATOSUS (FIG. 27.3)

- Photosensitive 'butterfly' rash over the malar areas and bridge of the nose (does not affect the nasolabial folds)
- The lesion will have erythema + edema during acute phase, and atrophy + telangiectasia in chronic phase

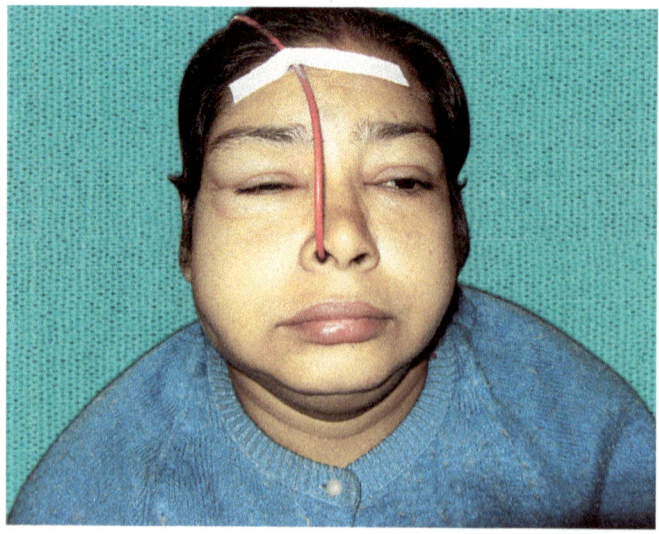

Fig. 27.8: Swelling of the face with periorbital oedema in nephrotic syndrome; the patient is in respiratory distress due to bilateral hydrothorax

- Patchy alopecia with 'lupus hairs' (short, broken hairs) seen above the forehead
- Ulcer in the oral cavity (especially, palatal ulcer).

Butterfly rash in systemic lupus erythematosus (SLE) is due to apoptosis of keratinized skin layer exposed to sunlight/ultraviolet (UV) light.

SCLERODERMA (SEE FIG. 35.1)

- Mask-like facies (lacking facial expression)
- Absence of normal wrinkling of skin ('ironed' out skin folds)
- Pinched-up nose or beaking of the nose
- Inability to open the mouth, i.e. microstomia (small mouth) with radial furrows or rhagades on closing (tobacco-pouch or fish-mouth appearance) the mouth
- Skin over the face seems taut and shiny
- Pigmentation, depigmentation and telangiectasia.

The typical face of scleroderma is known as *mauskopf* (mouse head) appearance.

MASKED FACIES

- Lack of facial expression (i.e. a blank look or hypomimia)
- Infrequent blinking with staring look (spontaneous ocular movements are lacking)
- Widened palpebral fissure.

Poverty of expression (i.e. Masked facies) is commonly seen in
- Parkinsonism
- Scleroderma
- Bilateral upper motor neuron (UMN) type facial nerve palsy
- Myxedema
- Depression
- Myasthenia gravis and facial myopathies (rare)
- Dementia
- Sometimes in pseudobulbar palsy.

MALAR FLUSH (SEE FIG. 30.2)

See Chapter 30.

PLETHORIC FACE (SEE FIG. 58.1)

Increased redness of face is confronted in clinical situations like:
- Chronic alcoholism
- Cushing's syndrome

- Polycythemia
- Superior vena caval (SVC) syndrome
- Chronic cor pulmonale
- Carcinoid syndrome.

MITRAL FACIES

It is rarely seen in India and is well appreciated in fair skinned individuals. There are pinkish purple patches on cheeks → it is due to:
- Low cardiac output in mitral stenosis → vsoconstriction → peripheral cyanosis in lips, tip of the nose and cheeks
- Vasodilatation (vascular stasis) in malar area leads to malar flush.

PARKINSONISM

It is a classical masked facies with all features present. Speech is monotonous, with bradylalia and hypophonia. The eye signs in parkinsonism are:
- Infrequent blinking with a staring look (akinetic face)
- Reptelian gaze
- Impaired pursuit movement of eyeball
- Hypometric saccades
- Oculogyric crisis (involuntary upward conjugate deviation of eyes)–in post-encephalitic variety
- Blepharoclonus (fluttering of eyelids on closing the eyes)
- Reversed Argyll Robertson pupil (post-encephlitic variety).

POLYCYTHEMIA (RUDDY CYANOSIS) (SEE FIG. 58.1)

Dusky-red (plethora + cyanosis) discoloration of nose, lips, malar prominence (facial plethora), ears and palpebral conjunctiva (i.e. suffused conjunctiva)

MYXEDEMA (SEE FIG. 41.1)

- Dull, espressionless, puffy face (periorbital puffiness with baggy lower eyelids)
- Coarse hair, patchy alopecia, thin and sparse eyebrows (loss of lateral 1/3rd of eyebrows—madarosis)
- Dry, rough skin with swollen lips
- Expressionless face, facial pallor (may have rose-purple malar flush) with macroglossia
- Deep and hoarse voice + bradylalia.

MYOTONIA (DYSTROPHICA) (SEE FIG. 67.1)

- Ptosis with ophthalmoplegia
- Long facial structure ('hatchet face' due to atrophy of temporalis + 'swan neck' due to atrophy of sternomastoid muscle)

- Frontal baldness
- Cataract
- Mental retardation (mild)
- A weak and expressionless face.

MYOPATHIC FACE (FACIOSCAPULOHUMERAL DYSTROPHY)

- Loose pout of lips at rest due to facial weakness
- A transverse smile (rire en travers)
- Ptosis (external ophthalmoplegia in ocular variety).

MYASTHENIC FACIES (SNARLING FACIES) (SEE FIG. 29.1)

- Uni- or bilateral (usual) ptosis; fluctuating ptosis → sustained upward gaze for 2 minutes leads to increase ptosis and injection of edrophonium corrects ptosis dramatically (Tensilon test)
- A peculiar smile (myasthenic snarl) where the lips elevate but do not retract
- Pupils are never affected
- Rarely, there may be complete paralysis of ocular movements.

LEONINE FACE (LEPROMATOUS LEPROSY) (SEE FIG. 19.1)

- Forehead lines become deeper; madarosis with thick eyebrows
- Depressed bridge of the nose, broad nose with nasal collapse (saddle-nose)
- Thickened skin of face + forehead, especially of infiltrated earlobes
- There may be perforated nasal septum
- Loosen upper central incisor teeth + hoarse voice.

ELFIN FACIES (IN SUPRAVALVULAR AORTIC STENOSIS)

- Broad forehead with pointed chin
- Cupid's bow-like upper lip with upturned nose
- Hypertelorism with low set ears.

- Elfin facies is seen in William's syndrome
- Monkey facies is found in marasmus and Gorilla-like face in acromegaly. Hurler's syndrome shows gargoyle facies.

CUSHING'S SYNDROME (CLASSICAL MOON FACE) (SEE FIG. 40.1)

a. Moon face
b. Dusky and plethoric face
c. Hirsutism.

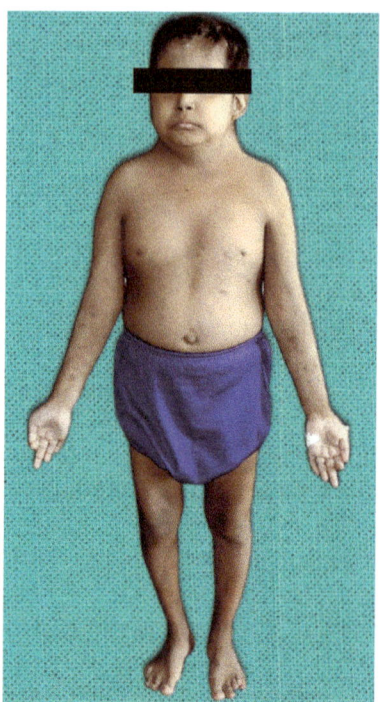

Fig. 27.9: Turner's syndrome with dwarfism, shield-like chest, cubitus valgus, low hair line, failure of development of secondary sexual character, short fourth metatarsal (left) and classical webbing of neck in a 18 years girl

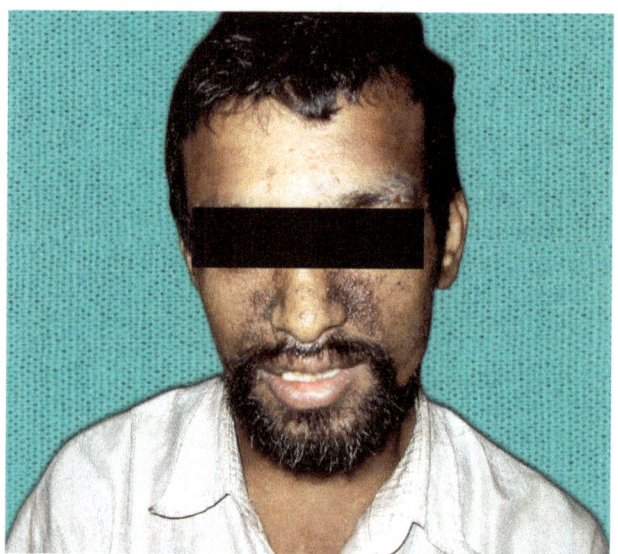

Fig. 27.10: Adenoma sebaceum (facial angiofibromas) with mental subnormality; a cut injury in left eyebrow reflects fall after epileptic convulsions – a patient of tuberous sclerosis (epiloia or Bourneville's disease)

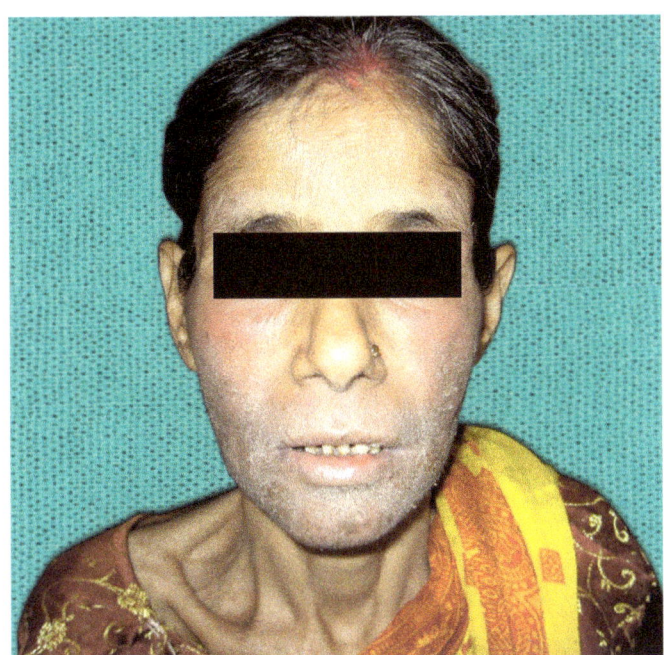

Fig. 27.11: Seborrheic dermatitis with facial cellulitis

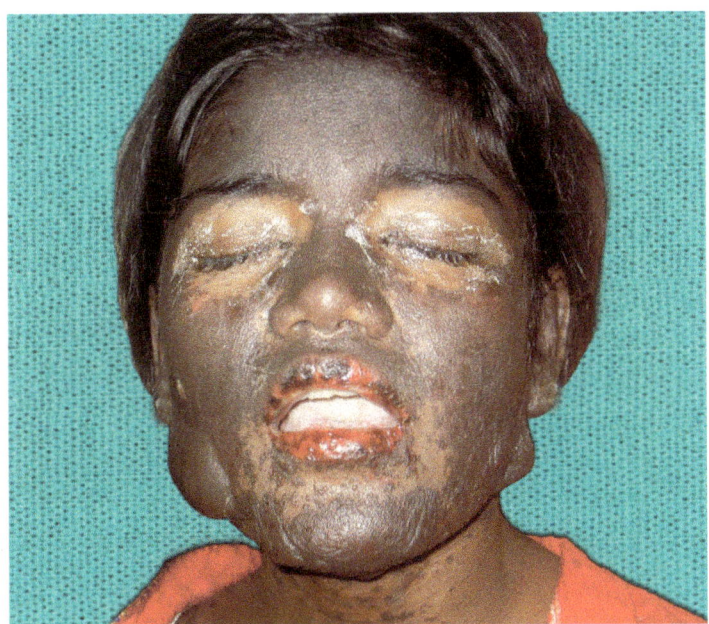

Fig. 27.12: Stevens-Johnson syndrome affecting skin and mucous membrane (ciprofloxacin-induced)

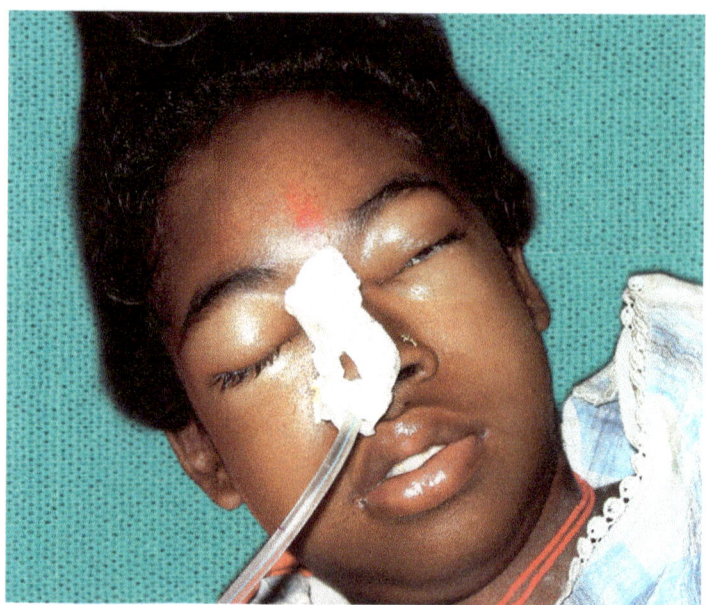

Fig. 27.13: Facial puffiness in a moribund patient of pyogenic meningitis

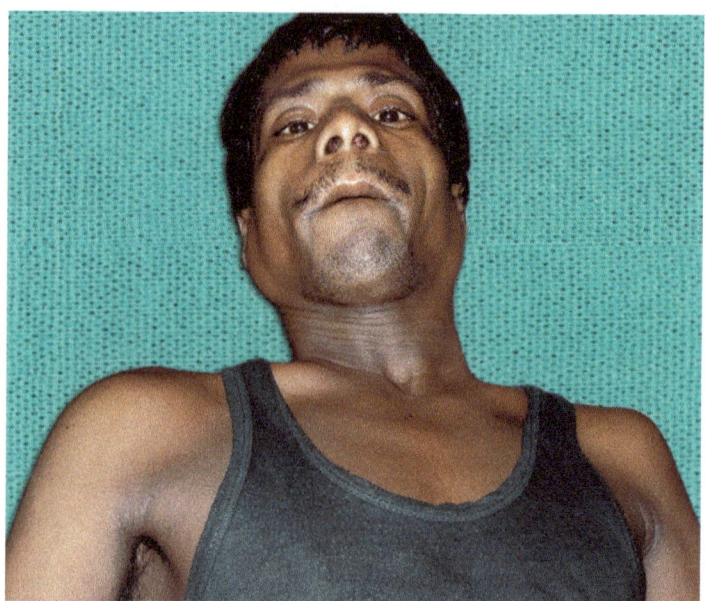

Fig. 27.14: Chorea (an involuntary movement)—choreiform movements started in face

Chapter 27 Face Reading

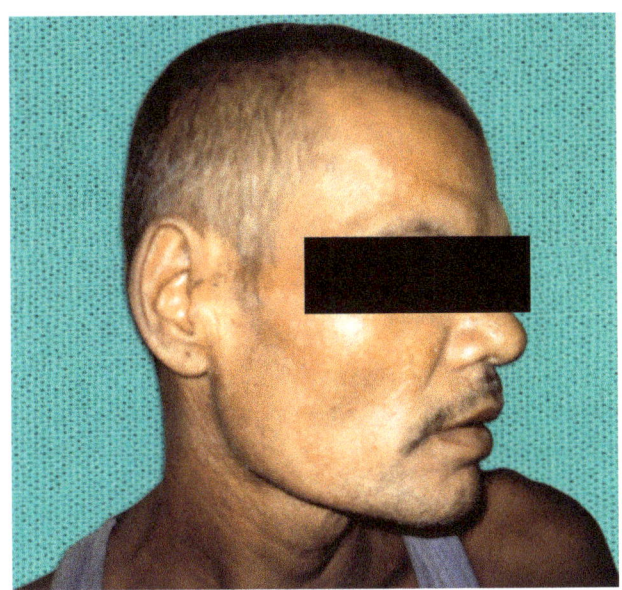

Fig. 27.15: Pityriasis versicolor – manifested by hypopigmented macules in right side of face

Note: Other than facial expression and different physical changes, one has to be very careful about alteration of facial contour, voluntary and involuntary movements of face, different eye signs and stigmata of acute illness reflected in the face (i.e. herpes labialis). Very often the clue to diagnosis remains in examination of tongue, pseudoptosis, mild exophthalmos, malar flush, masked appearance, small goiter in neck or asking the patient to show the upper teeth.

THE PEARLS

Facies is a distinctive facial expression or appearance associated with specific medical conditions. A clinician should try to read every patient's face in the first visit.

Facial Pain

PROLOGUE

Different pain-sensitive parts of face are teeth, gums, sinuses, temporomandibular joints, jaw and eyes; facial pain may be evoked by specific neurological conditions.

CLUE TO DIAGNOSIS

- Facial infection, cellulitis, abscess
- Chronic subclinical sinus infection
- *Trigeminal neuralgia (tic douloureux)*
  ↓
  - Never extends outside the Vth nerve territory
  - Mouth-ear zone and naso-orbit zone are commonly affected; ophthalmic division is involved rarely (5%)
  - (Female: male) F:M = 3:1; middle-aged or elderly
  - Strictly unilateral
  - Sudden, severe, stabbing/shooting/lancinating pain, for seconds which may be repetitive. Precipitated by touching the 'trigger zones' in face or by eating; usually no neurological sign present
  - Remit and relapse
  - May be related to disseminated sclerosis or posterior fossa tumor
- *Postherpetic neuralgia (Fig. 28.1)*
  ↓
  - Very elderly females more than males, over 70 years
  - Over ophthalmic division of Vth nerve (forehead) → most severe over eyebrows and may mimic headache of temporal arteritis
  - Very severe; often non-stopping type
  - Post-herpetic scars are anesthetic; normal skin between scars are tender
  - High suicidal tendency
- Trauma/post-traumatic neuralgia
- *Facial migraine syndrome*
  ↓
  - Males more than females; any age
  - Deep eye pain; often a feeling as if the mastoid is swollen

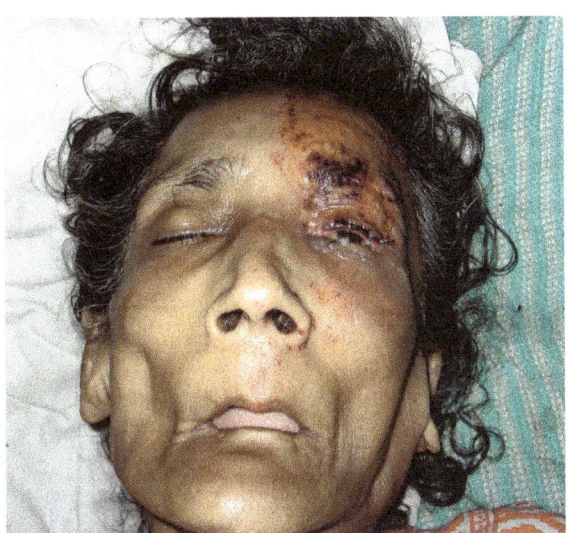

Fig. 28.1: Herpes zoster ophthalmicus on left side with impending danger of corneal ulcer and panophthalmitis; the patient may suffer from postherpetic neuralgia

- Throbbing type with lacrimation and conjunctival injection
- Alcohol aggravates the pain
- Probably a variety of **clusture headache**; previously called **ciliary neuralgia**, vidian neuralgia, petrosal neuralgia, sphenopalatine neuralgia or geniculate neuralgia are probably variants of facial migraine
- 'Sluder's lower-half headache' (rare)—bursting; near base of the nose, near mastoid, behind the eye with nasal congestion

■ *Atypical facial pain*
  ↓
- F > M; 30-50 years
- Continual, unbearable, deep bruning type pain; over either or both maxillary region; the patient clutches his face in pain
- May be associated with delusional overtones

■ *Temporomandibular osteoarthritis*
  ↓
- Usually in elderly females
- The site of pain is over the joint or just anterior to it
- May be mistaken with temporal arteritis
- Aggravates on chewing or yawning
- Severe aching type; only present on eating
- Or temporomandibular joint disorders (Costen's syndrome)

■ *Carotidynia*
  ↓
- Episodic throbbing type pain in neck

- Associated with swelling and tenderness of the carotid artery
- A little presure over carotid → pain ↑
- A firm presure over carotid → pain ↓
- According to some clinicians, it is a form of temporal arteritis
- ■ *Temporal arteritis (giant cell arteritis)*
  ↓
  - Intermittent claudication of jaw muscles and tongue; headache
  - Elderly; F > M = 4:1
  - Associated with scalp tenderness, fever, malaise, visual problems (from diplopia to permanent visual loss) or ptosis
  - Thickened, tortuous, nodular and tender temporal arteries
- ■ *Anginal pain*
  ↓
  - Along with central, stabbing chest pain with radiation to arms (left > right), there may be radiation of pain to neck and lower jaw
  - Sublingual isosorbide dinitrate relieves the pain
- ■ Somatization syndrome/anxiety
- ■ Glossopharyngeal neuralgia
- ■ Salivary gland infection (e.g. mumps)
- ■ Miscellaneous
  - Paget's disease
  - Carotid artery aneurysm
  - Cerebello-pontine angle tumor
  - Nasopharyngeal carcinoma
  - Tolosa-Hunt syndrome
  - Geniculate neuralgia
  - Dental abscess.

- To diagnose the facial pain variants, one should totally depend clinically on— history, age, sex, site of pain, character of pain and aggravating and relieving factors.
- There is no such special investigation which may pin-point the diagnosis.

PAIN IN THE EYES

- ■ Trauma
- ■ Conjunctivitis, blepharitis
- ■ Iritis, iridocyclitis, uveitis
- ■ Foreign body
- ■ Glaucoma
- ■ Clusture headache
- ■ Tic douloureux
- ■ Periorbital cellulitis
- ■ Xerophthalmia
- ■ Entropion
- ■ Retrobulbar neuritis
- ■ Cerebral tumor/aneurysm
- ■ Irritation from eye drops
- ■ Ultraviolet light.

LUMP IN THE FACE

- Parotid swelling (mumps, mixed parotid tumor)
- Preauricular lymphadenititis (tender lymph nodes in front of ear)
- Subcutaneous abscess (a tender and fluctuant swelling)
- Dental abscess (tenderness of underlying tooth on gentle tapping)
- Preauricular lymphoma (non-tender lymph nodes in front of ear)
- Melanoma (painless swelling with pigmented lesion), sebaceous cyst (swelling with central punctum)
- Basal cell carcinoma (painless ulcer with rolled edge)
- Nasopharyngeal carcinoma (swelling at root of nose, ophthalmoplegia)
- Angioneurotic edema (solid asymmetrical edema involving lips and eyelids)
- Facial hematoma (from trauma)
- Neurofibroma (single or multiple painless rubbery cutaneous tumor), lipoma, fibroma
- Nodules (from lepromatous leprosy).

THE PEARLS

It is said that 'nearer to the brain, more is the pain' and this is why a pain of caries tooth often becomes unbearable. Remember, different vascular headaches (i.e. migraine) or muscle spasm headache may give rise to pain in the face. To diagnose diverse causes of facial pain, the clinicians have to depend on history first, and then the specific clinical examination. Few of the features of facial pain are unique of its own, e.g. claudication of the jaw in temporal aretiritis or precipitation of stabbing facial pain after touching the specific trigger zone in face in trigeminal neuralgia.

Fatigue

DEFINITION
It is the excessive tiredness on exertion, and occurs in organic or functional ill-health. The severe form of fatigue is known as *exhaustion*. Fatigue literally means that the patient is *tired all the time*. It is one of the most distressing symptom to the patient.

COMMON CAUSES
- Physiological—overwork, insomnia, boredom
- *Pathological*
  - Nutritional deficiency, dyselectrolytemia (↓Na, ↓K, ↑Ca, ↓Mg)
  - Congestive cardiac failure (CCF), hepatic failure, uremia, malignancy, immunocompromized states [e.g. acquired immune deficiency syndrome (AIDS)], sleep-apnea syndrome
  - Myxedema, diabetes mellitus, Addison's disease, thyrotoxicosis
  - Tuberculosis, brucellosis, post-viral infectious states (e.g. influenza or infectious mononucleosis), collagen vascular diseases [e.g. systemic lupus erythematosus (SLE)]
  - Anemia, lymphoma and leukemias, terminally-ill patients
  - Multiple sclerosis, myasthenia gravis (Fig. 29.1), motor neuron disease myopathies, poliomyelitis
  - Functional—anxiety, sleep disorders, depression, chronic fatigue syndrome (CFS), fibromyalgia
  - Drugs—β-blockers, sedatives, corticosteroids, α-methyldopa, antihistamiics, antiepileptic drugs
  - Terminally ill patients—disseminated carcinomatosis.

At least in 50% cases, the cause is functional, i.e. depression, anxiety or somatoform disorders.

UNDERLYING MECHANISM
- Accumulation of lactic acid in muscles and circulation
- Deficiency of oxygen
- Creatinine depletion form muscles
- Tumor necrosis factor and cytokines.

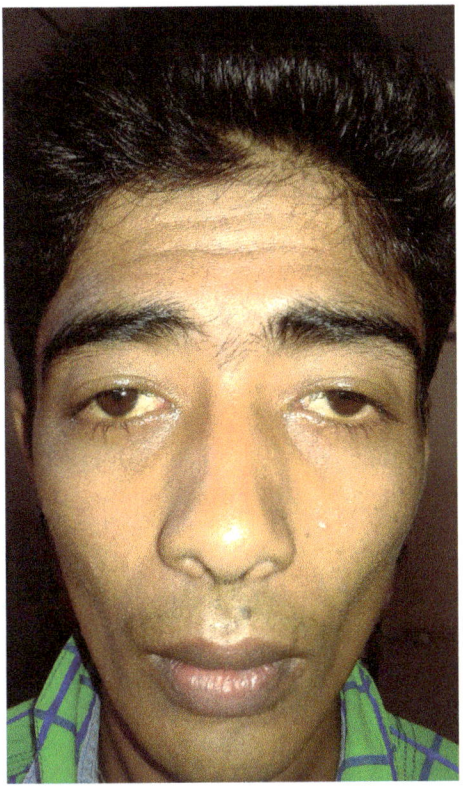

Fig. 29.1: Myasthenia gravis with bilateral partial ptosis and wrinkling of the forehead; the patient suffers from intense fatigue, especially towards the end of the day

FATIGUE IN CONGESTIVE CARDIAC FAILURE

- Inadequate systemic perfusion
- Sleep disturbance (due to paroxysmal nocturnal dyspnea, orthopnea, decubitus angina, nocturia)
- Side-effects of β-blockers
- Dyselectrolytemia due to diuretic therapy
- Systemic manifestations of subacute bacterial endocarditis (SBE; a potential cause of fatigue) which may lead to congestive cardiac failure (CCF).

DIAGNOSIS

Clinically examine for anemia, malnutrition, loss of weight, muscle bulk/wasting/power, tremor, fasciculations, delayed ankle jerk and hepatosplenomegaly. Test the power of shoulder girdle (to lift arms above shoulders), trunk muscles (to sit up from supine position), pelvic muscles (rise from squatting position).

Investigations like hemoglobin (Hb)%, erythrocyte sedimentation rate (ESR), total leukocyte count/differential leukocyte count (TLC/DLC) of white blood cell (WBC), serum sugar/urea/creatinine/electrolytes/creatine kinase (CK—MB/MM fraction), liver and thyroid function tests, serum cortisol and adrenocorticotropic hormone (ACTH), antinuclear antibody (ANA), electromyogram (EMG) and even muscle biopsy may have to be done to have a pin-point etiological diagnosis.

CLUE TO DIAGNOSIS

- Functional → more at rest, disappears on activity, clinically WNL, investigations NAD (WNL = within normal limit, NAD = no abnormality detected)
- Cachexia with loss of weight → tuberculosis, hematological or systemic malignancy
- Tremor + muscle cramps → dyselectrolytemia
- Females in their 20–50 years of age → fatigue after minimal exertion CFS (*see* Chapter 21)
- Hypotension + hyperpigmentation → Addison's disease
- ↑ Appetite + weight loss → thyrotoxicosis
- Polyuria + polyphagia + polydipsia → diabetes mellitus (fatigue may be presenting complaint)
- Frequent awakening at night + snoring + pauses in breathing during sleep + daytime sleepiness → sleep apnea syndrome
- Recent history of (H/O) viral illness + tiredness which goes away after few weeks or month → post-viral
- Early morning wake-up + tiredness maximum in the morning which persists all along the day + anorexia → depression.

ASSESSMENT

Fatigue is a subjective symptom and even objective changes like loss of body weight may be absent. So, clinically assessment should rely on self-reporting by the patient. Scales which measure fatigue, for example, Edmonton functional assessment tool, the fatigue self-report scales are useful in research rather than clinical purposes. The 'Karnofsky Performance Status' is a simple performance assessment clinical scale with questions like–"how much of the day does the patient spend in bed?" such a scale having grading, and allows assessment over time by third parties.

TREATMENT

- Reassurance for functional causes
- Graded exercise program and cognitive behavioural therapy for CFS
- Treatment of underlying etiology
- Psychotherapy (e.g. CFS)
- Antidepressants [e.g. selective serotonin reuptake inhibitors (SSRI)], tranquilizers, antianxiety drugs (e.g. clonazepam, buspirone), vitamins and electrolytes powder as and when necessary.

Chapter 29 Fatigue

TEN CAUSES OF 'FATIGUE' IN CLINICAL PRACTICE

- Diabetes mellitus
- Depression
- Hypothyroidism
- Anemia
- Post-viral illness
- Malnutrition
- Rheumatoid arthritis or SLE
- Malignancy
- Early renal failure (chronic)
- Chronic fatigue syndrome.

THE PEARLS

Fatigue is one of the most common symptom in medical science. Fatigue is the subjective experience of mental weariness, sluggishness and exhaustion. **Acute fatigue** should require immediate attention and medical evaluation to identify a cause. **Chronic fatigue** most commonly leads to a diagnosis of psychiatric illness or remains unexplained after evaluation. Chronic fatigue requires multidisciplinary treatment which may substantially improve quality of life.

Flushing of Face

DEFINITION

It is a slowly spreading erythema of the skin of face (often accompanied by neck and upper anterior chest) due to temporary capillary dilatation. Sometimes, it may be associated with light-headedness, tinnitus, tremulousness, nausea and a sense of suffocation. The flushing episode lasts from a few minutes to hours, depending on the etiology. Flushing is common in females in comparison to males.

CLUE TO DIAGNOSIS

Take history of (H/O) alcohol intake, sun-exposure, H/O treatment with disulfiram, intake of metronidazole while taking alcohol, menopause, emotional outburst (blushing), diabetes mellitus.

DIFFERENTIAL DIAGNOSIS

- Alcohol abuse
- Menopausal syndrome—hot flushes and perspiration
- H/O intake of alcohol, especially while on treatment with chlorpropamide, metronidazole or disulfiram
- *Carcinoid syndrome:* Classic triad is flushing, diarrhea and valvular heart disease; wheeze, telangiectasia → (also known as *flush syndrome*, and is due to the actions of serotonin, bradykinin and histamine produced by tumors arising from neuroendocrine cells)
- *Autonomic nervous system dysfunction* with special reference to diabetes mellitus
- Hormone-secreting tumors like pheochromocytoma (H/O episodic hypertension or fainting), medullary carcinoma of thyroid, vasoactive intestinal polypeptide-secreting tumors (VIPomas) or Zollinger-Ellison syndrome
- *Systemic mastocytosis* with pruritus, recurrent headache, lower abdominal crampy pain and palpitations
- Hypoglycemia
- *Rosacea:* Flushing after taking tea, coffee (usually postprandial) (Fig. 30.1)
- H/O drug intake (*see* page 130)
- Agnogenic flushing (i.e. of unknown cause).

Chapter 30 Flushing of Face

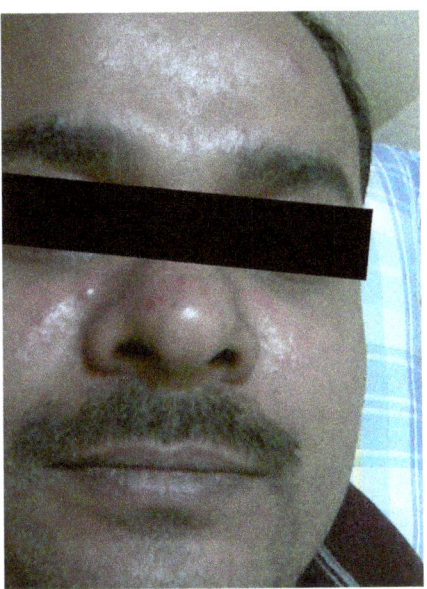

Fig. 30.1: A patient of rosacea who complains of flushing after taking tea

FLUSHED FACE APPEARANCE

- Menopause (Fig. 30.2), embarrassment, sunburn, fever, sexual intercourse, healthy normal persons
- High altitude
- Cushing's syndrome
- Myxedema
- Mitral stenosis
- Chronic alcoholism
- Polycythemia vera
- Thyrotoxicosis
- Carcinoid syndrome
- Systemic mastocytosis
- Systemic hypertension
- Pheochromocytoma
- Use of corticosteroid.

Blushing is the milder form of flushing

ROLE OF URINE EXAMINATION IN FLUSHING OF FACE

- Sugar—diabetes mellitus
- Alcohol—chronic alcohol abuse

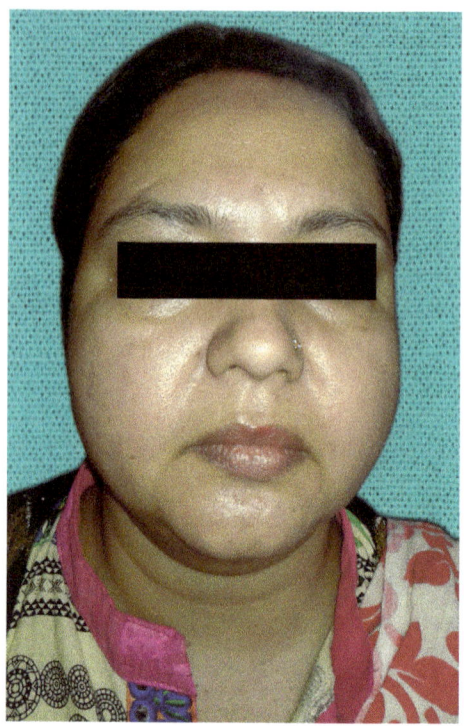

Fig. 30.1: Flushed face appearance in a female who attended menopause

- Hydroxyindoleacetic acid (5-HIAA)—carcinoid syndrome
- Vanillylmandelic acid (VMA)—pheochromocytoma.

DRUG-INDUCED/FOOD-INDUCED FLUSHING

Drug-induced

- Nicotinic acid
- Nifedipine
- Bromocriptine
- Amyl nitrite
- Diltiazem
- Levodopa
- Atropine poisoning
- Monosulfiram (tetmosol → anti-scabies)–after percutaneous absorption when used as soap.

Food-induced

Chinese restaurant syndrome after ingestion of monosodium glutamate (present in ajinomoto).

Alcohol-induced

Alcohol consumed with or without chlorpropamide, metronidazole or disulfiram.

 THE PEARLS

Flushing of face is a very specific symptom/sign of some diseases. In the day to day practice, the clinician should remember the physiological causes first, and then the rare disease entities.

31

Foul Breath

SYNONYM

- Halitosis
- Malodorous breath.

COMMON CAUSES

Normal breath should be devoid of any kind of odor. The causes of halitosis are as follows:
- Smoking, alcoholism, morning breath (after sleep)
- Decomposed food debris collected in between teeth (volatile sulfur compounds coming from bacterial decay of food)
- Consumption of onion, garlic, meats
- Stomatitis, gingivitis, septic tonsillitis, caries tooth, pyorrhoea alveolaris, diphtheria
- Vincent's angina
- Sinusitis
- Atrophic rhinitis
- Carcinoma of the tongue
- Achalasia cardia, stasis in pharyngeal pouch, pyloric stenosis
- Bronchiectasis, lung abscess, respiratory tract infections, pulmonary tuberculosis
- Gastrocolic fistula, intestinal obstruction
- Hepatic failure (Fig. 31.1)
- Diabetic ketoacidosis, starvation ketosis
- Uremia
- Septicemia, peritonitis
- Drugs like disulfiram, dimethyl sulfoxide
- Anxiety or depression (functional).

SPECIAL CHARACTERISTICS OF MALODOROUS BREATH (SMELL AS A PHYSICAL SIGN)

- **Diabetic ketoacidosis:** Sickly-sweet, fruity odor
- **Uremia:** Ammoniacal, fishy or urinary odor (e.g. unwashed lavatory)
- **Hepatic failure:** Sweetish-fecal small → fetor hepaticus (smell of a dead mouse)

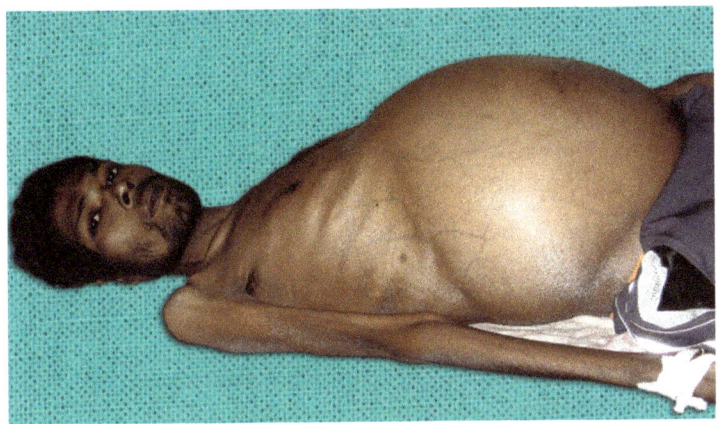

Fig. 31.1: Cirrhosis of liver with profound muscle wasting, thin limb, protuberant abdomen (mimics a 'spider man'), venous prominence and halitosis

- ***Gastrocolic fistula or intestinal obstruction:*** Feculent-foul smell
- ***Bronchiectasis/lung abscess/sinusitis/atrophic rhinitis:*** Putrid smell
- ***Gingivostomatitis/tonsillitis:*** Foul smelling offensive breath
- ***Pulmonary tuberculosis:*** Cinnamon-like breath
- ***Arsenic/thallium/phosphorous poisoning:*** Garlic-like (from body)
- ***Acute alcoholism:*** Ether like smell from breath
- ***Maple-syrup urine disease:*** Burnt sugar odor of urine (i.e. from body).

CLUE TO DIAGNOSIS

- History (smoking, diabetes mellitus, odynophagia, profuse expectoration, vomiting)
- Examination
    - Oral cavity (e.g. gingivostomatitis, caries, tartar, malignancy)
    - Nose (e.g. atrophic rhinitis, sinusitis)
    - Dehydration (e.g. diabetic ketoacidosis)
    - Cervical lymph nodes (e.g. carcinoma of the tongue)
    - Pallor (e.g. uremia, cirrhosis of liver)
    - Jaundice (e.g. hepatic failure)
    - Tremor (e.g. flapping → hepatic failure or uremia)
    - Edema (e.g. uremia, hepatic failure or diabetes mellitus)
    - Auscultation of respiratory system (e.g. bronchiectasis or lung abscess)
    - Auscultation of cardiovascular system (CVS) (e.g. pericardial rub from uremia)
    - Hepatosplenomegaly (e.g. cirrhosis of liver with hepatocellular failure)
    - Decreased ankle jerks (peripheral neuropathy from uremia, diabetes).

INVESTIGATIONS

- Blood for total leukocyte count (TLC), differential leukocyte count (DLC), erythrocyte sedimentation rate (ESR), atypical cells (e.g. leukemia with bad oral

hygiene), sugar (e.g. diabetes mellitus), urea and creatinine (e.g. uremia), liver function test (LFT) (e.g. hepatic failure)
- X-ray of sinuses, lung (e.g. bronchiectasis or lung abscess)
- Straight X-ray of abdomen (e.g. intestinal obstruction)
- Urine for ketone bodies and sugar (e.g. diabetic ketoacidosis), and routine examination (e.g. proteinuria and casts reflect intrinsic renal disease).

MANAGEMENT

- Often very difficult to treat; recalcitrant
- Treatment of etiology. Treatment of infection, if any
- Frequent gargling with some antiseptic solutions with tongue brushing (oral care)
- Keeping clove or elaichi within the mouth
- Dryness of the mouth can be alleviated by peppermints or pilocarpine
- A course of probiotics may be given.

Halitophobia (delusional halitosis): Patients with highly exaggerated concern of having bad breath, in the absence of any. It is a manifestation of olfactory reference syndrome.

🔬 THE PEARLS

Halitosis typically originates from the oral cavity and nasal passages. In some cases, the cause of halitosis remains undiscovered even after meticulous search where the clue may be hidden in 'poor oral hygiene' or the patient is suffering from functional disorder.

32

Genital Ulcer

PROLOGUE

Genital ulcer (or genital sore) may be infective or non-infective as well as ulcerative or non-ulcerative.

POSSIBILITIES

Infective

- Herpes simplex (genital herpes) → primary, recurrent
- Syphilis → primary chancre, secondary mucous patches, tertiary gumma
- Chancroid (soft sore)
- Lymphogranuloma venereum
- Granuloma inguinale
- Herpes zoster
- Condyloma acuminatum
- Scabies
- Others: Balanitis (by Vincent's organism), fungal infection, tuberculosis.

Non-infective

- Behçet's disease (Fig. 32.1)
- Malignancy
- Trauma
- Reactive arthritis (e.g. circinate balanitis)
- Toxic epidermal necrolysis
- Stevens-Johnson syndrome
- Others: Pemphigus vulgaris, lichen planus, psoriasis, functional (psychosis).

EVALUATION

Fever, pain, pruritus, malodour, genital swelling, joint pain, skin rash and eye symptoms should be enquired into. Ask for dysuria, hematuria and joint pain. Drug history and history of (H/O) allergy should be asked for. A detailed sexual history (number and types of sexual contacts) with partner's sex, regular/casual partner,

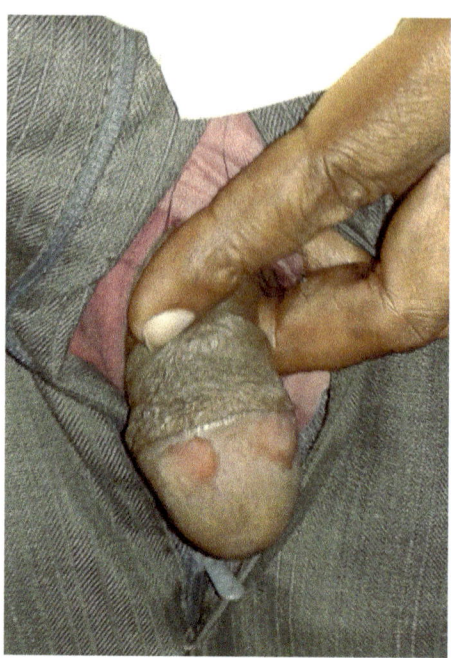

Fig. 32.1: Behçet's disease developing into ulcers in glans penis. The patient has painful aphthous ulcer-like lesions in oral cavity

use of condom/contraception, history of travel abroad, hepatitis B vaccination status should be explored.

On examination (O/E) → oral cavity, throat, skin, lymph nodes, inguinal, genital and perianal areas should be meticulously examined. Penile foreskin should be retracted, urethral meatus should be looked for any discharge and scrotal contents should be palpated for consistency of the testes. If history of anal intercourse is obtained, a rectal examination or proctoscopy should be performed.

BREAK-UP

- **Syphilis:** The **primary chancre** is caused by *Treponema pallidum* with an incubation period of 9 to 90 days. Usually, one ulcer present over the coronal sulcus or glans penis (or any part of penis) → sharply demarcated, oval, regular with dull, non-purulent, relatively non-vascular base. Induration +, may bleed on palpation. Inguinal nodes are firm and non-tender (bilateral affection). The ***secondary syphilitic lesion*** appears 6–8 weeks after the primary one → dull red, painless, indurated and is the most infectious form. ***Gumma (tertiary syphilis)*** occurs 3–10 years after the primary lesion → non-tender, oval, punched-out ulcers often associated with a wash leather slough.
- **Chancroid:** It is caused by *Haemophilus ducreyi* with an incubation period of 1–14 days. Single or multiple (usually) ulcers, few millimeter to 2 centemeter, tender

and painful with shaggy undermined edge which bleeds easily; prepuce, frenum and external meatus are commonly involved. Inguinal lymph nodes (unilateral affection usually) are tender and may suppurate.
- **Lymphogranuloma venereum (LGV):** It is caused by *Chlamydia trachomatis* with an incubation period from 3 days to 6 weeks. Usually single oval, non-indurated ulcer of 2–10 mm size is present on coronal sulcus, glans penis, prepuce or shaft of the penis. Chains of enlarged inguinal lymph nodes **(buboes)** above and below the inguinal ligament (the "sign of the groove") may be seen.
- *Granuloma inguinale (donovanosis):* It is caused by *Klebsiella → Calymmatobacterium granulomatis* with an incubation period of 1–4 weeks. Single or multiple ulcers are seen which are preceded by papule and vesicle. Ulcers are non-tender and of variable size with irregular edge, elevated and velvety; they bleed readily on touch. The lesion may spread to other areas by autoinoculation **(kissing lesion)**. Inguinal lymphadenopathy is uncommon though **pseudobubo** may be seen ('bubo' is seen in plague, tularaemia and lymphogranuloma venereum).
- *Herpes genitalis:* It is caused by *herpes simplex* virus type 2 and have an incubation period of 2–7 days. It commences as an oval vesicle with surrounding erythema over glans and shaft of the penis → ultimately the vesicle breaks down to develop into multiple, superficial erosions. The base of the erosions are serous, erythematous and non-vascular. Induration is absent; very often bilateral, firm, tender lymphadenopathy is present in the inguinal region.

POSSIBLE CAUSES OF GENITAL DISCHARGE (FEMALE)

- *Psychological:* Cervical mucus (i.e. excessive normal secretion), vaginal transudation
- Pregnancy
- Sexual response
- Infection *(Candida, Trichomonas)*
- Cervical erosion
- Foreign body, e.g. tampon, cervical cap, ring pessary
- Malignancy of cervix (or cervical polyp)
- Intrauterine contraceptive device (IUCD)
- Fistula (Crohn's disease, rectovaginal fistula)
- Chemical irritation (e.g. spermicide).

URETHRAL DISCHARGE

- Urethritis (gonococcal, chlamydial, trichomonal, ureaplasma urealyticum)
- Cystitis, prostatitis, vaginitis (e.g. candidiasis)
- Trauma (e.g. masturbation, foreign body, cycle riding)
- Urethral stricture
- Meatal chancre *(Treponema pallidum)*
- Idiopathic.

DIFFERENTIAL DIAGNOSIS OF INGUINAL SWELLING (LUMP IN THE GROIN)

- Hernia (inguinal, femoral) → impulse on coughing, reducible
- Inguinal lymphadenopathy (bubo, pseudobubo, lymphoma)
- Femoral artery aneurysm or pseudoaneurysm → expansile pulsation
- Undescended, ectopic or retractile testis → recognized by its shape, feel and testicular sensation
- Saphena varix → disappears on lying down, non-pulsatile and presence of varicose veins in legs; impulse on coughing +
- Cold abscess → may result from tuberculosis of the hip joint
- Psoas abscess → much larger swelling than femoral hernia or saphena varix; fluctuation present
- Tumors of the spermatic cord
- Hidradenitis of inguinal apocrine gland
- Miscellaneous—cellulitis, lipoma (↑mobility), sebaceous cyst (with central punctum), fibroma, hematoma (iatrogenic during drawing blood from femoral vein) may occur in the groin as elsewhere; varicocele or hydrocele.

THE PEARLS

Usually the patients with genital ulcer are very shy to disclose their problems to the physician, especially the females. Chancroid and syphilis are not very common nowadays because of widespread use of broad-spectrum antibiotics but LGV, donovanosis and herpes infection continue to cause genital ulceration in some developing countries. Clinical grounds and epidemiological considerations can usually guide the initial management.

Gingival Bleeding

PROLOGUE

The connective tissue of gum is highly supplied by capillaries. Bleeding from gingiva may be due to physical injuries (e.g. brushing, trauma), thermal injuries (e.g. consumption of hot tea) or may be precipitated by various infections (e.g. gingivitis). **Platelet plug** formation at the bleeding site is the most important hemostatic mechanism which comes to halt bleeding. Coagulation disorders are usually associated with delayed hemorrhage; in clinical practice, severe degree of clotting factor deficiencies and platelet disorders result in gum bleeding. Connective tissue disorders hampering the supporting tissues of gingival capillaries may result in gum bleeding in day to day practice.

PROBABLE ETIOLOGY

- *Thrombocytopenias:* Idiopathic or immune thrombocytopenic purpura (ITP), aplastic anaemia, acute leukemias
- *Platelet functional defects:*
  - Adhesion defect, e.g. von Willebrand's disease, Bernard-Soulier syndrome
  - Aggregation defect, e.g. thrombasthenia (Glanzmann's syndrome).
- *Coagulation disorders*, e.g. hemophilia, Christmas disease, afibrinogenemia, vitamin K deficiency, disseminated intravascular coagulation (DIC), anticoagulation therapy.
- *Vessel wall disorders:* Scurvy, Cushing's syndrome, Henoch-Schönlein purpura, dysproteinemias (e.g. multiple myeloma), Ehlers-Danlos syndrome, pseudoxanthoma elasticum.
- *Gingival bleeding due to gum inflammation*, e.g. gingivitis/periodontitis, pregnancy, Vincent's angina, ill-fitted dentures, poor oral hygiene.

- In clinical practice, thrombocytopenia, as the first cause (e.g. ITP) of gum bleeding, comes in the mind of clinicians (Fig. 33.1).
- Ehlers-Danlos syndrome and pseudoxanthoma elasticum are connective tissue disorders.

CLINICAL CLUE

- Bleeding from other sites—platelet disorder, coagulation disorder
- Profuse and induced bleeding—platelet disorder

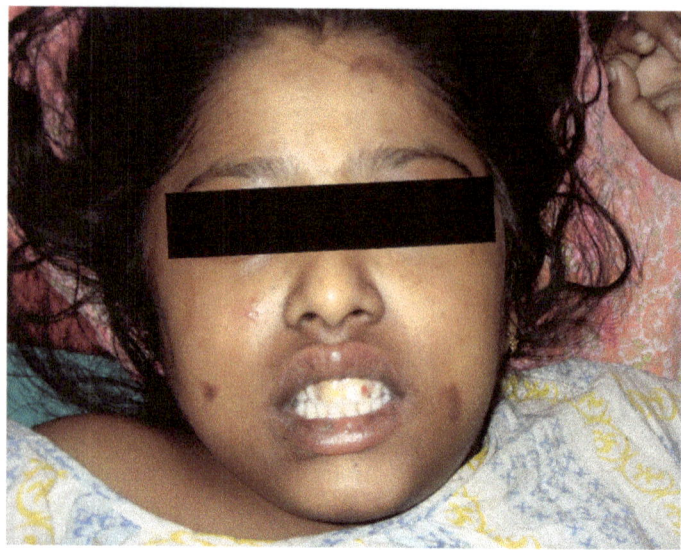

Fig. 33.1: Gum bleeding (recovering) in a patient of immune thrombocytopenic purpura (ITP)

- Persistent bleeding—coagulation disorder
- Associated gum hypertrophy—probable causes mentioned in chapter 34
- Splenomegaly—acute myeloid leukemia (AML), acute lymphoblastic leukemia (ALL), blast crisis of chronic myeloid leukemia (CML) and chronic lymphocytic leukemia (CLL), systemic lupus erythematosus (SLE), hypersplenism, lymphoma, myelofibrosis
- Absence of splenomegaly—aplastic anemia, ITP, coagulation disorder
- Sternal tenderness—acute leukemias, CML
- Associated hemarthrosis or muscle hematoma—coagulation disorder.

In ITP, spleen is enlarged in less than 10% patients and if palpable, it is more or less 1 cm enlarged below left costal margin.

CLUE TO DIAGNOSIS BY INVESTIGATIONS

- Increased bleeding time → thrombocytopenia → low platelet count
- Platelet functional defects → platelet count within normal limit (WNL)
- Increased clotting time → coagulation factor disorders
- Bone marrow examination
  - Hypocellular—aplastic or hypoplastic anaemia
  - More than 30% blast cells—acute leukemias
  - Normal or increased megakaryocytes—ITP
  - Normal or hypercellular—hypersplenism
- Vitamin C level estimation in white blood cell (WBC)—scurvy (low level).

TREATMENT

- Apply pressure directly on the gums with a gauze pad soaked in ice water
- Treatment of etiology, e.g. antibiotics for gingivitis, platelet transfusion for platelet number and function disorders, specific clotting factors to be given in coagulation disorders
- Vitamin C 100 mg, tds orally in scurvy
- Maintenance of good oral hygiene by frequent gargling/application of boroglycerine in gum as and when necessary. Avoid brushing the teeth in active bleeding
- Try to avoid aspirin
- For *linear gingival erythema* [human immunodeficiency virus (HIV) gingivitis] chlorhexidine and nystatin rinses may be used.

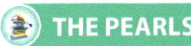
THE PEARLS

Do not carry out occult blood test in stool in the presence of gum bleeding. Though, initially looks harmless, gum bleeding may come out to be a serious illness.

34

Gum Hypertrophy

PROLOGUE

True hypertrophy of gum is rare. Gingival hypertrophy may be due to infiltration by (1) fibrous tissue and (2) cellular elements. The most common cause of gum hypertrophy is infection associated with the dental structures. There is elevation of gum papillae in between the gums. The gums are hypertrophied and may be spongy.

CLUE TO DIAGNOSIS

- **With gum bleeding**
    - Scurvy (soft, red, spongy and hypertrophied)
    - Acute monocytic leukemia (e.g. M5 variety of acute myeloid leukemia)
    - Poor oral hygiene (e.g. caries tooth)
    - Pregnancy
    - Cyanotic congenital heart disease (spongy and hemorrhagic).
- **Without gum bleeding**
    - Phenytoin therapy in epileptics (firm and hypertrophied)
    - Nifedipine or amlodipine therapy in systemic hypertension
    - Cyclosporine therapy
    - Idiopathic familial gingival fibromatosis, epulis (benign tumor over gingival mucosa)
    - Infiltration of gum by hemangioma
    - Mouth breathers since childhood
    - Ill-fitted dentures.

GUM BLEEDING (COMMONLY SEEN IN DAY TO DAY PRACTICE)

- Gingivitis, periodontitis, injury, tartar, pyorrhoea
- Idiopathic or immune thrombocytopenic purpura (ITP)
- Acute leukemias
- Aplastic anemia
- Hemophilia
- Vincent's angina (painful ulcero-membranous gingivitis due to spirochaete and fusiform bacillus infection)
- Anticoagulant therapy
- Hyperviscosity syndrome.

GRAY LINE IN THE GUM

- Tartar on teeth
- Bismuth therapy.

DARK LINE IN THE GUM

Mercury poisoning.

BLUE LINE IN THE GUM

Chronic lead poisoning (Burtonian line).

> If a piece of white paper is inserted between the gum and the teeth, the stippled line due to lead poisoning will be more pronounced whereas color change due to tartar on the teeth will disappear.

STRAWBERRY GUM

Red, purplish granular gingivitis seen in granulomatosis with polyangiitis (Wegener's granulomatosis).

GUM PIGMENTATION

- People with dark complexion
- Addison's disease
- Peutz-Jeghers syndrome
- Nelson's syndrome
- Human immunodeficiency virus (HIV) disease
- Melanoma
- Chronic betel-leaf chewer, chronic smoker.

PYORRHOEA ALVEOLARIS

Gingivitis → bleeding → swollen interdental papillae → as time progresses food debris, bacteria and pus collect between the teeth and the gum margin → pyorrhea alveolaris→ tender, swollen gum with halitosis → pus may be aspirated and lead to pneumonia → teeth loosen, and may be aspirated and obstructed within bronchus (non-resolving pneumonia) → transient bacteremia from pyorrhoea alveolaris may lead to infective endocarditis in a patient with valvular heart disease.

> Healthy gums are pink, adhere to teeth and have a sharp border. In gingivitis, gums are retracted and sometimes pus can be squeezed on pressing the gum (pyorrhea alveolaris).

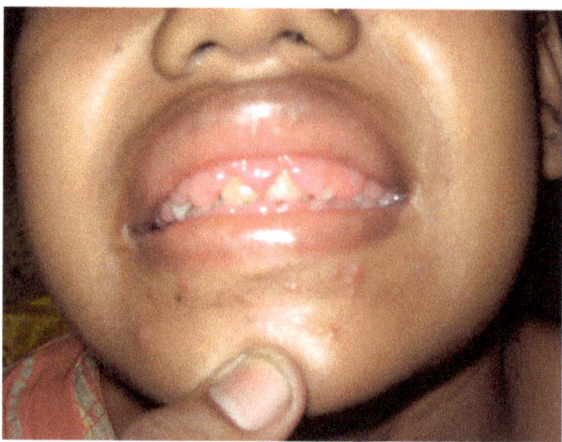

Fig. 34.1: Gum hypertrophy in acute myeloid leukemia

THE PEARLS

Gum hypertrophy is commonly seen in chronic phenytoin therapy in epileptics. Usually the etiologies are benign except the M5 variety of acute myeloid leukemia (AML) (Fig. 34.1).

35
Hardness (Thickening) of Skin

COMMON POSSIBILITIES

- Scleroderma and morphea (localized form of progressive systemic sclerosis) (Figs 35.1 and 35.2)
- Lymphedema (may be in the background of carcinomatous or lymphomatous metastasis into skin, or filariasis; peau d'orange-like skin) (Fig. 35.3)
- Vascular insufficiencies (chronic)
- Recurrent cellulitis associated with venous stasis
- Lipoid proteinosis (hyaline deposition into skin and mucous membrane, firm tongue which is difficult to protrude, hoarseness of voice; face/dorsum of hand and feet, and eyelid margins are commonly involved)
- Carcinoid syndrome (in carcinoid tumor of lung or gut, there may be violaceous cyanosis-like discoloration of skin)
- Porphyria cutanea tarda (presence of fragility of sun-exposed skin)
- Chronic lyme disease
- Chronic graft-versus-host disease
- Eosinophilia-myalgia syndrome (as a result of L-tryptophan therapy)
- Bleomycin or polyvinyl chloride-induced

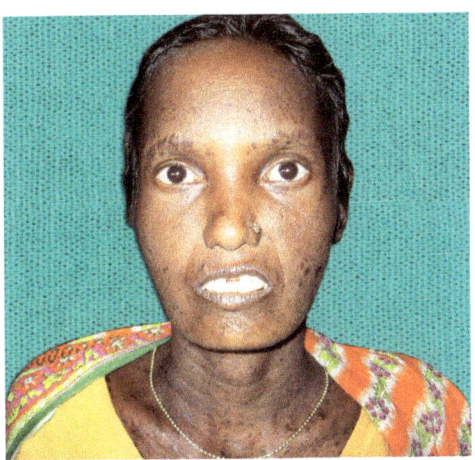

Fig. 35.1: Mask-like face, absence of normal wrinkling of skin, microstomia, loss of eyebrows and pigmentation—facies of scleroderma

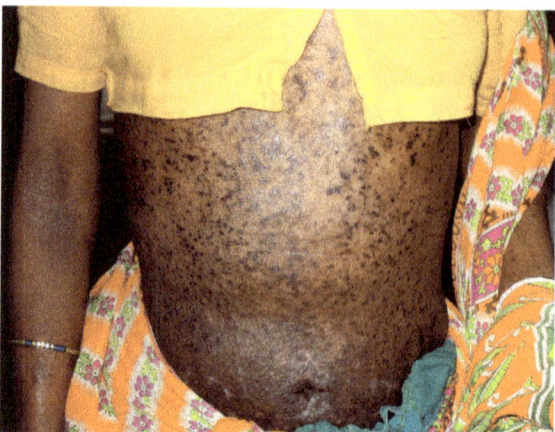

Fig. 35.2: Calcinosis cutis in progressive systemic sclerosis

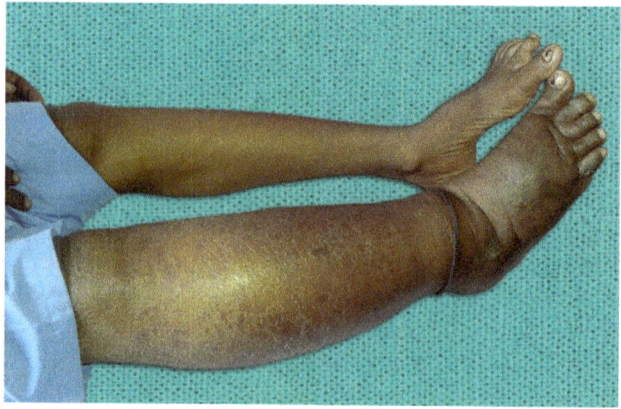

Fig. 35.3: Lymphedema of right leg with nonpitting edema producing thickening of skin (filariasis); ichthyosis-like (fish-scale skin) dermatological changes are present

- Pseudoscleroderma (amyloidosis, acromegaly, scleredema, scleromyxedema)
- Keloid—localized hardening
- Nephrogenic systemic fibrosis (uremic patients on hemodialysis—gadolinium-induced)
- Diabetes mellitus (scleroderma-like skin over shoulders and upper back).

Stiff and Firm Tongue on Palpation

- Primary amyloidosis
- Mucopolysaccharidosis, e.g. Hurler syndrome
- von Gierke's disease (glycogen storage disease)
- Cretinism, acromegaly and myxedema (when associated with macroglossia)
- Carcinoma of the tongue
- Lipoid proteinosis.

DIFFERENTIAL DIAGNOSIS OF SCLERODERMA (THICKENING OF SKIN)

- **Disorders associated with skin thickening in fingers and hands:**
  - Digital sclerosis of diabetes mellitus (cheiroarthropathy)
  - Vinyl chloride-induced
  - Bleomycin-induced
  - Chronic reflex sympathetic dystrophy
  - Mycosis fungoides
  - Adult celiac disease
  - Vibration disease
  - Amyloidosis.
- **Disorders associated with generalized skin thickening but sparing fingers and hands:**
  - Scleredema adultorum of Buschke
  - Scleromyxedema
  - Eosinophilic fasciitis
  - Eosinophilia-myalgia syndrome
  - Pentazocine-induced
  - Chronic graft-versus-host disease
  - Porphyria cutanea tarda
  - Amyloidosis.
- **Disorders associated with asymmetric skin change:**
  - Linear scleroderma
  - Morphea (localized disease)
  - En coup de sabre (linear scleroderma affecting face in children).

WHAT IS SCLEREDEMA ADULTORUM OF BUSCHKE?

Scleredema adultorum of Buschke is painless, edematous, sclerotic induration of face, neck, trunk and proximal extremities (sparing hands and feet), which occurs commonly in children. This may be associated with previous streptococcal infection in some cases; diabetes mellitus and monoclonal gammopathy are known causes. Sparing of hands/feet and absence of Raynaud's phenomenon differentiate this condition from scleroderma. Histopathology shows minimal epidermal changes with markedly thickened dermis as well as accumulation of proteoglycan, hyaluronic acid and collagen.

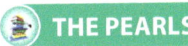
THE PEARLS

Scleroderma (i.e. progressive systemic sclerosis) is the most common disease in clinical practice with hardness of skin. There are many scleroderma mimickers (described above) which are to be differentiated at the first visit.

Head-nodding

DEFINITION

The to and fro movement of head is known as head-nodding. It is a gesture where the head is tilted up and down along the sagittal plane.

POSSIBLE ASSOCIATIONS

- May be a part of tics (habit spasm). Tics are brief, sudden, rapid, intermittent and stereotyped movements (motor tics) or sounds (vocal tics)
- Physiologic: Mannerisms, gestures
- Mental retardation, autism
- Creutzfeldt-Jacob disease, encephalitis
- Titubation: Head-nodding in anteroposterior ('yes-yes') or side-to-side ('no-no') direction, and is found in midline cerebellar disorder
- de Musset's sign: To and fro head-nodding synchronous with carotid pulsation, and is seen in aortic regurgitation (named after a French poet)
- Parkinsonism
- Drug-induced: Anticonvulsants, levodopa, cocaine, dopamine-receptor blocking drugs
- Benign or familial disorder of tremor.

COMMON MOTOR TICS

- Blinking
- Facial grimace
- Shoulder movement
- Nose-twitching
- Sniffing
- Head-shaking/jerking
- Torticollis.

HEAD TILT

- Extension of head (head tilt) done along with lifting of chin (chin lift) in maintenance of airways in basic life support (BLS) of cardiopulmonary resuscitation (CPR)

- Head is tilted (head tilt) towards the direction of action of weak extraocular muscle (e.g. in right-sided IVth cranial nerve or superior oblique palsy, head is tilted to the left) to overcome diplopia
- In cerebellar hemispheric lesion, the patient may have head tilted towards the side of the lesion.

HEAD RETRACTION

- Severe meningitis and meningism
- Subarachnoid hemorrhage
- Asphyxia especially in children with bronchiolitis, bronchopneumonia or foreign body in larynx
- Intermittent retraction:
  - Tetanus
  - Rabies
  - Strychnine poisoning
  - Spasmodic torticollis (wry neck) and torsion spasm.
- Cerebellar pressure cone syndrome [resulting from intracranial space occupying lesion (ICSOL), hematoma, cerebral abscess, cerebral edema or hydrocephalus]—lumbar puncture may result in death
- Spinal disorder involving upper part of spine.

All of the above (head retraction) produce stiffness of neck when examined for neck rigidity.

THE PEARLS

Head-nodding, head tilt and head retraction are important bedside tools for a clinician, though in the era of hightech medicine, these signs are losing their importance.

37

Heel Pain

ETIOLOGY

- **Dermatological**
  - Ulcer
  - Fissure
  - Keratosis
  - Verruca.
- **Connective tissue-related**
  - Panniculitis
  - Plantar fasciitis
  - Bursitis
  - Enthesopathy
  - Gout
  - Spondyloarthropathy (SpA) (Fig. 37.1)
  - Stress fracture
  - Osteopenia
  - Malignant bone tumor

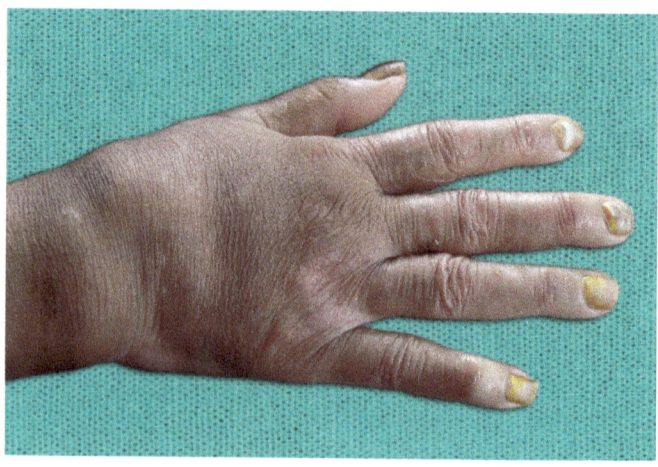

Fig. 37.1: Psoriatic arthropathy (a variety of spondyloarthropathy)—synovitis, skin changes and nail changes are present; there is heel pain too

- Paget's disease
- Calcaneal spur
- Plantar nerve entrapment
- Painful peripheral neuropathy
- Tarsal tunnel syndrome.
- **Miscellaneous**
  - Acute osteomyelitis
  - Plantar bursitis
  - Plantar abscess
  - Foreign body
  - Psychogenic
  - Idiopathic.

COMMON CAUSES OF HEEL PAIN

- *Plantar fasciitis:* It is an enthesitis at the tendon insertion into calcaneum. Pain and tenderness occur in the midline during standing or walking. It may occur as an isolated entity or associated with seronegative SpA. Radiology may show soft tissue clacification. Treatment modalities are sensible restriction of activity, gentle stretching exercise, nonsteroidal anti-inflammatory drugs (NSAIDs), ultrasonography (USG)–guided local steroid or lignocaine injection, lifting of heel, soft shoe, night brace and daytime cast brace. It is usually a self-limiting disease.
- *Calcanean spur:* It is traction lesion at the insertion of plantar fascia; painful after trauma.
- *Calcaneal bursitis:* It is a pressure-induced bursa and compression of the heel pad from sides become painful (ref: midline pain in plantar fasciitis).

PAIN BEHIND THE HEEL

- *Achilles tendonitis:* It is an enthesitis at tendon insertion into calcaneum. Heel raising reduces pain; usually traumatic or may be associated with seronegative SpA. Steroid injection may be beneficial.
- *Achilles tendinosis:* A painful and tender swelling may be present few centimeters above the tendon's insertion. Ultrasonography is helpful and local steroid injection may result in rupture of tendon. Advise to avoid jumping and walking barefooted.
- *Achilles bursitis:* It lies anterior to the tendon; steroid injection is beneficial and can be done safely.
- *Sever's disease:* It is a traction apophysitis of Achilles tendon; affects young people.

PAIN IN THE BALL OF THE GREAT TOE

- Osteoarthritis of 1st metatarsophalangeal (MTP) joint—most common
- Gout (Fig. 37.2)
- Hallux rigidus (a stiff, dorsiflexed great toe)

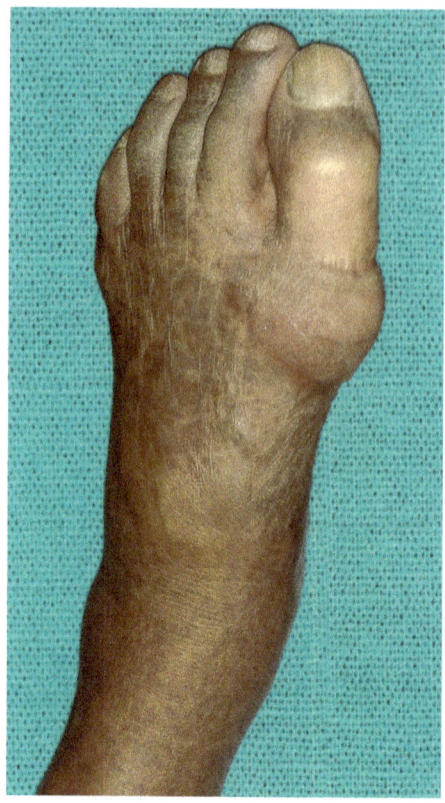

Fig. 37.2: Patient with pain in the ball of the great toe—gout (podagra)

- Hallux valgus
- Metatarsalgia (as a result of high heel, trauma or rheumatoid arthritis)
- Pressure-induced bursa, corn or callosities
- Septic arthritis of 1st MTP joint
- *Miscellaneous:* Pseudogont, psoriatic and reactive arthritis (sausage toe), tendonitis (turf toe), damage in the sesamoids in the flexor hallucis brevis tendon (misdiagnosed as a problem in joints).

PAIN IN THE SHIN BONE

- Blunt trauma
- Referred pain from above (e.g. osteoarthritis of knee joint or sciatica)
- Periostitis due to any cause, trauma, osteomyelitis
- Hypertrophic pulmonary osteoarthropathy (HPOA)
- Tabes dorsalis (lightning pain, stabbing in nature)—rare
- Associated with erythema nodosum (panniculitis)
- *Compartment syndrome:* There is little room within leg for expansion as the lower leg muscles are enclosed in a fascial compartment. The compartment syndrome

may be acute and severe (e.g. collection of blood within leg muscles in Viperidae snake bite in leg), and immediate surgical decompression is done to prevent muscle necrosis. Chronic compartment syndrome may occur after exercise with leg pain.

 THE PEARLS

Treatment of heel pain is unsatisfactory. They are often self-limiting. Plantar fasciitis, calcaneal spur, gout and SpA are common in the community as the causes of heel pain.

Usually the pain is felt when the first step is given on floor after taking rest (e.g. post-sleep). The heel pain may be very nagging.

Herpes Labialis

SYNONYMS

Fever blisters, cold sore (as associated with respiratory infection).

DEFINITION

Herpes labialis refers to small, grouped, closely set vesicles on an erythematous base found on the skin of the face innervated by cutaneous branches of the maxillary and mandibular divisions of the Vth cranial nerve, particularly around the lips (Fig. 38.1) and it is due to herpes simplex virus-type 1.

CHARACTERISTICS

- Often recurrent
- Usually no constitutional symptoms

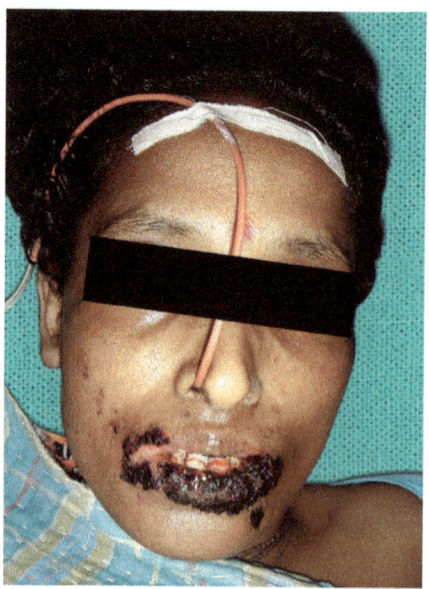

Fig. 38.1: Extensive herpes labialis with crusting in a moribund patient

Chapter 38 Herpes Labialis

- Starts with prodromal symptoms like pain, burning, tingling or itching
- Usually lasts for 6–48 hours
- Rapid vesiculation, pustulation and crusting with local lymphadenopathy
- Complete healing takes about 10 days
- Heals without residue
- It is caused by herpes simplex virus-type 1
- Tongue, gum and palate may be involved
- ***Trigger factors***
  - Fever
  - Sunlight
  - Stress
  - Menstruation
  - Local trauma.

Vesicle is small (< 5 mm), usually clear fluid-containing elevated lesion, whereas **bulla** are large vesicles (> 5 mm).

CLINICAL ASSOCIATIONS

- Influenza
- Acute lobar pneumonia (often gives clue to the side affected, e.g. left side of the lip is affected in left lung involvement)
- Meningococcal meningitis
- Malaria
- Weil's disease
- *Mycoplasma pneumoniae* infection
- Acquired immunodeficiency syndrome (AIDS).

DIFFERENTIAL DIAGNOSIS

- Herpes zoster infection (does not recur in the same site as herpes labialis)
- Hand, foot and mouth disease caused by coxsackievirus (vesicular eruptions in hands and feet as well)
- Impetigo (may be confused with herpes labialis infected by *Staphylococcus*).

TREATMENT

Usually no treatment is necessary. Paracetamol is used to reduce pain. If treatment is needed, acyclic antivirals are the drug of choice and the therapy should be started in the first 48 hours of appearance of first sign of the blisters. Acyclovir (200 mg, 5 times daily), famcyclovir (250 mg, 8 hourly daily), or valacyclovir (500 mg, 12 hourly daily) may be given for 5 days. Acyclovir cream is applied five times daily for recurrent mild facial pain. Solution of 5-iodo-2-deoxyuridine (IDU) may be applied.

CLINICAL FEATURES OF HERPESVIRUS HOMINIS [HERPES SIMPLEX VIRUS (HSV)]

HSV-1

- Acute gingivostomatitis, herpes labialis
- Rhinitis
- Keratoconjunctivitis
- Meningoencephalitis
- Eczema herpeticum (Kaposi's varicelliform eruption)
- Traumatic herpes (includes herpetic whitlow, generalized cutaneous herpes simplex and herpes gladiatorum)
- Erythema multiforme (HSV-1 is the most common identifiable infective cause of erythema multiforme)
- Esophageal ulceration or interstitial pneumonia in immunosuppressed patients.

HSV-2

- Vulvovaginitis (HSV-2 infection is the most common cause of genital vesicles/ulcer in women)
  - Associated with increased risk of carcinoma of the cervix
  - Tzanck smears (a cytologic technique) are positive
  - Differential diagnosis with cytomegalovirus (CMV), varicella-zoster virus, variola virus, drugs or contact dermatitis, or Behçet's disease-induced genital vesicles/ulcers
  - Treated with acyclovir.
- Aseptic meningitis
- Mild hepatitis.

CHEILOSIS OR CHEILITIS

It is the development of cracks and fissures at mucocutaneous junction of the lip.
- Iron-deficiency anemia
- Riboflavin, nicotinic acid, folic acid, vitamin B12 or pyridoxine deficiency
- Solar or actinic cheilitis:
  - Uncommon
  - Cracked lower lip
  - Yellow-white thickenings
  - Scaling and crusting
  - May be a manifestation of light eruption, xeroderma pigmentosum or secondary to use of lipsticks
  - Long-standing cheilitis → warty lesions → may become malignant.
- May be a part of stomatitis.

SORE MOUTH

- Aphthous ulcers
- Infections: Candidiasis, Vincent's angina, dental sepsis, HSV-1, herpangina, coxsackievirus
- Traumatic ulcers due to ill-fitted dentures
- Angular stomatitis
- Sore tongue from vitamin B-complex or iron deficiency, malignancy, glossitis
- *Miscellaneous:* Drug allergy (sulfonamides, penicillins, cytotoxics), recurrent gingivitis from blood dyscrasia, persistent ulceration from agranulocytosis, Behçet's disease, inflammatory bowel disease and dermatological conditions like pemphigoid, erythema multiforme, pemphigus vulgaris and lichen planus.

SORE THROAT

A very common presentation in clinical practice and most of the cases are viral in origin (pharyngitis), self-limiting and need no specific treatment. The clinician should be careful so that any serious underlying life-threatening condition is not overlooked. The common causes are:

- Viral: Adenovirus, herpes simplex, Epstein-Barr virus (all producing pharyngitis)
- Acute follicular tonsillitis (streptococcal commonly)
- Infectious mononucleosis
- Candidiasis (thrush) of buccal or esophageal mucosa
- Vincent's angina (spirochaetes and fusiform bacilli)
- Diphtheria
- Agranulocytosis, acute leukemias, aplastic anemia.

Sore throat may be associated with odynophagia (painful swallowing).

Note: While evaluating sore throat, at the first hand, the clinician should distinguish between benign (common: Viral or streptococcal) and dangerous (less common: Diphtheria) causes of sore throat. Associated symptoms like rhinitis, cough and hoarseness (indicating involvement of larynx) usually suggest a viral upper respiratory tract infection but it has to be remembered that a more serious infection like epiglottitis may give rise to hoarseness of voice too.

Danger signs in sore throat are:

- Persistence of symptoms more than 1 week in spite of treatment
- Odynophagia
- Respiratory distress, especially associated with stridor
- A palpable mass in the neck
- Increased salivary secretion (drooling).

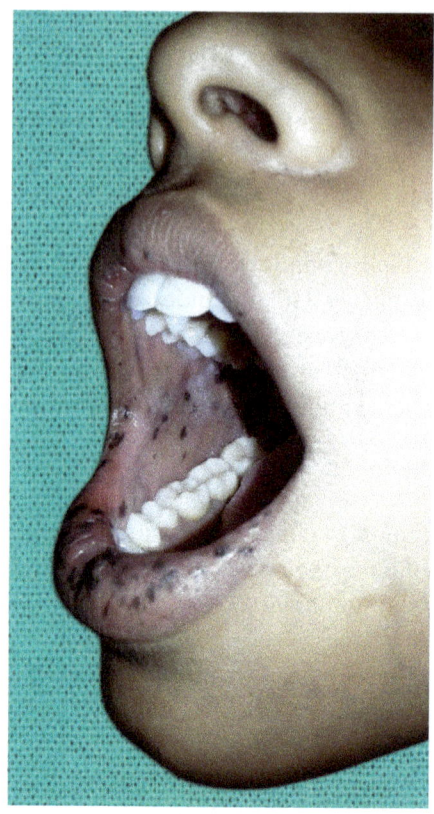

Fig. 38.2: Oral and perioral pigmentation in Peutz-Jeghers syndrome, presented with hematochezia due to bleeding polyps in the intestine

PIGMENTATION OF ORAL CAVITY

- Racial
- Addison's disease
- Peutz-Jeghers syndrome (Fig. 38.2)
- Melanotic macule
- Chloasma
- ***Drug reaction:*** Chlorpromazine, busulfan, quinacrine
- ***Miscellaneous:*** Lead line, amalgam tattoo, neurofibromatosis.

HERPES ZOSTER (SHINGLES)

It is a disease caused by reactivation of varicella-zoster virus (chickenpox) (Fig. 38.3). Following the primary infection, the chickenpox virus becomes latent in the dorsal root ganglia and re-emerges when there is immune compromization (e.g. diabetes, malignancy, AIDS). Pain localized to a dermatome → with constitutional symptoms (fever, malaise) → erythematous maculopapular rashes → evolve in groups into

Chapter 38 Herpes Labialis 159

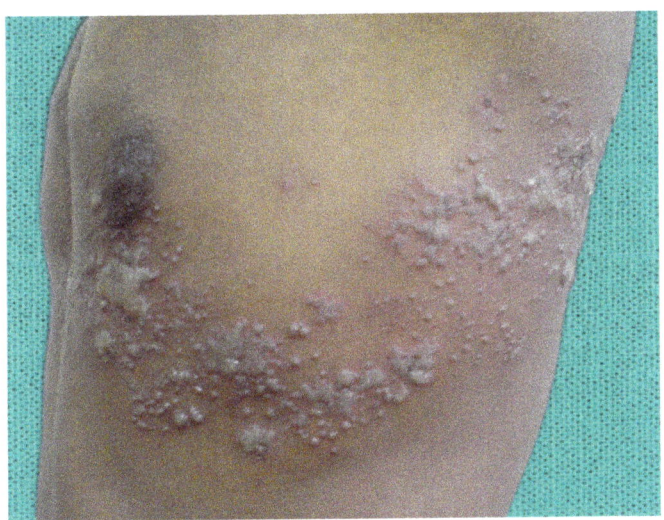

Fig. 38.3: Herpes zoster infection (shingles) involving the thoracic dermatomes (due to reactivation of latent varicella-zoster virus from the dorsal root ganglion of sensory nerves)

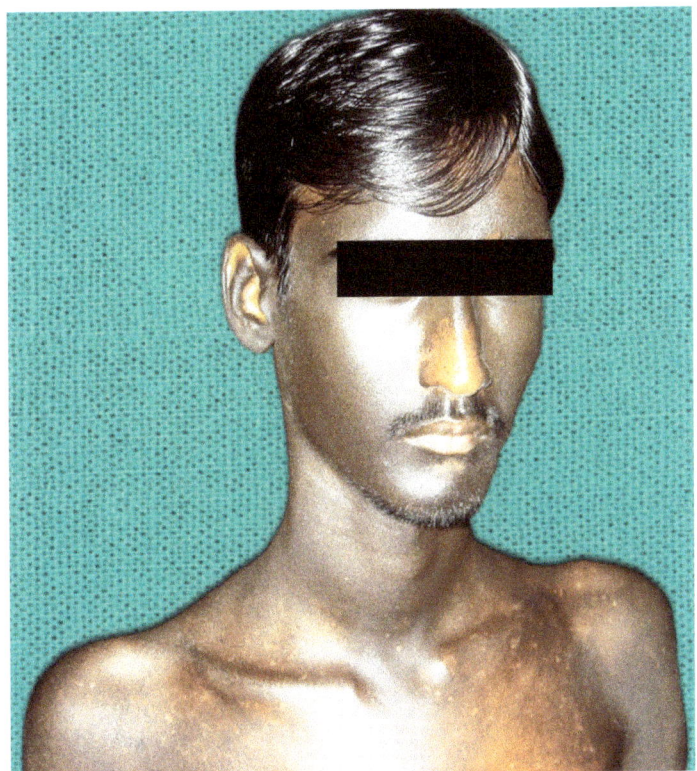

Fig. 38.4: Intensive blackish pigmentation in Addison's disease; the patient also suffers from asthenia and hypotension

vesicles/pustules by the 3rd or 4th day, and are of various sizes (herpes simplex have vesicles which are uniform in size). The anterior and lateral chest wall are commonly affected. Viral cultures and Tzanck smear diagnose the patients with atypical presentation. Postherpetic neuralgia is a nagging problem. Acyclovir (800 mg, 5 times daily), famcyclovir (500 mg, 8 hourly daily), or valacyclovir (1000 mg, 8 hourly daily) may be given for 7 days.

 THE PEARLS

Both the herpes viruses may be serious, especially in an immunocompromized patient. Common Bell's palsy may occur due to herpes simplex infection, whereas herpes zoster may affect the ophthalmic division of trigeminal nerve (herpes zoster ophthalmicus), or the geniculate ganglion of facial nerve (Bell's palsy; Ramsay Hunt syndrome).

39

Hiccough

SYNONYMS

Hiccup, singultus.

DEFINITION

It is the abrupt, involuntary, synchronous contraction of the diaphragm and the inspiratory intercostal muscles, followed by immediate closure of the glottis—the glottic closure is responsible for the characteristic inspiratory sound and associated discomfort. Though hiccough is a normal, benign and transient physiological phenomenon, many a time persistent hiccough pose problem in management.

POSSIBLE ASSOCIATIONS

- *Transient:* Ingestion of chilli/irritant spicy food in a quick succession, gastric distension after a rapid meal, sudden excitement or emotion, ingestion of alcohol, esophageal obstruction or sudden change in temperature.
- *Persistent:*
  - *Central nervous system disorders (CNS):* Cerebrovascular accident (CVA), lateral medullary syndrome, encephalitis, multiple sclerosis, posterior fossa space occupying lesion (SOL) or lower brainstem lesion
  - *Thoracic disorders:* Basal pneumonia (diaphragmatic pleurisy), acute myocardial infarction (MI) (mainly in inferior wall involvement), pleurisy (e.g. diaphragmatic), empyema thoracis, pericarditis, aneurysm of the aorta, diaphragmatic herniation or irritation (e.g. subphrenic abscess), mediastinal tumor
  - *Metabolic disorders:* Uremia, hyperventilation
  - *Abdominal disorders:* Acute gastritis [e.g. nonsteroidal anti-inflammatory drug (NSAID)-induced], gastric ulcer/carcinoma, acute hepatitis, amebic liver abscess, intestinal obstruction, acute pancreatitis, acute peritonitis
  - *Miscellaneous:* Psychogenic, idiopathic, surgery, general anesthesia, irritation of external auditory canal, drug-induced (benzodiazepines, barbiturates), epidemic hiccough (viral infection related to influenza and encephalitis, occurring in epidemics), high pyrexia, septicemia.

COMMON CAUSES OF HICCOUGH IN CLINICAL PRACTICE

- Overdistension of stomach
- Acute gastritis
- Alcohol excess
- Chronic renal failure (uremia)
- Diaphragmatic pleurisy (e.g. basal pneumonia)
- Excitement
- Idiopathic.

MANAGEMENT OF INTRACTABLE HICCOUGH

Recurrent hiccough is very distressing to the patient and difficult to manage:
- **Reassurance:** The patient along with the relatives should be reassured
- **Simple household remedies:** Divert patient's attention (e.g. by conversation, sudden slapping), intake of ice-cold water, series of deep breath holding, Valsalva maneuver, lifting uvula with cold spoon, breathing in and out in a plastic bag for 5 minutes, induction of vomiting by pharyngeal stimulation, spray of ethyl chloride under the costal margins, swallowing rapidly one teaspoonful of dry granulated sugar or dry bread, drinking water without taking any breath; coughing, sneezing
- **Local measures:** Intake of local anesthetic viscus, e.g. lignocaine, nasogastric suction followed by ice-cold stomach wash or alkaline stomach wash through a Ryle's tube
- **Antacids/H_2-RA/proton pump inhibitor:** Any liquid antacid (preferably containing oxethazaine) is given 2–4 tsf, 6–8 hourly daily, orally, or ranitidine 150 mg BDAC, or omeprazole 20 mg ODAC, orally. It is often advised to take the tablets with little or no water and irritation of the pharynx may end a bout of hiccough in a stubborn case.
- **Drugs or pharmacotherapy:** Chlorpromazine (probably best tried first, as an intravenous (IV) bolus; 25 mg, orally tds or 25 mg/IV bolus stat), baclofen (10 mg, orally tds), metoclopramide [10 mg intramuscular (IM), tds], haloperidol (5 mg, IM stat or 0.25 mg, orally, tds), clonazepam (2 mg, orally, tds), amitriptyline, amantadine, quinidine (200 mg, orally, tds), ondansetron (4 mg, IV, tds), anticonvulsants like phenytoin sodium, carbamazepine, valproic acid are worth trying in resistant cases. Baclofen (beta-agonist) is an effective drug in the treatment of intractable hiccough.
- **Surgery:** In a recalcitrant case, phrenic nerve block by bupivacaine or nerve section may be effective.
- Treatment of the underlying cause.

PROBABLE CAUSES OF BELCHING (ERUCTATION)

It is the forceful regurgitation (expulsion) of air from the stomach or esophagus.
- Consumption of carbonated beverages, hurried eating habit, gum chewing, ill-fitted dentures.

- Addictions like smoking, chewing betel nut/pan; mouth breather.
- *Abdominal disorders:* Acute gastritis or duodenitis, hiatus hernia, chronic cholecystitis, irritable bowel syndrome, intestinal obstruction.
- Psychogenic conditions like anxiety, emotional disturbances, depression.

Avoidance of addiction and faulty habits as well as intake of conventional antacid containing methylpolysiloxane (MPS) many a time relieve the person from belching.

THE PEARLS

Hiccough, a benign disorder, may be recurrent or intractable. The patient feels exhausted in persistent hiccough. One should take the opinion of a physician if it persists for few hours. Simple household remedies often work wonder. Many a time overview of the etiology of hiccough gives clue to the clinician.

Hirsutism

HIRSUTISM

Hirsutism is the growth of terminal hair in women in a pattern characteristic of men. In females, excess hair growth is seen in sides of the face, moustache and beard area (Fig. 40.1) (upper lip and chin), in between the breast, periareolar region, over the abdomen and in the extemities. There is upward extension of pubic hair too. It usually affects 10% women in the community.

VIRILIZATION

The characteristic features are:
- Frontal baldness
- Increase in size of shoulder girdle muscles
- Coarsening of voice
- Acne and seborrhea
- Hirsutism

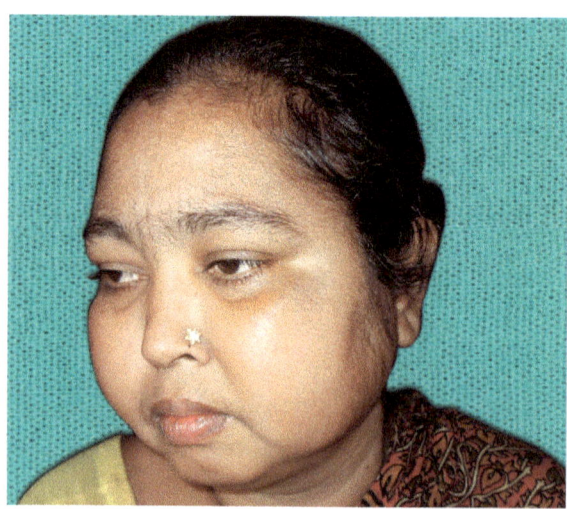

Fig. 40.1: Moon face (Cushingoid features—facial plethora, hirsutism) after prolonged corticosteroid therapy in nephrotic syndrome

- Clitoromegaly
- Increased libido.

> Congenital adrenal hyperplasia is the most common cause of virilization (associated with ↑ androgens with ↓ or normal glucocorticoids and mineralocorticoids).

DEFEMINIZATION (DIMINISHING FEMALE CHARACTERISTICS)

- Decrease in breast size
- Loss of female body contours
- Amenorrhea.

HYPERTRICHOSIS

It is the excessive hair growth in both sexes and is commonly due to malnutrition, hypothyroidism, dermatomyositis, porphyria cutanea tarda, drugs (e.g. minoxidil, cyclosporin, phenytoin, diazoxide), underlying malignancy, anorexia nervosa and Cushing's syndrome.

Hypertrichosis in the male ears (hairy ears) is a Y-linked disorder (Fig. 40.2).

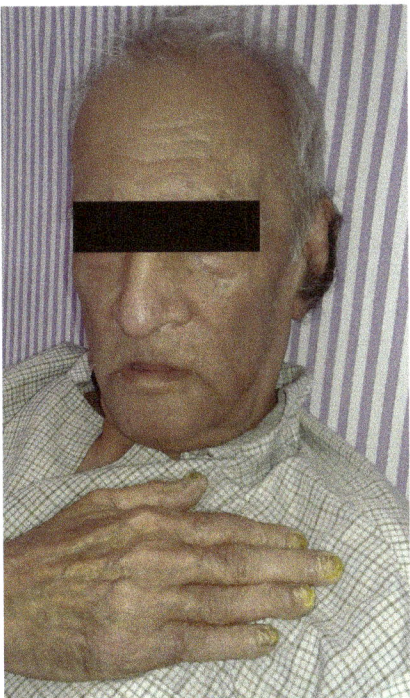

Fig. 40.2: Hairy ear (hypertrichosis) in a male subject is the only Y-linked single gene disorder; the patient has onychodystrophy due to fungal infections

Some Basics

Certain races (e.g. Mediterranean and Asian) have more male pattern hair growth which is not due to androgen excess but happens to be as a result of genetically determined altered sensitivity to androgens. Fetal hair is known as ***lanugo hair***. Hair can be categorized into two types—***vellus*** (fine, soft and nonpigmented) and ***terminal*** (long, coarse and pigmented). In the lifetime, the number of hair follicle does not increase but the follicle size and type of hair change in response to multiple factors, e.g. androgens (it can transform vellus hair into a terminal hair).

Three phases in the cycle of hair growth have been observed:
1. Anagen (growth phase) = has six stages like pro-anagen (1–5), met-anagen (6) stages.
   Met-anagen to catagen phase = 2–10 years
2. Catagen (involution or transition phase) = 6 weeks
3. Telogen (rest phase) = 3 months.

HORMONAL INFLUENCES ON GROWTH OF HAIR

- Eyebrows, eyelashes, and vellus hair—androgen-sensitive.
- Axillary and pubic hair—sensitive to low levels of androgens.
- Hairs on face, chest, upper abdomen, and back—needs high level of androgens and thus seen in males.

> In women, vellus hair covers face, chest, back and gives the impression of ***hairless skin***; in most of the men, terminal hair covers face and body. Terminal hair cover scalp, pubic and armpit in both sexes.

Note: Nonsexual or neutral hairs are under the control of growth hormone, e.g. hairs on the scalp, eyelashes, forehead and lower part of the body in both sexes; whereas ambisexual hair, in both sexes, are under the influence of testosterone. The axillary and pubic hair in females are under the control of adrenal androgen and thus hair loss in those regions are seen in Addison's disease, whereas this does not occur in males because testosterone alone maintains the growth of hair in axilla and pubic region.

Remember 'androgen excess underlies most of the cases of hirsutism'. Androgen excess in females lead to increased growth of hair in most of the androgen-sensitive sites (3rd bullet above) except in the scalp region. In females, androgens are derived from ovaries and adrenal glands, as well as from peripheral conversion—hence, etiology lies either in adrenal or in ovary.

POSSIBLE ASSOCIATIONS OF HIRSUTISM

- Familial and racial
- Possible ↑ sensitivity to androgens (idiopathic or simple hirsutism)
- Menopause

- Polycystic ovarian syndrome (Stein-Leventhal syndrome)
- Cushing's syndrome, hyperprolactinemia, virilizing ovarian tumor (e.g. arrhenoblastoma or hilus cell tumor), acromegaly, congenital adrenal hyperplasia, adrenal androgen secreting tumor (adenoma, carcinoma), true hermaphroditism
- Obesity (in the adipose tissue, estrogens are converted into androgens)
- Drug-induced: phenytoin, oral contraceptive pills, androgens, diazoxide, cyclosporine, minoxidil, psoralens, anabolic steroids, penicillamine, corticosteroids.

CLINICAL PRESENTATION

- *Hirsutism with virilization:*
  - Severe polycystic ovarian syndrome [ultrasonography (USG) of ovary, ↑luteinizing hormone (LH), ↑androgens]
  - Congenital adrenal hyperplasia (↑17-hydroxyprogesterone)
  - Ovarian tumor (USG/laparoscopy).
- *Hirsutism without virilization:*
  - Idiopathic or simple hirsutism (with normal menstruation, normal ovaries/adrenals)
  - Familial (positive family history of hirsutism in mother or grandmother)
  - Mild polycystic ovarian syndrome (same as above)
  - Drugs [hypertrichosis mainly, history of (H/O) specific drug intake]
  - Congenital adrenal hyperplasia (late onset)–↑17-hydroxyprogesterone, after adrenocorticotropic hormone (ACTH) injection
  - Adrenal tumors [computed tomography (CT) scan of adrenals].

OUTLINE OF INVESTIGATIONS IN HIRSUTISM

- Serum androgens (very high in adrenal neoplasm or congenital adrenal hyperplasia)
- Other hormones: thyroid-stimulating hormone (TSH), ACTH, LH, follicle-stimulating hormone (FSH) and cortisol; a short ACTH stimulation test is helpful in congenital adrenal hyperplasia, and LH:FSH ratio more than 3:1 very often suggests polycystic ovarian disease
- Serum insulin level and glucose tolerance test in polycystic ovarian disease—diagnose insulin resistance
- Pelvic USG of ovaries (e.g. polycystic ovarian disease); CT or magnetic resonance imaging (MRI) scan of adrenal glands or pituitary gland
- Laparoscopy or laparotomy (for diagnosis of ovarian pathology)
- Biopsy of the ovary (e.g. ovarian neoplasm).

TREATMENT OF HIRSUTISM

- *Nonpharmacological*
  - Bleaching
  - Shaving
  - Chemical treatment (depilatory creams)
  - Epilatory treatment (plucking, waxing, electrolysis and pulsed laser therapy)

- Electrolysis usually removes hairs permanently, especially in the hand of a skilled electrologist but the process is lengthy as well as expensive.
- At first hand, stop the offending drug, if drug-induced.

- **Pharmacological**
  - Oral contraceptive pills to suppress androgen production
  - Spironolactone (100–200 mg/day) is a weak anti-androgen; may be used in combination with oral contraceptives; bromocryptine and cimetidine have no value
  - Cyproterone acetate (50–100 mg/day) is given on days 1 to 15, and ethinyl estradiol (50 µg/day) is given on days 5 to 26 of menstrual cycle; cyproterone is a prototypic anti-androgen
  - Eflornithine cream is novel treatment for removal of facial hair in women
  - Flutamide (nonsteroidal anti-androgen) may be used; finasteride (5 mg/day), a 5 α-reductase inhibitor has also been shown to be effective
  - Low dose dexamethasone, prednisolone (to suppress ACTH), ketoconazole are also tried. Metformin is reserved for insulin-resistant cases.

GRAYING OF HAIR (CANITIES)

- Aging
- Hereditary
- Over a patch of vitiligo
- Albinism
- Pernicious anemia
- Thyrotoxicosis
- Chloroquine toxicity.

THE PEARLS

Most of the **hairy women** have no underlying disease and only face cosmetic problems.

Every doctor concerned should do a meticulous physical examination with special reference to voice, acne, striae, acanthosis nigricans, body habitus, galactorrhea, signs of virilization and defeminization, and abdominal and pelvic examinations. Hirsutism is both an endocrine (androgen excess; total testosterone may be normal but free testosterone is elevated) and cosmetic problem for patients. It is essential to search for an adrenal tumor.

Pituitary tumor with hirsutism may have associated visual field defects

41

Hoarseness of Voice

DEFINITION

It is the rough and harsh voice due to abnormality in vocal cords, and may range from slight huskiness to complete aphonia.

ETIOLOGY

Congenital

Laryngeal web, dermoid cyst, cystic hygroma, lipoma, fibroma or hemangioma of larynx.

Acquired

- *Traumatic*
  - **Overuse of voice:** Singer's nodule, hawker's voice
  - Anesthetic intubation injury, strangulation or post-cough injury
  - Tobacco, irritant gases, inhaled steroid
- *Inflammatory*
  - **Specific:** Diphtheria, tuberculosis, leprosy, lupus, syphilis of the larynx
  - **Nonspecific:** Simple infective laryngitis, acute laryngotracheobronchitis, edema of the larynx, chronic simple laryngitis, tracheitis, croup, epiglottitis
- *Neoplastic:* Papilloma, squamous cell carcinoma, polyp, lipoma, angioma, fibroma, leiomyoma of larynx
- *Paralytic (as a result of recurrent laryngeal or vagus nerve palsy):* Bronchogenic carcinoma, cardiac surgery, post thyroidectomy/parathyroidectomy, chest surgery, mediastinoscopy, pulmonary hypertension
- *Neurological*
  - Cerebrovascular accidents (CVA), parkinsonism, Guillain-Barré (GB) syndrome, disseminated sclerosis, bulbar palsy, amyotrophic lateral sclerosis
  - Hysteria [often with history of (H/O) recurrence under stress; coughs normally; no abnormality in laryngoscopy]
- *Systemic*
  - Myxedema (very common medical cause in clinical practice)
  - Leprosy

- Rheumatoid arthritis (cricoarytenoid joint affection)
- Poliomyelitis (bulbar)
- Angioneurotic edema
- Wegener's granulomatosis
- Systemic lupus erythematosus (SLE)
- Mitral stenosis (Ortner's syndrome)
- Puberty/menopause
- Lipoid proteinosis
- Acromegaly
- Sicca syndrome.

OLIVER'S SIGN (TRACHEAL TUG) + HOARSENESS

Aneurysm of aorta.

BOVINE COUGH + STRIDOR + HOARSENESS

Recurrent laryngeal nerve palsy.

HORNER'S SYNDROME + HOARSENESS

Mediastinal mass.

MOON FACE + PLETHORIC FACE + HOARSENESS

Superior mediastinal syndrome (e.g. bronchogenic carcinoma producing recurrent laryngeal nerve palsy).

- Right sided recurrent laryngeal nerve remains high up. Left sided recurrent laryngeal nerve is usually compressed by a mediastinal mass (e.g. hilar adenopathy from bronchogenic carcinoma, lymphoma, etc.) → *indirect laryngoscopy* shows the position of the left vocal cord in paramedian or cadaveric position during phonation → a method of quick diagnosis of mediastinal mass-induced (from bronchogenic carcinoma or lymphoma) hoarseness in clinical practice.
- In health, during phonation the vocal cords become adducted and during respiration the cords are abducted.

COMMON CAUSES OF HOARSENESS IN CLINICAL PRACTICE

- Chronic simple laryngitis (H/O recurrent acute laryngitis, inflamed vocal cord at laryngoscopy, benign in nature)
- Carcinoma of the larynx (progressive hoarseness, smoker, confirmed by laryngoscopy with biopsy)
- Paralytic (having H/O surgery or stigmata of superior vena caval (SVC) syndrome, confirmed by laryngoscopy with cadaveric position of vocal cord)

- Myxedema (gradual hoarseness over months, tiredness, obesity, constipation, menorrhagia, swollen vocal cords at laryngoscopy)
- Singer's nodule (positive occupational history like singer, orator, hawker or teacher as a result of voice abuse; vocal cord shows nodules at laryngoscopy)
- Granuloma, i.e. tuberculosis, sarcoidosis, Wegener's granulomatosis (onset over months, confirmed by laryngoscopic biopsy).

MECHANISM

Normal voice is produced as a result of vibration as well as movement of vocal cord. If the vocal cord is affected by edema, inflammation, infiltrative diseases, tumor or compression over recurrent laryngeal nerve → hoarseness of voice results.

CLUE TO DIAGNOSIS OF MEDICAL CAUSES OF HOARSENESS

Look for:
    Dull expressionless puffy face + madarosis + delayed relaxation of ankle jerk → Myxedema (Fig. 41.1)
    ↓
    Thickened ulnar nerve + leonine facies → Leprosy
    ↓

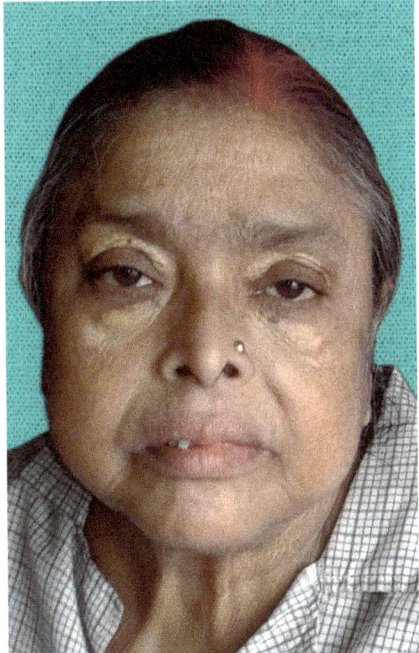

Fig. 41.1: Expressionless face of myxedema with xanthelasma around the eyes; the patient presented with hoarseness of voice

H/O sudden choking sensation + presence of giant hives → Angioneurotic edema
↓

Butterfly rash in face of a female, patchy alopecia, arthralgia + H/O Raynaud's phenomenon → SLE
↓

Swan-neck and button-hole deformity of the hand along with spindle-shaped fingers, and restricted + painful joint movement → Rheumatoid arthritis
↓

Destruction of nose and nasal septum, H/O Raynaud's phenomenon + features of vasculitis like digital infarction, digital ulceration, nail-fold thrombi, splinter hemorrhage → Wegener's granulomatosis
↓

Dry mouth and eyes over months + arthritis + deglutition difficulty → Sicca syndrome
↓

Recurrences at times of stress. Variable symptoms and the patient (usually a female) coughs normally → Functional hoarseness

THE PEARLS

Persistent hoarseness of some weeks' or months' duration may have some deadly causes that need urgent attention as well as intervention. H/O smoking should be taken (smoking-induced, bronchogenic carcinoma, carcinoma of larynx), and a chest X-ray and laryngoscopy should be done at the first visit, if suspected for sinister causes.

42 Hyperkeratosis of Palms

CLUE TO DIAGNOSIS

- Manual laborer
- Phrenoderma (vitamin A or essential fatty acid deficiency)
- Arsenic poisoning (dry, gray, irregular, hyperkeratotic papules) (Fig. 42.1)
- Psoriasis (usually bilaterally symmetrical)
- Tylosis palmaris et plantaris (congenital hyperkeratosis, and pitting of palms and soles believed to be associated with carcinoma of the esophagus)
- Secondary to rash of secondary syphilis or keratoderma blennorrhagica (Reiter's syndrome)
- Drug-induced, e.g. β-blockers

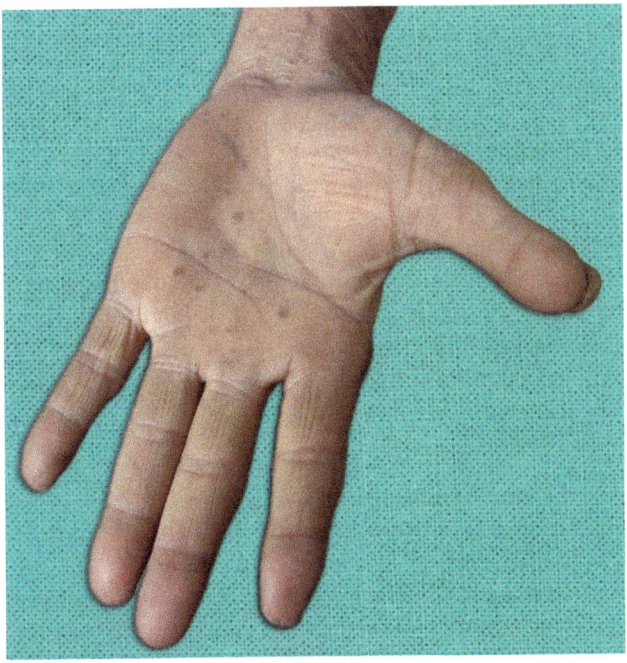

Fig. 42.1: Hyperkeratosis of palm from arsenic toxicity

- Eczematous dermatitis (e.g. hands of housewives)
- Ichthyosis (especially from Hodgskin's disease)
- Florid cutaneous papillomatosis (a paraneoplastic syndrome)
- **Miscellaneous:** Corn and callosity, warts, palmoplantar keratoderma, pityriasis rubra pilaris, tyrosinemia, Papillon-Lefèvre syndrome, fungal infection.

HYPERKERATOSIS

It is the thickening of horny layer of skin usually resulting from retention and increased adhesion of epidermal cells often associated with the presence of an abnormal quantity of keratin.

DERMATOLOGICAL CHANGES OFTEN ASSOCIATED WITH INTERNAL MALIGNANCY

- Dermatomyositis (in ovarian/breast/colon carcinoma, lymphoma)
- Acanthosis nigricans (in gastric carcinoma, lymphoma)
- Ichthyosis (adult-onset)
- Alopecia mucinosa (in mycosis fungoides)
- Pachydermoperiostosis (acquired; in bronchogenic carcinoma)
- Erythema gyratum repens (concentric, arcuate lesions look like the grain of a soft wood)
- Intractable pruritus without any skin lesion
- Hypertrichosis lanuginosa acquisita (acquired in malignancy of breast, lung, colon)
- Migrating thrombophlebitis (related to carcinoma of the pancreas)
- Multiple irritable seborrheic warts (sign of Leser-Trelat).

POMPHOLYX

- An endogenous eczema
- Bilaterally symmetrical, recurrent vesicular eruptions in palms (cheiropompholyx) and soles
- Sago-grain like, excruciatingly itchy; may be painful
- Affects young adults; in summer; multifactorial; provoked by heat or stress
- Hyperhydrosis
- Spontaneous resolution with scaling
- Treatment by topical corticosteroids.

PALMAR XANTHOMA

- Yellowish discolorations of the palmar digital creases
- Seen in familial dysbetalipoproteinemia (accumulation of remnant-like particles in plasma)
- Associated with fulminant atherosclerosis and premature coronary artery disease
- Often associated with obesity, diabetes mellitus or hypothyroidism
- Histology includes xanthoma cells (i.e. lipid-laden foam cells), Touton giant cells with admixture of inflammatory cells.

PALMAR ERYTHEMA (BRIGHT RED PALM)

The thenar and hypothenar eminences, base and pulp of the fingers turn red in:
- Cirrhosis of liver *(liver palms)*
- Alcoholics
- Pregnancy
- Rheumatoid arthritis (long-continued)
- Thyrotoxicosis
- Hyperdynamic circulation, e.g. pyrexia, pregnancy
- Polycythemia
- Rarely in normal persons (familial).

BLACK PALMAR CREASES

Addison's disease.

CHEIROARTHROPATHY

It is the limited joint mobility of hands in long-standing diabetes mellitus. The patient cannot extend finger/fingers at metacarpophalangeal or interphalangeal joints—resulting in painless stiffness in hands—the classical *prayer sign* (mild, fixed curvature of fingers making it impossible to appose both hands as done in prayer). This is due to excessive nonenzymatic glycosylation of collagen in skin, vessels and periarticular structures, and to decreased collagen degeneration and removal.

SWELLING/NODULES IN HAND

- Osler's node (tender papule in pulp—subacute bacterial endocarditis)
- Heberden's node (bony nodules at dorsal aspect of distal interphalangeal (DIP) joint—osteoarthritis)
- Bouchard's node (bony nodules at dorsal aspect of proximal interphalangeal (PIP) joint—osteoarthritis)
- Gouty tophi (over dorsal aspect of PIP and DIP joints)
- Rheumatoid nodule or nodule formation in leprosy
- Calcinosis (in scleroderma)
- Ganglion, neurofibroma and lipoma (of surgical interest).

THREE 'PS' OF UNDERLYING MALIGNANCY

- Pallor
- Pigmentation
- Pruritus.

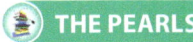
THE PEARLS

Hyperkeratosis of palms is also a clinical window through which a clinician can view some known diseases, which may be benign or malignant. This chapter reflects the importance of **hand examination** in clinical medicine.

Hypertelorism/Hypotelorism

HYPERTELORISM

Definition

This is synonymous with widely set (spaced) eyes (Figs 43.1 and 43.2). When the distance between inner canthus of two eyes is greater than half of the interpupillary distance, hypertolorism is said to be present. Quantitatively, it is defined as the ratio between the inner canthal distance over the outer canthal distance and if it is more than 0.38, it is known as hypertelorism; or the interpupillary distance more than 85 mm (hypertelorism) where the average normal value is 60 mm.

Hence, the root of the nose appears broad and the distance between the eyes seems to be increased.

Possible Causes

- Mild hypertelorism may be seen in normal children
- Racial

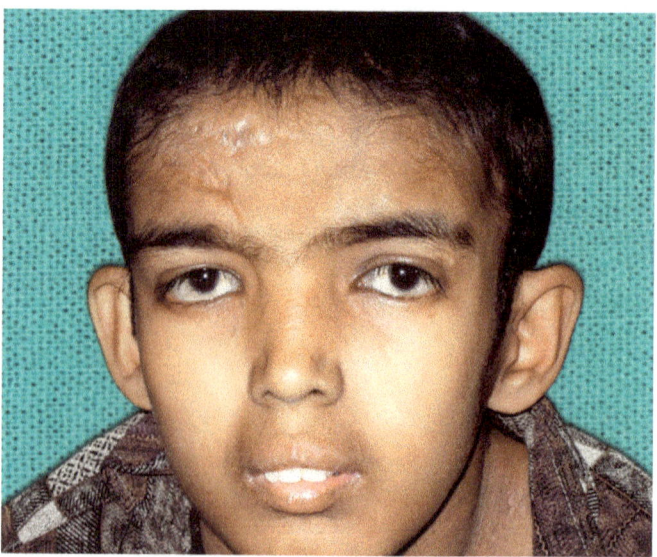

Fig. 43.1: Hypertelorism (widely set eyes) in Ehlers-Danlos syndrome with mild blue sclera

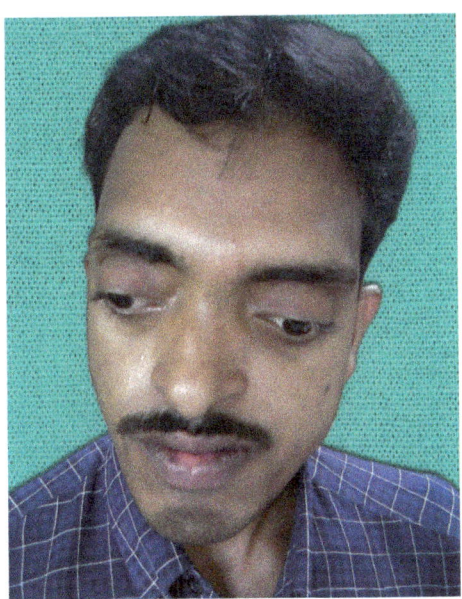

Fig. 43.2: Hypertelorism in a patient of craniostenosis (Crouzon syndrome)

- Down's syndrome
- Thalassemia major
- Cretinism
- Craniostenosis, e.g. Crouzon syndrome (Fig. 43.2)
- Turner's syndrome, Ehlers-Danlos syndrome, Noonan syndrome
- Elfin facies seen in congenital supravalvular aortic stenosis
- Associated with congenital pulmonary stenosis
- Associated with mental retardation
- Carpenter syndrome
- LEOPARD syndrome.

- Probable pathology—due to hyperplasia of lesser wing of sphenoid bone (e.g. thalassaemia).
- Hypertelorism literally means increased distance between paired organs (e.g. between two kidneys).

HYPOTELORISM

Eyes being located too close to each other with decreased interpupillary distance.

Why Hypotelorism Occurs?

When the brain has not divided into two hemispheres and there exists a single ventricle (holoprosencephaly), hypotelorism is said to be exist. Common examples are trisomy 13 (Patau syndrome), ethmocephalus, cebocephaly; may be familial (Fig. 43.3).

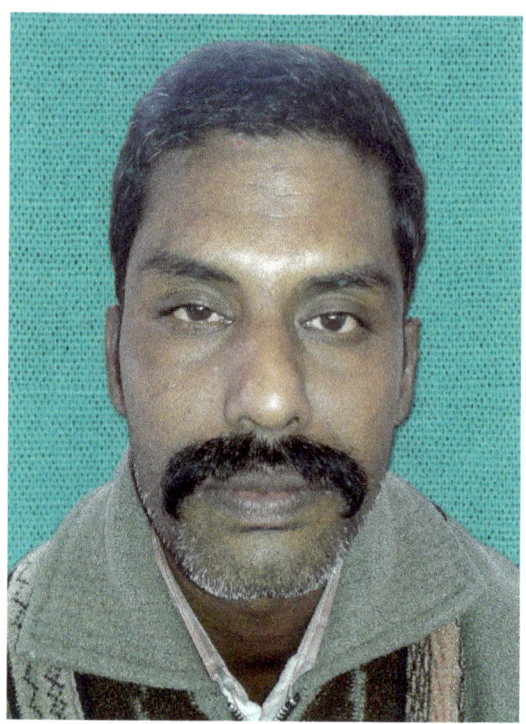

Fig. 43.3: Hypotelorism (familial)

Low Set Ears

In health, if an arbitrary horizontal line is drawn from the outer canthus of the eye to the ipsilateral pinna, about one-third of the pinna is seen above the line. In low set ears, less than one-third of total length of pinna lies above the line. It is seen in disorders like:
- Down's syndrome
- Trisomy 18 (Edward's syndrome)
- Trisomy 13 (Patau syndrome)
- Mental retardation
- Elfin facies.

Diagonal Crease in Ear Lobule (Frank's Sign)

Very often a prominent horizontal crease is seen over the lobule of the ear—designated as a marker for ischemic heart disease (IHD) (Fig. 43.4).

Chapter 43 Hypertelorism/Hypotelorism

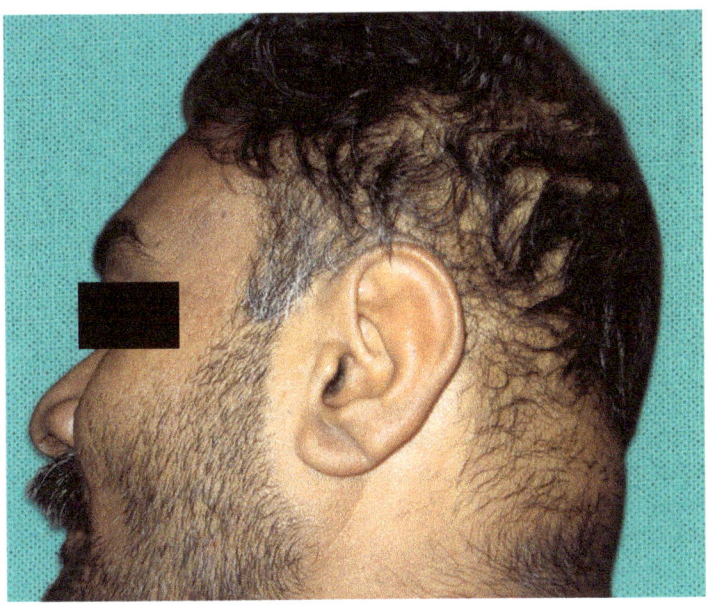

Fig. 43.4: Diagonal ear lobe crease (Frank's sign), a strong morphological feature of ischemic heart disease

THE PEARLS

Hyper- and hypotelorism are clusters of syndromes of which many of them are noncurable diseases though these (hyper- and hypotelorism) are regarded as very important unmistakable physical signs in clinical medicine.

Indigestion (Dyspepsia)

DEFINITION

A vague and nonspecific term—meaning changes from patient to patient. It may mean a number of abdominal symtoms like abdominal fullness, gaseous distension, nausea, heartburn, epigastric discomfort, belching, bloating, heartburn, flatulence, port-prandial fullness (with early satiety), presence of undigested food materials in stool or loose motion.

POSSIBLE ASSOCIATIONS

- Gastroesophageal reflux disease (GERD)
- Gastritis
- Functional dyspepsia (anxiety/stress)
  - Reflux-like → acid reflux and heartburn
  - Ulcer-like → epigastric pain+nocturnal pain → relieved by vomiting/food/antacid
  - Dysmotility-like → nausea, eructation, bloating and early satiety
- **Drugs:** Nonsteroidal anti-inflammatory drugs (NSAIDs), corticosteroid, nitroimidazoles (e.g. metronidazole)
- Lactose intolerance
- Cholecystitis
- Chronic pancreatic insufficiency
- Peptic ulcer disease or non-ulcer dyspepsia
- Dietary—consumption of fat, spicy food, cabbage, radish, onion, legumes
- *Miscellaneous:* Aerophagia, magenblase, gas entrapment syndrome, gastroparesis (e.g. autonomic neuropathy from diabetes), constipation, malignancy or lymphoma of stomach, irritable bowel syndrome, psychological disorders, chronic renal failure, congestive cardiac failure, cirrhosis of liver, mouth breathing, betel nut chewing.

AEROPHAGIA (AIR SWALLOWING)

Approximately 20–60% of intraluminal gas (seen in fluoroscopy) is swallowed air. Aerophagia can also be called as *eructation* or *belching*. It may happen to occur with/without the patient's awareness → some people attempt to do it in a false hope to relieve abdominal pain/distension/discomfort. It is seen under certain circumstances, e.g.

- Chronic anxiety
- Poor eating habit (e.g. rapid ingestion of food)
- Consumption of food in supine position
- Gum chewing, ill-fitted dentures
- Comsumption of cabbage, onion, peppers or carbonated beverages
- Cholecystitis, hiatus hernia, non-ulcer dyspepsia
- Any organic intestinal disease (aerophagia may increase in magnitude day by day).

NON-ULCER DYSPEPSIA

- Symptoms suggestive of dyspepsia and peptic ulcer but no evidence of ulcer on endoscopy
- Probably a combination of mucosal + motility + psychiatric disorders
- Young (< 40 years); female: male (F:M) = 2:1
- Complains of (C/O) nausea, bloating, incomplete rectal evacuation, irritable bowel syndrome like symptoms
- Many have *Helicobacter pylori* infection and often associated with prolonged gastric emptying time
- Endoscopy is necessary to exclude mucosal disease. Ultrasonography (USG) should be performed to detect gallstones, if any
- Management is done by reassurance, prokinetics and anti-*H. pylori* regimen.

MAGENBLASE

Synonym → **gastric bubble syndrome**. It is the acute gastric distension due to aerophagia, resulting in sharp precordial pain mimicking angina pectoris. It is a perplexing situation in older patients with coronary artery disease, who may experience true postprandial angina from time to time.

SPLENIC FLEXURE SYNDROME (GAS ENTRAPMENT SYNDROME)

Swallowed air may be trapped in the splenic flexure of colon, if not eructed out orally. The person may complain of left upper quadrant fullness and pressure with radiation to the left side of the chest → relief may be obtained with defecation or expulsion of flatus. It can be diagnosed by increased tympanicity on percussion over the extreme left lateral portion of the upper abdomen.

FLATULENCE (WIND)

Flatulence or excess gas in the abdomen is one of the most common complaint encountered in clinical practice. The patient may present in three ways like (1) excessive belching, (2) intestinal distension, bloating or meteorism, and (3) the passage of excessive flatus.

The meaning of flatulence varies from patient to patient like repeated belching → abdominal fullness → offensive rectal flatus → borborygmi (i.e. audible intestinal peristaltic sounds). Intestinal gas (have three sources) may be derived from swallowed air + colonic bacterial fermentation of poorly absorbed carbohydrates + a very small quantity from diffusion from the blood into the gut lumen; the normal volume of flatus varies from person to person, i.e. 200–2000 mL/day. The composition of intestinal gas is basically by N_2, O_2, H_2 and CO_2 (99%) though a small quantity of methane may be present. Increased flatus formation may be due to aerophagia, lactase deficiency, malabsorption or small bowel dysmotility. Obstipation or absolute constipation (absence of stool + flatus per rectally) is seen in acute intestinal obstruction. Excessive wind formation may result in social embarrassment.

ABDOMINAL DISTENSION

- *Acute or sudden onset:* Intestinal perforation, intestinal obstruction, paralytic ileus, post-pneumoperitoneum (e.g. after peritoneoscopy)
- *Gradual:* Ascites [cirrhosis, congestive cardiac failure (CCF), hypoproteinemia with anemia, nephrotic syndrome, constrictive pericarditis, pericardial effusion, tuberculous or malignant peritonitis], cystic swelling (pseudopancreatic, hepatic, splenic, mesenteric, ovarian), pregnancy or any visceromegaly.

Never forget 7 F's, i.e. fat (obesity), feces (gut obstruction), fetus (pregnancy), flatus (gaseous distension), fluid (ascites or any cystic swelling), full bladder (urinary) and fibroid (or any huge mass) as causes of abdominal distension.

FEW TERMINOLOGY

- Nausea → A subjective feeling of vomiting
- Vomiting → Expulsion of upper gastrointestinal (GI) contents orally
- Regurgitation → Effortless passage of gastric contents into the mouth
- Water brash → Salivary hypersecretion, i.e. filling of the mouth suddenly with a clear but slightly salty fluid, secreted by the salivary glands. It may be a transient episode in normal individuals
- Heartburn (pyrosis) → Substernal sensation of warmth or burning, and is usually due to reflux of gastroesophageal contents
- Rumination → Repeated regurgitation of contents of stomach which are often rechewed and reswallowed
- Eructation (belching) → Forceful regurgitation of air from the stomach or esophagus
- Retching → Laboured and rhythmic contraction of respiratory and abdominal muscles preceding vomiting
- Dysphagia → Difficulty in deglutition
- Odynophagia → Painful deglutition

- Phagophobia → Fear of swallowing (e.g. rabies, tetanus, or psychogenic)
- Appetite → Pleasurable desire to eat
- Hunger → unpleasant sensation produced as a result of empty stomach as well as peristaltic contractions
- Satiety → A sensation of satisfaction after taking food.
- Anorexia → loss of appetite

THE PEARLS

Dyspepsia (indigestion) is very common and 80% of the population may suffer from this at some time of their life. It is 'alarming' and has to be investigated if associated with dysphagia, loss of weight, profound anorexia, vomiting, or hematemesis/melena.

Profound anorexia is common in psychogenic (anxiety, depression, anorexia nervosa), endocrine/gastrointestinal disorders (e.g. Addison's disease/acute viral hepatitis), carcinoma (e.g. carcinoma of stomach), medication (e.g. chloroquine, metronidazole), or infectious disorders (e.g. tuberculosis).

45
Intermittent Claudication

DEFINITION

It is a cramp-like pain associated with tightness, numbness and extreme fatigue in muscles, and occurs most commonly in calf muscles on walking. The pain is relieved by rest and reappears when the person starts walking. The pain during walking may be so intense that the patient is bound to halt immediately.

The pain is due to muscle ischemia which is felt on walking. The actual distance a patient can walk before the onset of intermittent claudication is known as *claudication distance*, which is a good index of severity of arterial occlusion. Later, the pain becomes constant and aching in nature, and persists even on rest, i.e. *rest pain*, which is due to ischemic changes in the somatic nerves (so called, cry of the dying nerves).

POSSIBLE CAUSES

- **With vascular insufficiency (i.e. narrowed arteries)**
  - Atheroma or embolism of lower limb arteries (Fig. 45.1)
  - Buerger's disease (thromboangiitis obliterans; young and heavy-smoker males)
  - Arteritis (e.g. syphilitic, aortoarteritis)
  - Coarctation of aorta
  - Leriche's syndrome (embolism at branching of common iliac arteries, i.e. claudication of thigh and leg muscles, and impotence)
  - Aortoiliac occlusion
  - Diabetes mellitus.
- **Without vascular insufficiency (i.e. normal arteries)**
  - Overexertion (e.g. marathon runner)
  - Severe anemia
  - McArdle's disease (muscle phosphorylase deficiency)
  - Venous claudication [bursting pain on walking, previous history of (H/O) deep vein thrombosis (DVT)]
  - Lumbar canal stenosis (i.e. neurogenic claudication).

NEUROGENIC CLAUDICATION

It is also known as *claudication of cauda equina* or *lumbar canal stenosis*. This entity is the end result of combination of disc lesion and a congenital narrowing of

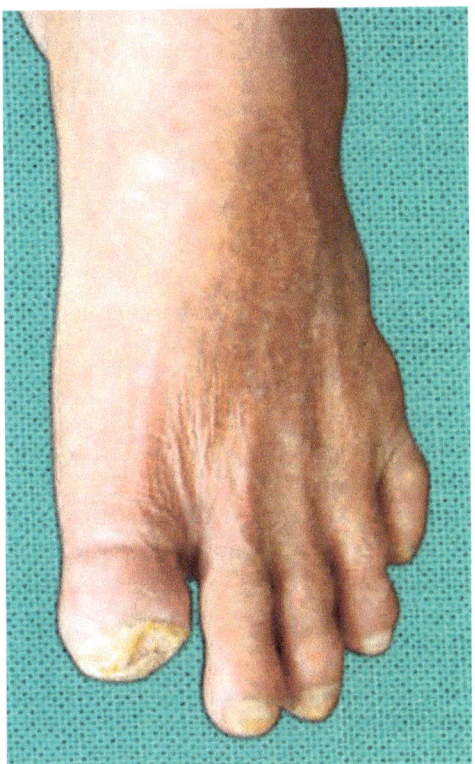

Fig. 45.1: Loss of pulp tissue in the left great toe in a patient of severe atherosclerosis. The patient has history of intermittent claudication with loss of pedal pulse

lumbar theca. The disease is made worse at middle age due to degenerative changes, especially between L_4 and L_5 vertebra. Walking or prolonged standing interferes with the blood supply to the cauda equina which leads to root pain, weakness of legs, paresthesia and even foot drop (pulse remains normal). Ankle jerk may be diminished or absent; rest pain never occurs in contradiction to vascular claudication. The patient usually relieves by ***rest*** or ***stooping forward position***.

EXAMINATION

- ***Color:*** Pale to pink on leg raising at 45°. Trophic changes present.
- ***Palpation:*** Determination of arterial occlusion by careful palpation of pulses; cold extremities (lower). Calf muscle may be tender on palpation.
- ***Auscultation:*** For bruit in distal aorta, femoral or iliac arteries; auscultate heart for source of embolism.
- ***Examination of motor function:*** At rest, motor functions (nutrition, tone, power, coordination) are normal. After exercise, pulses (arteria dorsalis pedis) may be diminished or absent, which is an important diagnostic clue in obstructive arterial disease.

Ankle jerk may be diminished in neurogenic claudication; pregangrenous conditions may develop (i.e. with vascular decompromise) after exercise.
- **Ophthalmocopy:** It is done for search of atherosclerotic retinal vessels, hemorrhage, etc.

INVESTIGATIONS

- Peripheral color Doppler studies of both legs
- Ankle brachial pressure index (ABPI), which in heath is ≥ 1.0 in supine position, ≤ 0.8 in claudication and < 0.4 in critical limb ischemia. Detection of ABPI needs a hand-held Doppler and a sphygmomanometer
- Arteriography (the gold standard investigation)
- Impedence plethysmography
- Ultrasonography/computed tomography (USG/CT) scan of abdomen to detect cause of vascular occlusion/aneurysm, etc.
- Biopsy of artery (to diagnose Buerger's disease, arteritis)
- X-ray of lumbar spine, nerve conduction velocity (NCV), magnetic resonance imaging (MRI) scan of lower spinal cord to diagnose lumbar canal stenosis.

At the bedside, palpation of peripheral pulses and measurement of lower extremity blood pressure (BP) after exercise often clinches the diagnosis of vascular claudication.

TREATMENT

- Abstinence form smoking or consumption of tobacco in any form
- Treatment of diabetes, hypertension and hyperlipidemia, if present. Aspirin 150 mg ODPC may be prescribed
- Vasodilators (e.g. nifedipine 5 mg OD/BDS) or hemorrheology modifier (e.g. pentoxifylline 400 mg BDS/TDS) may be used
- Analgesics or vitamin E (400 mg BDS) may be helpful
- Treatment of specific diseases (e.g. amputation for Buerger's disease, transluminal balloon angioplasty for severe atherosclerosis; gabapentin or pregabalin along with neurosurgical opinion in neurogenic claudication)
- Amitriptyline 25-50 mg at bedtime may be used in rest pain/nocturnal pain.

ACROPARESTHESIA

It is the feeling of tingling and numbness (described by the patient as ***pins and needles***) or often burning sensation in the tip of the fingers and toes. The common etiologies considered in clinical practice are:
- Cervical (in fingers) or lumbar spondylosis (in toes)
- Cervical rib
- Lesion in brachial plexus

- Carpal tunnel syndrome
- Peripheral neuropathy (leprosy, alcohol, diabetes mellitus)
- ***Physiological:*** Prolonged sitting over the front rod of a bicycle (foot and toes), arms compressed by body due to malposition while sleeping (hand and fingers)
- ***Functional:*** Often complained by middle-aged female patients as a manifestation of weakness.

WORK-UP

Palpate peripheral leg arteries (popliteal, posterior tibial or arteria dorsalis pedis).

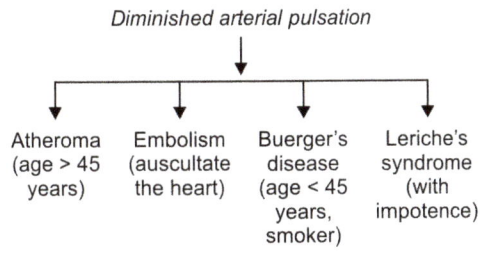

LEG PAIN: INCREASE ON STANDING AND DECREASE BY LYING

The two common diseases in clinical practice are:
1. Varicose veins (or peripheral venous disease)
2. Prolapsed intervertebral disc.

> A patient of arterial disease in legs (e.g. severe atheroembolism) sleeps with legs hanging down, i.e. over edge of the bed or in a chair.

THE PEARLS

Claudication (Latin meaning 'to limp') means leg pain brought on by exertion and relieved by rest. It is analogous to angina where pain occurs in the chest. Approximately 70% patients suffering from peripheral arterial disease will have concomitant coronary artery disease (CAD). Claudication is often considered as a marker for generalized atherosclerosis.
- ***Vascular claudication:*** cold legs, pallor, color change, trophic changes (hair loss, non-healing ulcer), feeble/absent pulse
- ***Neurogenic claudication:*** Paresthesia, limb weakness, diminished ankle jerk, normal pulse.

46

Joint Pain

MONOARTHRITIS

- Septic arthritis (*Staphylococcus aureus, Neisseria gonorrhoea*, meningococci, *Staphylococcus pneumoniae*, gram-negative infections)—extremely tender
- Crystal-induced arthritis (gout, pseudogout, calcium oxalate or hydroxyapatite crystals)
- Traumatic joint injury
- Osteoarthritis
- Tuberculosis of the joint (e.g. knee)
- Hemarthrosis (traumatic)
- Monoarticular flare of polyarticular rheumatic diseases [e.g. rheumatoid arthritis (RA) (Figs 46.1 and 46.2), systemic lupus erythematosus (SLE), psoriasis, reactive arthritis (Fig. 46.3)]

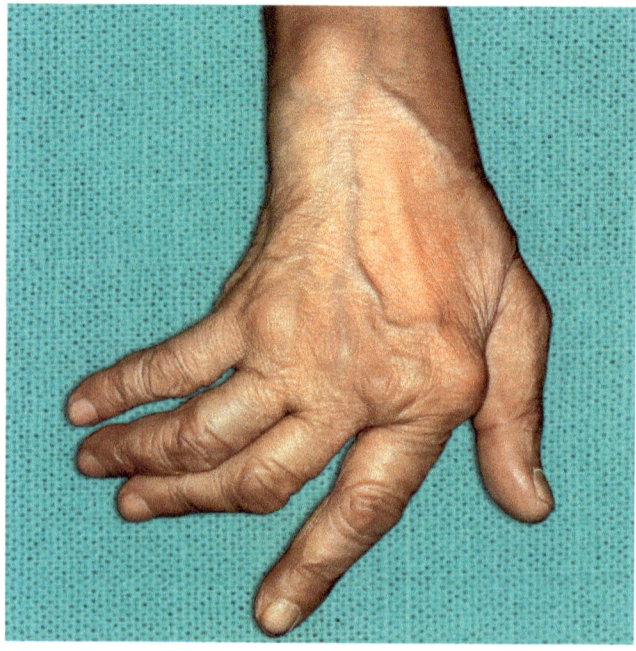

Fig. 46.1: Swelling of wrist and metacarpophalangeal joints, radial deviation of wrist with ulnar deviation of digits ('zigzag' deformity) in rheumatoid arthritis

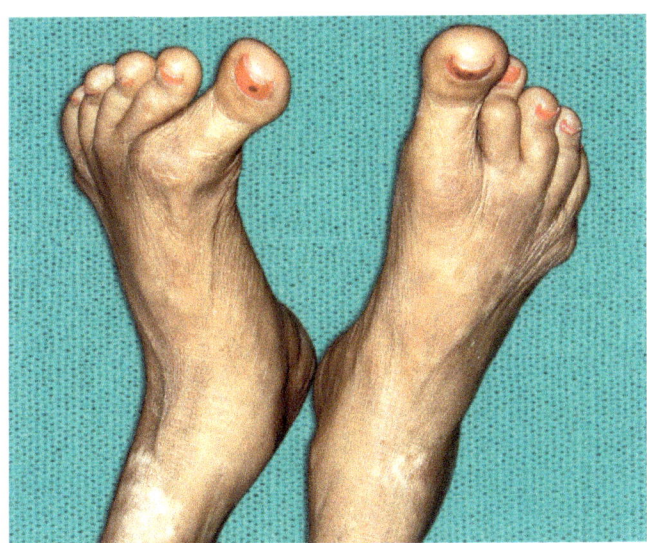

Fig. 46.2: Hallux varus deformity, widening of the forefeet with cock-up great toes in rheumatoid arthritis

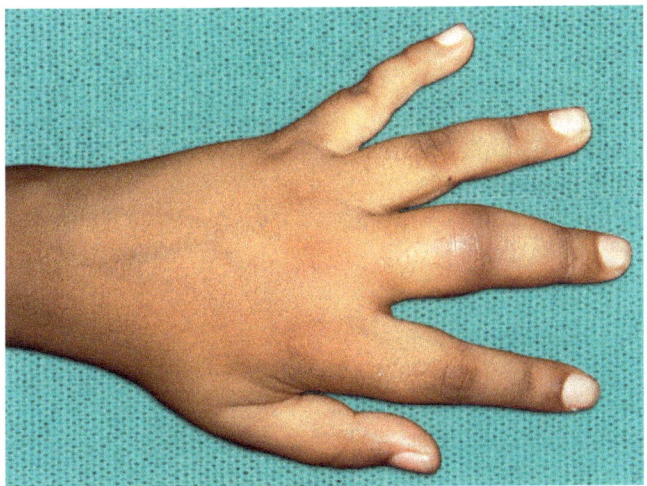

Fig. 46.3: Fusiform swelling of entire left middle finger (dactylitis or sausage digit)—often a clinical clue in reactive arthritis

- Palindromic rheumatoid arthritis
- Charcot joint (neuropathic joint from diabetes, leprosy, syringomyelia or tabes dorsalis)
- Hemophiliac joint (e.g. knee), acute leukemias, Henoch-Schönlein purpura
- Pigmented villonodular synovitis

Note: As any delay in the treatment of septic arthritis would lead to joint destruction, it is prudent to start antibiotic therapy empirically before laboratory reports give

a definitive diagnosis. Urgent synovial fluid examination is mandatory in acute monoarthritis for
- Crystals (under polarized light microscopy)
- Pathogens (Gram staining and microbial culture)
- White blood cells (WBCs) (> 2000/mm^3 is diagnostic of inflammatory joint disease).

Charcot's joint and pigmented villonodular sinovitis give rise to chronic monoarthritis.

POLYARTHRITIS

- RA, juvenile idiopathic arthritis (JIA)
- SLE and other connective tissue diseases
- Psoriatic arthritis
- Spondyloarthropathy (e.g. ankylosing spondylitis)
- Palindromic rheumatism
- Rheumatic fever, subacute bacterial endocarditis (SBE), Lyme arthritis
- Reactive arthritis
- Crystal-induced arthritis (e.g. gout)
- Adult-onset Still's disease (AOSD) (rare)
- Drug hypersensitivity (e.g. serum sickness)
- HIV, hepatitis B, parvovirus B19, chikungunya or rubella infection
- **Miscellaneous:** Generalized osteoarthritis, lymphoma, leukemia, sarcoidosis, Behçet's disease, Whipple's disease, Henoch-Schönlein purpura, neuropathic joint, HPOA (hypertrophic pulmonary osteoarthropathy), relapsing polychondritis, malignancy, poststreptococcal reactive arthritis (PSRA) and amyloidosis.

FEW TERMINOLOGY

- Arthralgia—only pain in the joints
- Arthritis—pain + swelling in the joints
- Monoarthritis—affection of single joint
- Oligo- or pauciarticular arthritis—affection of 2-4 joints
- Polyarthritis—affection of 5 or more joints
- Enthesitis—inflammation of site of tendon or ligament insertion in bone.

DURATION OF JOINT PAIN

- Acute (< 6 weeks)
- Chronic (> 6 weeks).

PATTERN OF INVOLVEMENT

- Axial (spine, sacroiliac, anterior chest wall, shoulder and hip joint)
- Appendicular (peripheral joints)

Chapter 46 Joint Pain

Shoulder and hip joints are known as root joints.

CLINICAL PARAMETERS OF INFLAMMATORY JOINT DISEASES
- Significant early-morning stiffness (usually > 30 minutes)
- Symptomatic improvement on gentle use of joint
- Spontaneously up-and-down course (i.e. spontaneous flare)
- Constitutional symptoms (e.g. fatigue, low appetite, low body weight, low-grade fever, night sweats).

COMMON LABORATORY INVESTIGATIONS PERFORMED IN JOINT DISEASES
- Acute phase reactants (confirm inflammatory nature of the disease):
  - Erythrocyte sedimentation rate (ESR)
  - Platelet count
  - Albumin-globulin ratio
  - C-reactive protein (CRP)
  - Alkaline phosphatase.

All of the above are raised and albumin-globulin ratio is reversed in active inflammatory arthritis.

- Rheumatoid factor (RF)
- Antinuclear antibody (ANA) and its subsets, e.g. anti-dsDNA, anti-RNP, etc.
- Complement C_3 and C_4
- Antibodies to cyclic citrullinated peptide (anti-CCP) to diagnose early rheumatoid arthritis
- Antistreptolysin 'O' (ASO) antibody titer
- Antineutrophil cytoplasmic antibody (ANCA, i.e. c- or p-ANCA)
- Synovial fluid analysis
- Serum uric acid level
- **Others:** HLA-B27 screening, Ca, PO_4, alkaline phosphatase, protein electrophoresis (for multiple myeloma), antiphospholipid antibody, arthroscopy, synovial fluid analysis, details of radiology [from X-ray to positron emission tomography (PET) scan; Dexa scan for osteoporosis], electromyography (EMG) and nerve conduction velocity (NCV), biopsy (synovium, or sural nerve for vasculitis).

PATIENTS COMPLAINING OF STIFF/PAINFUL MUSCLES
- ***Strenuous exercise:*** [History of (H/O) unaccustomed exercise 24–48 hours before]
- Ankylosing spondylitis (young, low backache, progressive loss of spinal movement)

- Polymyositis/dermatomyositis (proximal muscle weakness increases)
- Polymyalgia rheumatica (elderly, fatigue, painful proximal muscle)
- Fibromyalgia (females with specific tender points all over the body associated with anxiety and/or depression)
- Rheumatoid arthritis (middle-aged female, morning stiffness in active disease, metacarpophalangeal (MCP) and proximal interphalangeal (PIP) joints involved in hands)
- Myxedema (middle-aged female, obese, hoarse voice, cold intolerance, constipation, and with muscle weakness)
- Early manifestation of occult malignancy (onset over weeks or months with loss of weight and anorexia).

DRUGS PRODUCING ARTHRALGIA/ARTHRITIS

- Sulfonamides
- Penicillin
- Hydralazine
- Procainamide
- Phenytoin
- Iodides.

ARTHRITIS ASSOCIATED WITH

- ***Murmurs in the heart***
  - Acute rheumatic fever
  - Ankylosing spondylitis
  - SBE
  - RA
  - SLE (Libman-Sacks endocarditis)
  - Atrial myxoma
  - Relapsing polychondritis
- ***Subcutaneous nodules***
  - RA
  - Gout
  - Acute rheumatic fever
  - Sarcoidosis
  - Erythema nodosum
  - SLE
  - Xanthoma
  - Amyloidosis
  - Reticulohistiocytosis (multicentric)
  - Whipple's disease.
- ***Rash***
  - Vasculitis
  - SLE

- Dermatomyositis
- Psoriasis
- Still's disease
- Chronic urticaria
- Sarcoidosis
- Leprosy
- Viral infection (parvovirus B19, rubella).

■ ***Enthesopathy***
- Ankylosing spondylitis
- Psoriatic arthritis
- Reactive arthritis
- Viremia or bacteremia
- Drugs (e.g. ciprofloxacin)
- Disseminated idiopathic sketelal hyperostosis (DISH).

■ ***Involvement of the eye***
- Spondyloarthropathy (e.g. uveitis)
- Sjögren's syndrome (e.g. xerophthalmia)
- Rheumatoid arthritis (e.g. episcleritis) (Fig. 46.4)
- Vasculitis, Wegener's granulomatosis (e.g. proptosis)
- Reactive arthritis (e.g. conjunctivitis)
- Behçet's syndrome (e.g. uveitis)
- Sarcoidosis (e.g. bilateral uveitis).

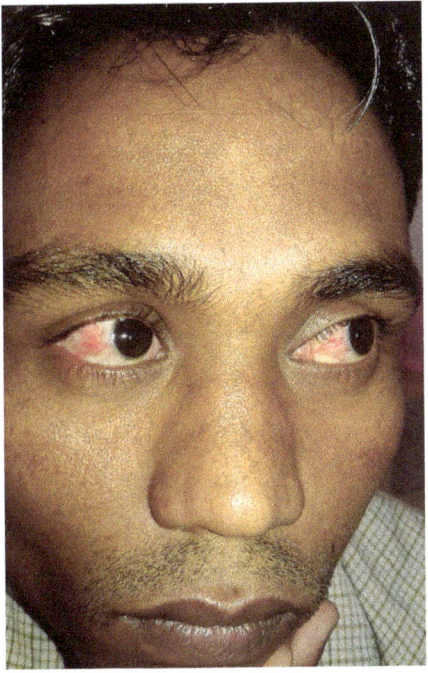

Fig. 46.4: Episcleritis in a patient of rheumatoid arthritis

COMMON CAUSES OF POLYARTHRITIS IN HANDS

- RA (MCP, PIP)
- Nodal osteoarthritis [DIP but spares MCP; affects 1st carpometacarpal joints (base of thumb)]
- Psoriatic arthritis (commonly DIP)
- Chronic tophaceous gout (MCP, interphalangeal)
- SLE (Jaccoud's arthritis; MCP joints commonly)
- Viral arthritides (all joints).

MCP = metacarpophalangeal, PIP = proximal interphalangeal, DIP = distal interphalangeal, IP = interphalangeal.

DIFFERENTIAL DIAGNOSIS OF ACUTE MONOARTHRITIS PRESENTING AS RED HOT JOINT

- ***Infections (septic arthritis):*** Bacterial (e.g. nongonococcal/gonococcal), viral
- ***Crystal-induced:*** Gout, pseudogout
- Acute exacerbation of RA, reactive arthritis, psoriatic arthritis and palindromic rheumatism (monoarticular RA lasting 24–48 hours)
- Hemophilia (Fig. 46.5)
- Traumatic.

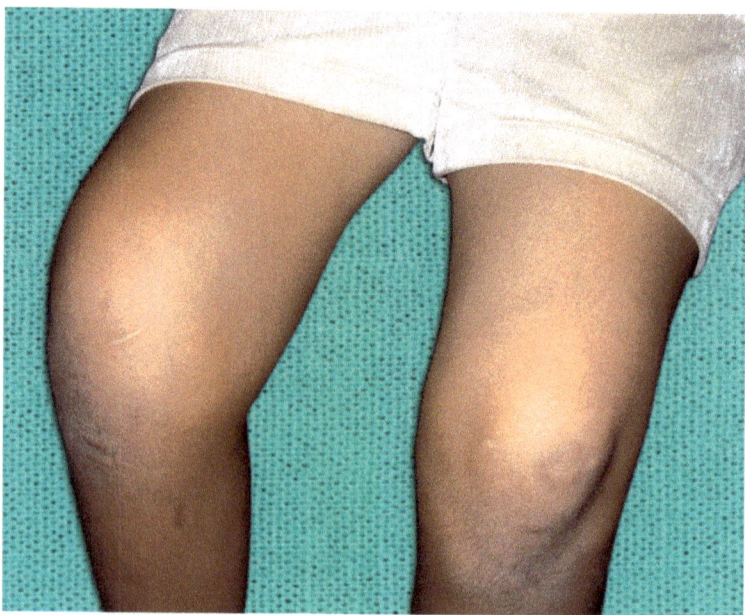

Fig. 46.5: Painful and swollen right knee (monoarthritis) in a patient of hemophilia

DISEASE COURSE OF POLYARTHRITIS

A.
- ***Intermittent:*** Gout, relapsing polychondritis
- ***Progressive:*** Classical RA

B.
- ***Migratory*** (as the inflammation of one joint is subsided, other tends to become affected, i.e. usually one joint is affected at a time for about 3 days): Rheumatic arthritis (i.e. from acute rheumatic fever), SLE, drug reaction/serum sickness, arthritis following gonococcal or meningococcal septicemia, viral arthritis (Lyme arthritis, chikungunya), following inflammatory bowel disease/Whipple's disease, seroconversion in AIDS, septicemia, sarcoidosis, following intestinal by pass surgery.
- ***Additive:*** RA, ankylosing spondylitis, reactive arthritis.

AGE AND SEX-RELATED ARTHRITIDES

- ***Age:***
  - Children   : Rheumatic arthritis, JIA, hemophilia, trauma
  - Adolescents   : RA, spondyloarthropathy, trauma, JIA, poststreptococcal reactive arthritis (PSRA)
  - Young   : Trauma, gonococcal
  - Adults   : Spondyloarthropathy, reactive arthritis, psoriasis, SLE, gout
  - Middle age   : RA, gout, osteoarthritis, scleroderma.
- ***Sex:***
  Arthritides predominant in males are:
  - Gout
  - Ankylosing spondylitis
  - Reiter's syndrome (i.e. reactive arthritis)
  - Polyarteritis nodosa.

All other arthritides are common in females except those four mentioned above.

ARTHRITIDES AFFECTING DIP JOINTS

- Osteoarthritis (with Heberden's node)
- Psoriatic arthritis
- Scleroderma
- Sarcoidosis
- Gout
- Adult-onset Still's disease (AOSD)
- Enteropathic arthritis (e.g. from ulcerative colitis or Crohn's disease).

JACCOUD'S ARTHRITIS

Ulnar deviation of MCP joints due to subluxation may develop from:
- Rheumatic arthritis
- SLE
- Progressive systemic sclerosis
- Sjögren's syndrome.

STOOPED POSTURE (INCREASED THORACIC KYPHOSIS)

- Ankylosing spondylitis
- Parkinsonism
- Osteoporosis of the spine with collapse (widow's stoop).

THE PEARLS

The clinician first determines whether it is arthralgia, or arthritis, or soft-tissue rheumatism. A detailed history with meticulous local (the joint) and systemic examination are mandatory to have a diagnosis. Judicious order of investigations (e.g. specific autoantibody or radiology) often clinches the diagnosis. Remember, a good rheumatologist is always a good internist.

47

Leg Ulceration

ETIOLOGY

- ***Venous diseases:*** Varicose ulcer, deep vein thrombosis (DVT), deep venous obstruction from pelvic growth, incompetent valves
- ***Arterial insufficiency:*** Atherosclerosis, Buerger's disease, vasculitis
- ***Small vessel diseases:*** Diabetes mellitus (Fig. 47.1), vasculitis
- ***Neuropathy:*** Diabetes mellitus, leprosy, tabes dorsalis, syringomyelia, peripheral neuropathy
- ***Hemorheological:*** Sickle cell disease, hereditary spherocytosis, thalssaemia major, cryoglobulinemia, immune complex diseases, cold agglutinin disease, macroglobulinemia
- ***Tumor:*** Squamous cell carcinoma, Kaposi's sarcoma, malignant melanoma, basal cell carcinoma, mycosis fungoides, metastasis
- ***Traumatic ulcer:*** Burns, cold injury, factitial
- ***Tropical ulcer*** (a chronic form of callous ulcer with its edge raised and undermined, and very often refuses to heal)
- ***Trophic ulcer*** (affecting sole of foot, especially over the heel or ball of the great toe → diabetes mellitus, leprosy, syringomyelia and tabes dorsalis) → painless ulcer
- ***Chronic atopic eczema***

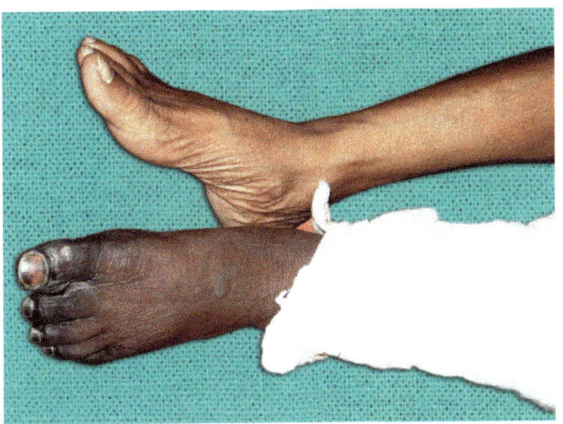

Fig. 47.1: Diabetic foot with dry gangrene in left foot

- **Miscellaneous:** Pyoderma gangrenosum (ulcerative colitis, rheumatoid arthritis, immunodeficiency), gout, necrobiosis lipoidica diabeticorum (diabetes; over shins, yellowish plaque-like lesion with a brownish border), tuberculous ulcer, actinomycosis, panniculitis, malingering, Bazin's disease, bullous pemphigoid, filariasis.

CLUE TO DIAGNOSIS

- **Surface temperature**
  Normal → Venous disease or neuropathy, and others
  Cold → Arterial insufficiency
- **Site of ulcer**
  Venous → lower leg, ankle (over medial malleolus with pigmentation) (Fig. 47.2)
  Arterial → shin, foot
  Vasculitis → shin, upper leg (painful), often punched-out
  Neuropathy → heel, ball of the great toe (painless)
- Peripheral arterial pulsation, e.g. feel the pulsation of arteria dorsalis pedis/ posterior tibial artery
  ↓
  ↓ pulsation in arterial insufficiency, vasculitis
- Homan's sign (forcible dorsiflexion of the foot with the knee extended elicits pain in calf muscles) and Moses' sign (squeezing of the calf muscles from side to side is painful) present: DVT

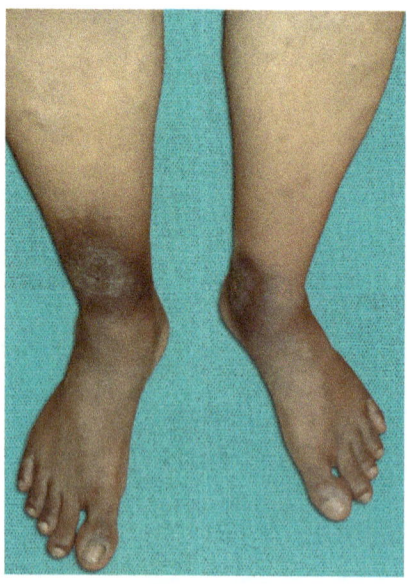

Fig. 47.2: Venous ulcers with pigmentation seen over lower part of legs in a patient with varicose veins

- Ankle jerk ↓ in neuropathy
- Vibration sense ↓ in neuropathy with special reference to diabetes mellitus
- *Edema (may be non-pitting):* Commonly in venous diseases
- *Thickened peripheral nerves:* Present in leprosy (with peripheral neuropathy)
- *Anesthetic patches (e.g. leprosy)*
- *Trendelenburg test:* Positive in varicose veins
- *Blood pressure:* Hypertensive in atherosclerosis, diabetes mellitus
- *Local cyanotic hue:* Especially in arterial insufficiency.

BASIC INVESTIGATIONS PERFORMED

- *Blood:* Peripheral smear examination for anemia, blood dyscrasias; venereal disease research laboratory (VDRL), sugar and lipid profile; antinuclear factor (ANF), antineutrophil cytoplasmic antibody (ANCA)
- *Urine:* For sugar
- *Bacterial swab:* For detection of pathogens
- *Doppler ultrasound:* For documentation of arterial insufficiency
- *Ankle brachial pressure index (ABPI)*
- *Venography:* For venous diseases
- *Nerve conduction study:* For peripheral neuropathy.

BAZIN'S DISEASE

- Erythema induratum
- Uncommon, bilateral, painful and tender duskey-red nodules usually over calves
- Females > males
- Recurrent, irregular edges, heals with scar
- May need prolonged anti-tuberculosis treatment.

THE PEARLS

When the leg ulcers are present on the lower leg, it is usually due to vascular disease.

It is the clinician's duty to examine the patient for tenderness, peripheral arterial pulses, blood pressure, ankle jerk, vibration sense, edema, local cyanotic hue and thickened peripheral nerves.

The basic outlines of treatment for leg ulcer are stoppage of smoking, control of diabetes/hypertension/dyslipidemia, local care, judicious use of antibiotics in infections, advice of chiropodist and surgery (balloon dilatation of artery) or amputation in selected cases.

48

Lockjaw

SYNONYM

Trismus (inability to open the mouth).

MECHANISM

Develops as a result of sustained involuntary spasm of masseter and temporalis muscles leading to closure of the jaws so that the mouth cannot be opened.

POSSIBILITIES

- Tetanus (a cause par excellence of trismus with positive spatula test)
- Strychnine toxicity (often a late manifestation)
- Tetany
- Drug-induced dyskinesia (e.g. metoclopramide, phenothiazines)
- Temporomandibular joint osteoarthritis or ankylosis
- Impacted wisdom teeth
- Peritonsillar abscess (quinsy), dental abscess, Ludwig's angina, dislocation of jaw, cyanide poisoning.
- Acute follicular tonsillitis
- Parotitis, mumps
- Hydrophiidae group of snake bite
- Hysterical or malingering (during sleep, muscles relaxes completely)
- Stiff-man syndrome (progressive fluctuating muscular rigidity)
- Rabies (rare)
- Anesthesia-induced malignant hyperthermia.

> In temporomandibular joint dislocation, the patient cannot close the **opened mouth**.

SPATULA TEST

In healthy patient, if the posterior pharyngeal wall is touched by a spatula, it produces reflex opening of mouth. In tetanus, the mouth closes paradoxically in such a way that the spatula cannot be taken out easily. Spatula test is positive in tetanus and negative in others.

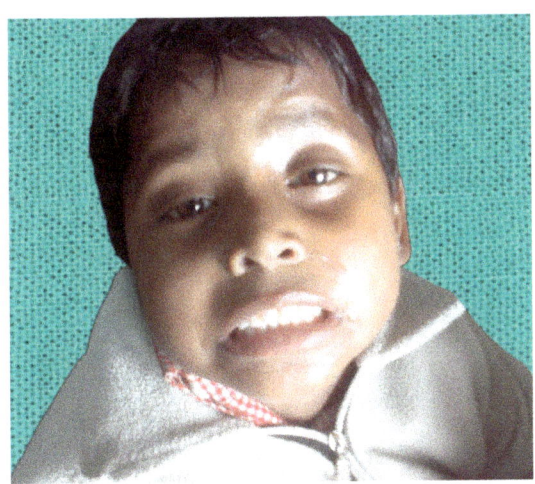

Fig. 48.1: Tetanus with a fixed sardonic smile (risus sardonicus or smile of 'Satan') with lockjaw

RISUS SARDONICUS

When more and more muscles are involved in tetanus, rigidity becomes generalized, and sustained contractions of facial muscles give rise to a characteristic expression → a fixed sardonic smile, i.e. **smile of 'Satan' or devil** (where the smile does not reach the eyes) → risus sardonicus (Fig. 48.1).

- In tetanus, trismus is an early sign (convulsions lately)
  In strychnine poisoning, trismus is a late sign (convulsions early)
- In scleroderma and submucosal fibrosis of oral cavity, the patient may find difficulty in opening the mouth; but this is not true trismus (pseudotrismus).

MANAGEMENT

- Reassurance
- Treatment of the etiology
- Maintenance of nutrition by feeding through side of the mouth/Ryle's tube/intravenous fluid
- In severe cases, air entry may be maintained by tracheostomy
- Analgesics and anti-inflammatory drugs with muscle relaxants
- Role of injectable corticosteroids at the site/surgery should be considered in selected cases.

THE PEARLS

To a clinician, for all practical purposes, lockjaw is synonymous with tetanus but examination in an open mind often pin-points other diagnosis. Examination of the neck is important (e.g. lymphadenopathy in painful oral pathology or edema in Ludwig's angina). Diphtheria does not give rise to trismus.

49

Lump in Right Iliac Fossa

ASSOCIATIONS (LUMP IN RIGHT ILIAC FOSSA)

- Ileocecal tuberculosis
- Amebic typhlitis (inflammation of cecum)
- Appendicular lump
- Carcinoma of cecum or ascending colon
- Tubo-ovarian mass
- Crohn's disease (granuloma)
- Intussusception
- Impaction of roundworms
- Dropped or unascended right kidney
- Lymphoma
- Carcinoid syndrome
- Iliac aneurysm, psoas abscess
- Malignant undescended testicle
- Transplanted kidney.

LUMP/MASS IN OTHER PARTS OF ABDOMEN

- *Left iliac fossa*
  - Amoebic colitis
  - Carcinoma of colon
  - Diverticulitis
  - Tubo-ovarian mass
  - Colon loaded with hard stool (scybala—pits on pressure)
  - Dropped or unascended left kidney
  - Lymphoma, psoas abscess.
- *Mid-abdomen*
  - Abdominal tuberculosis
  - Lymphoma
  - Pregnancy
  - Full bladder
  - Mesenteric cyst or lymphadenitis
  - Retroperitoneal growth

- Ovarian cyst
- Omental mass.

Epigastrium (Figs 49.1 and 49.2)
- Carcinoma of stomach
- Carcinoma of head of pancreas
- Enlargement of left lobe of liver (abscess, hepatoma)
- Pseudopancreatic cyst
- Growth in transverse color
- Omental mass
- Aortic aneurysm
- Epigastric hernia

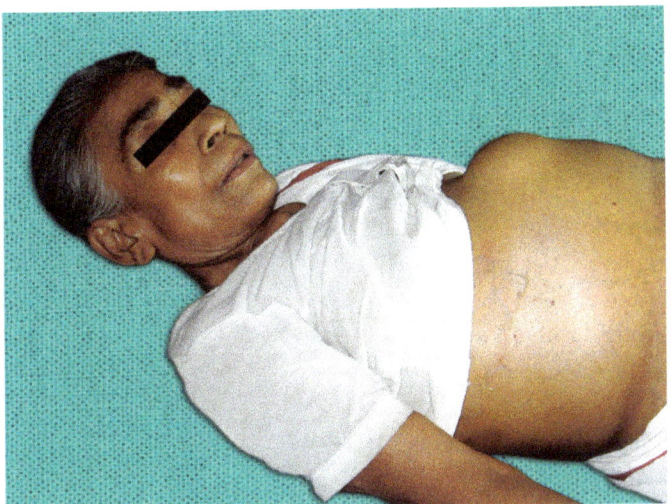

Fig. 49.1: Visible lump in epigastrium: A case of hepatocellular carcinoma (hepatoma)—imprints of leukoplast straps after liver biopsy is seen here

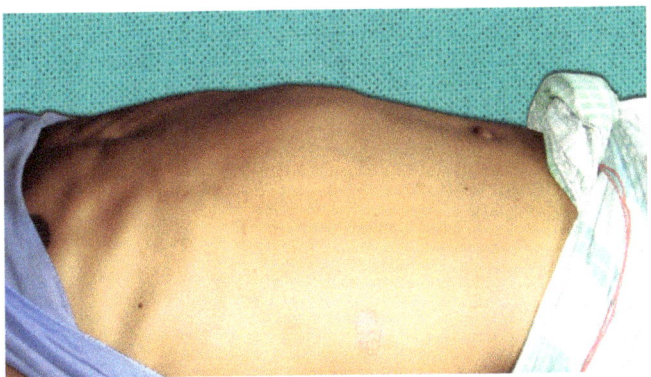

Fig. 49.2: Visible fullness in epigastrium and left hypochondrium: Splenic mass in a patient of chronic myeloid leukemia

- ***Right hypochondrium***
  - Hepatic mass (carcinoma, abscess, cyst)
  - Gallbladder lump
  - Colonic mass
  - Carcinoma of head of pancreas
  - Renal lump (right)
  - Omental mass.

RIGHT LOWER QUADRANT ABDOMINAL PAIN

- Acute appendicitis
- Crohn's disease or ileocecal tuberculosis
- Meckel's diverticulitis
- Incarcerated hernia
- Ectopic pregnancy
- Salpingitis
- Tubo-ovarian abscess
- Endometriosis
- Torsion of ovarian cyst
- Perforated ulcer of cecum
- Intestinal obstruction
- Renal or ureteral calculi
- Psoas abscess/hematoma
- Leaking aortic aneurysm
- Mittelschmerz (i.e. 'ovulation pain')
- Cecal diverticulitis
- Trauma.

So, a proper history-taking may solve the mystery of Pandora's box (i.e. abdomen).

PERIUMBILICAL ABDOMINAL PAIN

- Small bowel obstruction (Fig. 49.3)
- Mesenteric thrombosis (abdominal angina)
- Intestinal amebiasis
- Roundworm infestations
- Dissecting aneurysm of aorta
- Acute pancreatitis
- Early phase of acute appendicitis
- ***Miscellaneous:*** Diabetic ketoacidosis, uremia, trauma.

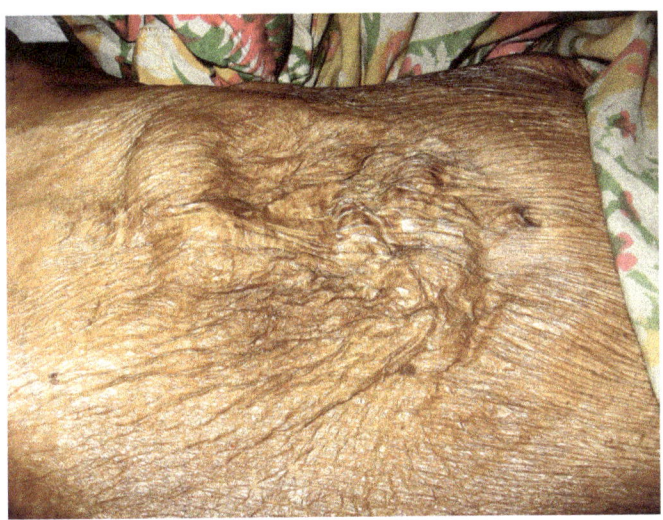

Fig. 49.3: Visible peristalsis (step-ladder pattern) of small gut is seen in a woman of 76 years

POSSIBLE CAUSES OF ACUTE SCROTUM

- Torsion of testis
- Epididymitis (filarial, tuberculous)
- Testicular malignancy
- Orchitis (e.g. mumps)
- Incarcerated hernia
- Trauma
- Hydrocele, hematocele, spermatocele, varicocele
- Fournier gangrene (Fig. 49.4).

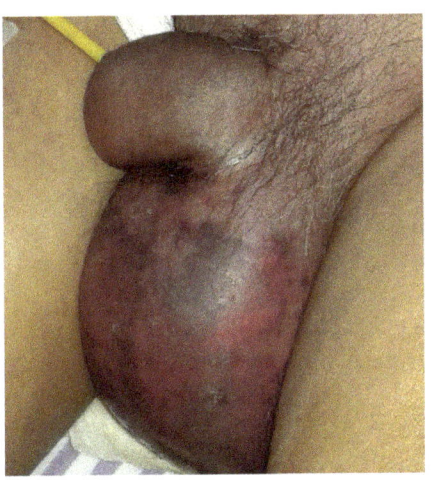

Fig. 49.4: Fournier gangrene of scrotum in an aged diabetic patient

DISCHARGING SINUSES OVER THE ABDOMEN

- Fecal fistula
- Tuberculosis of the intestine
- Intra-abdominal malignancy
- Crohn's disease
- Scrofuloderma or trauma
- Actinomycosis.

LYMPH NODE LUMPS IN THE ABDOMEN

- Mesenteric lymph node tuberculosis
- Lymphoma (commonly pre- and paraaortic nodes)
- Metastasis from neighboring carcinoma
- Metastasis from carcinoma of testis
- Filariasis (retroperitoneal lymphadenitis; rare).

PAIN ABDOMEN REFERRED FROM EXTRA-ABDOMINAL SOURCES

Thorax: Pneumonic consolidation, basal pleurisy, acute myocardial infarction (inferior wall)
↓
referred to upper abdomen

Spine: Arthritis, radiculitis
↓
referred to upper, mid or lower abdomen according to level of lesion in spine

Genitalia: Torsion of testis or ovary
↓
referred to lower abdomen

METABOLIC CAUSES OF PAIN ABDOMEN

- Diabetic ketoacidosis (polyuria, dehydration, Kussmaul's breathing)
- Acute intermittent porphyria (family history present, ↑ blood pressure (BP), peripheral neuropathy)
- Uremia (anorexia, pallor, oliguria)
- Lead poisoning (anorexia, headache, metallic taste)
- Addison's disease (an endocrine cause with asthenia, pigmentation, hypotension)
- Hypercalcemia (e.g. hyperparathyroidism—lethargy, confusion, polyuria).

DIARRHEA ALTERNATING WITH CONSTIPATION

- Intestinal tuberculosis
- Irritable bowel syndrome

- Carcinoma of colon
- Diverticulosis of colon.

MEDICAL CAUSES OF PAIN ABDOMEN

- Basal pneumonia (i.e. basal pleurisy)
- Acute myocardial infarction (commonly inferior wall infarction)
- Diabetic ketoacidosis (may be due to acute gastric dilatation)
- Intercostal herpes zoster (radicular pain)
- Henoch-Schönlein purpura (vasculitis)
- Sickle cell anemia (vaso-occlusive crisis)
- Acute intermittent porphyria (autonomic neuropathy)
- Caries spine/cord compression/collapse of vertebra (radicular pain)
- Lead poisoning (colic)
- Torsion of testis
- Polyarteritis nodosa (vasculitis)
- Tabetic crisis (probably due to autonomic neuropathy; rare)
- Allergic pain (C_1 esterase inhibitor deficiency)
- Functional
- ***Miscellaneous:*** Peptic ulcer, acute pancreatitis, acute hepatitis, hyperlipidemia, hypercalcemia.

ABSOLUTE 'WATERY' DIARRHEA

Dehydration commonly develops in this setting from:
- Enterotoxigenic *Escherichia coli* infection (incubation period 12–72 hours)
- Traveller's diarrhea (history of recent travel)
- Cholera (fever, vomiting, severe watery diarrhea)
- Rotavirus (in children mainly)
- Norwalk virus (in older children and adults).

THE PEARLS

The clinician should have a clear-cut idea of nine distinct areas of abdomen, when the abdomen is divided by two horizontal (i.e. subcostal and inter-tubercular lines) and two vertical (line joining mid-inguinal point below to midclavicular point above, on both the sides) lines. It is essential to know the specific contents (i.e. organs) occupying each area for a specific diagnosis of area-wise mass or pain in abdomen. As abdomen is a 'mystery box', there may be overlap of area-wise causes of mass or pain.

50. Macroglossia

CLUE TO DIAGNOSIS

Ask the patient to protrude the tongue
↓
Enlarged tongue with indentation of teeth at the margins
↓
Macrosomia with prognathism—***acromegaly*** (*see* Fig. 27.4)
↓
Mental retardation—***cretinism, Down's syndrome (Figs 50.1 to 50.3)*** (with furrowed tongue), ***Hurler syndrome*** (mucopolysaccharidosis)
↓
Expressionless puffy face, baggy lower eyelids along with madarosis (loss of hair in lateral one-third of eyebrow)—***myxedema*** (*see* Fig. 41.1)
↓
Tongue feels stiff and firm to palpation with hepatosplenomegaly and lymphadenopathy—***primary amyloidosis***

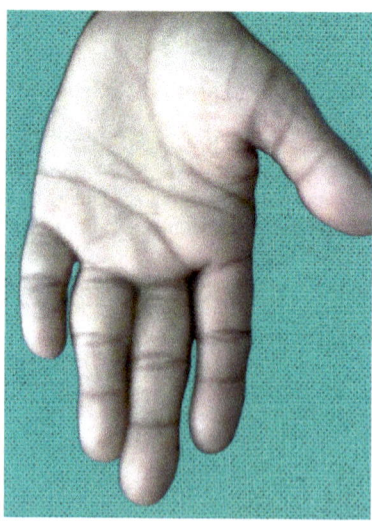

Fig. 50.1: Clinodactyly—absent (or hypoplastic) middle phalanx as well as one crease in the little finger (produces incurved little finger) in Down's syndrome

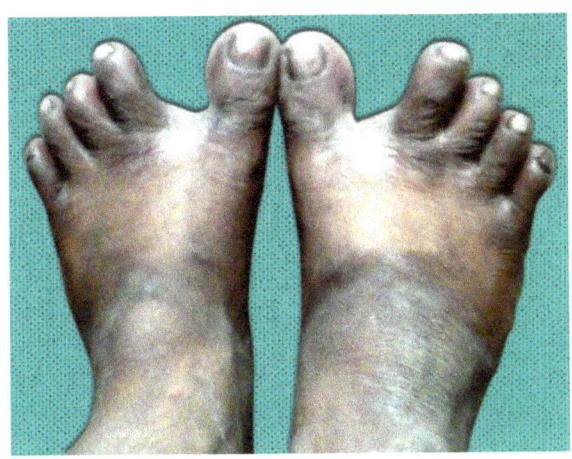

Fig. 50.2: Sandal gap, i.e. increased gap between great toe and second toe in Down's syndrome

↓

'Doll-like' facies with retarded physical growth in a child—***von Gierke's disease***

↓

Facial palsy (bilateral), edema of lips, plication as well as deeply furrowed tongue—Melkersson's syndrome

↓

Surgical conditions like **lymphangioma** or **hemangioma of tongue**—color changes, very large tongue, and may have localized swelling

↓

Angioneurotic edema of tongue (may be with patchy swelling of lips).

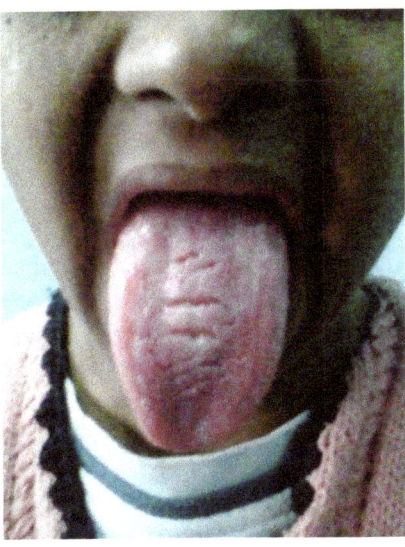

Fig. 50.3: Macroglossia with grossly fissured/furrowed tongue in mongolism

Macroglossia is large tongue and microglossia is small tongue.

MICROGLOSSIA

- Motor neuron disease (MND)
- Bulbar (flaccid) and pseudobulbar (spastic) palsy
- Wasting of the tongue (lower motor neuron lesion of XIIth cranial nerve)
- Cerebral diplegia.

DIFFERENT MOVEMENTS OF TONGUE

- Tremor (fine; in anxiety neurosis, thyrotoxicosis, chronic alcoholism)
- Fasciculation (MND or bulbar palsy)
- Chewing tongue (athetosis)
- Lizard tongue—tongue is protruded momentarily and taken back within the oral cavity instantaneously (chorea)
- Jack-in-the-box tongue (Sydenham's chorea from rheumatic fever)
- Trombone tongue [rapid forward and backward movement of tongue in general paresis of insane (GPI)]
- Irregular and continual rotatory movement (dyskinesia, mainly drug-induced or extrapyramidal syndromes)
- Rolling movements (Down's syndrome, cretinism)
- Lingual myoclonus, tics or forced deviation of tongue (as part of focal seizure).

Method of examination: For tremor—ask to protrude the tongue, for fasciculation—ask to keep the tongue in floor of the mouth, other movements—can be examined by opening the mouth.

SIALORRHEA (PTYALISM OR EXCESSIVE SALIVATION)

- Carcinoma of the tongue or mouth (with cervical lymphadenopathy)
- Caries tooth, stomatitis
- Wilson's disease (drooling of saliva with Kayser-Fleischer ring in cornea)
- Post-encephalitic parkinsonism (past history of encephalitis, mental retardation, rigidity > tremor, plantar response may be extensor; seborrhea)
- Bulbar palsy (history is important; dysphagia, dysarthria, dysphonia with nasal regurgitation; small, wasted tongue)
- Pregnancy
- Hydrophobia (history of dog bite)
- Schizophrenia, mania

- Arsenic, mercury or lead poisoning (area of residence, occupation or history of poisoning); acid or alkali poisoning
- Smell and sight of spicy food.

See 'Xerostomia' from Chapter 55. Xerostomia is opposite to ptyalism.

DROOLING (DRIBBLING) OF SALIVA

Common examples in clinical practice are as follows:
- Mental retardation
- Stomatitis
- Facial palsy
- Wilson's disease
- Epilepsy
- Acid or alkali poisoning (accidental or suicidal ingestion)
- During sleep (often embarrassing).

SCROTAL TONGUE

- Tongue shows deep horizontal fissures where debris may collect
- It is of no clinical importance.

DIFFERENTIAL DIAGNOSIS OF ACUTE SWELLING OF TONGUE

- Angioneurotic edema or giant urticaria in tongue
- Hemophilia or bleeding disorder
- Pemphigus (a fatal 'blistering' disease)
- Tongue bite (accidental or during convulsions) or bee-stings
- Infection (e.g. associated with stomatitis)
- Corrosives or acute irritant applications
- Effect of drugs—mercury, aspirin (rare).

Acute swelling of tongue may compromise with breathing.

🔖 THE PEARLS

Tongue should be examined in all the patients. The examination of the tongue, many a time, have a placebo effect on the patient. Though previously considered as a mirror of gastrointestinal tract, tongue is now regarded as mirror of dysfunction of all the systems of the body.

51

Nerve Thickening

NERVE THICKENING COMMONLY ASSOCIATED WITH

- Leprosy (commonly in tuberculoid variety)
- Neurofibromatosis (Fig. 51.1)
- Acromegaly
- Charcot-Marie-Tooth (CMT) disease (juvenile)
- Amyloidosis (primary)
- Chronic Guillain-Barré (GB) syndrome or chronic inflammatory demyelinating polyneuropathy (CIDP)
- Sarcoidosis
- Dejerine-Sottas type neuropathy or Refsum's disease
- Idiopathic hypertrophic neuropathy
- Roussy-Levy syndrome.

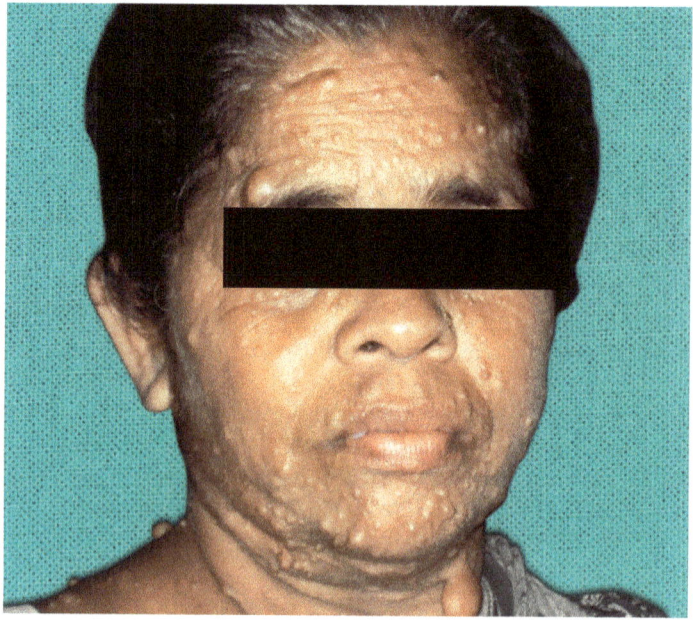

Fig. 51.1: Multiple neurofibromatosis

Chapter 51 Nerve Thickening

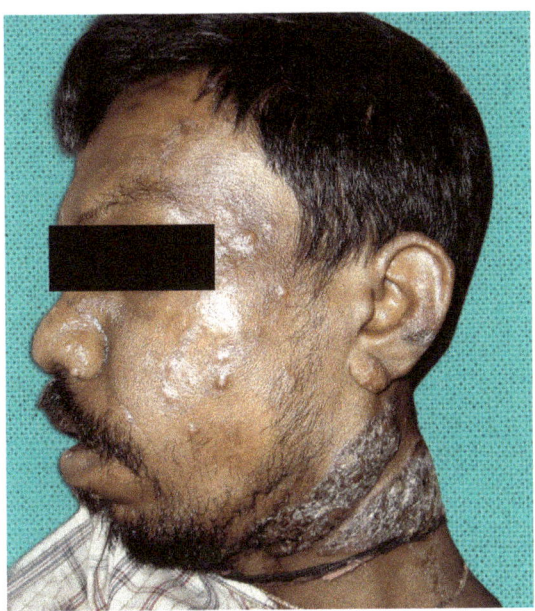

Fig. 51.2: Nodular infiltrative lesions in leprosy with scrofuloderma in neck (simultaneous *Mycobacterium leprae* and *Mycobacterium tuberculosis* infections in a single patient)

PERIPHERAL NERVES COMMONLY THICKENED (ESPECIALLY IN LEPROSY) (FIG. 51.2)

- Great auricular nerve in the neck across the sternomastoid muscle—the nerve stands out by turning the head to opposite side
- Ulnar nerve at elbow
- Common peroneal nerve at the neck of fibula.

CLUE TO DIAGNOSIS

- Cafe-au-lait spots + kyphoscoliosis → neurofibromatosis (Fig. 51.3)
- Anesthetic and hypopigmented patch → leprosy (Fig. 51.4)
- Hepatosplenomegaly → amyloidosis, leprosy
- Lymphadenopathy → sarcoidosis, amyloidosis
- Parotid swelling, uveitis → sarcoidosis
- Ichthyosis, deafness, retinitis pigmentosa → Refsum's disease
- Facial palsy → leprosy, chronic GB syndrome, sarcoidosis
- Prognathism, facial enlargement → acromegaly
- Macroglossia → acromegaly, amyloidosis
- **Nerve biopsy:** Onion bulb formation → Dejerine-Sottas type neuropathy or Refsum's disease.

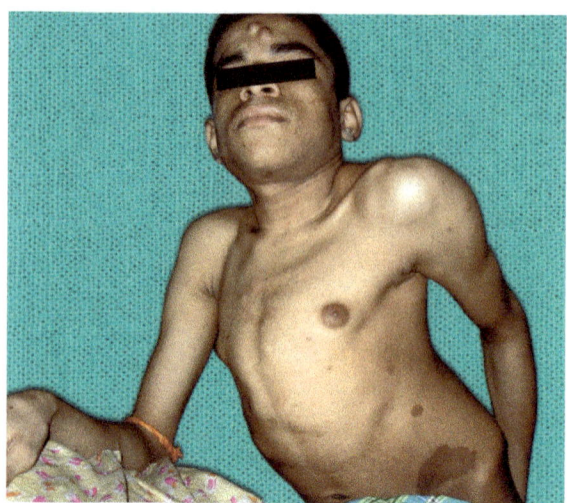

Fig. 51.3: Pectus carinatum, café-au-lait spots (light brown macules) in abdomen and chest, spinal deformity (kyphoscoliosis), and neurofibroma in forehead—a patient of von Recklinghausen's disease

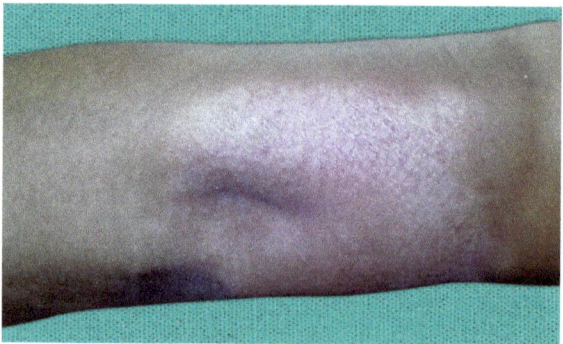

Fig. 51.4: Hypopigmented and anesthetic patch over skin in leprosy

THE PEARLS

The most common cause of peripheral thickening of nerve is leprosy (tuberculoid variety). So, if we think in the other way—one has to examine the patient for nerve thickening in the mentioned sites, if he/she presents with hypopigmented and anesthetic skin patches. In leprosy, the patient may suffer from peripheral neuropathy (lepromatous variety). Always test the nerves for thickening, nodularity and tenderness, as well as its motor and sensory functions.

52

Night Blindness

SYNONYM

Nyctalopia

ASSOCIATIONS

- Vitamin A deficiency
- Retinitis pigmentosa
- Peripheral chorioretinitis
- Chronic simple glaucoma associated with marked contraction of visual field
- Myopic degeneration in the periphery of retina (i.e. congenital high myopia)
- Detachment of the retina
- Zinc deficiency
- Malingering.

DETECTION

Done by history (e.g. poor vision at night especially in feeble illumination), clinical examination (signs of vitamin A deficiency, e.g. Bitot's spot or xerophthalmia; ophthalmoscopy), and clinical detection by an instrument called 'adaptometer'. Nyctalopia results from either damage to the rods or due to deficient regeneration of visual purple.

DAY BLINDNESS (HEMERALOPIA)

Here, the vision is poor in bright light but better in dim light. Pupil dilates in dim light, and the peripheral retina is used for vision (rods are normal but cones are at fault). The patient has photoaversion (i.e. dislike of light) rather than photophobia. It is the exact opposite of nyctalopia. The common causes are:
- Pathological changes in macula (e.g. cone dystrophy)
- Central opacity of cornea or lens
- Polar cataract
- Congenital, when associated with color blindness; albinism.

The retina is covered with two kind of photoreceptors—rods and cones. An owl's eye has far more rods than cones, and thus owls can see clearly in dark but not in day light.

AMBLYOPIA

It means partial loss of vision, e.g. in suppression of macular function, and often associated with squinting eye in the child.

AMAUROSIS FUGAX

It means sudden but 'temporary' complete loss of vision (usually monocular), e.g. as on rising suddenly from sitting position, migraine (from spasm of retinal arteries), multiple sclerosis, etc.

AMAUROSIS

It is the complete loss of vision. 'Acute' loss of vision is found in:
- *Painful*
   - Acute angle-closure glaucoma
   - Uveitis
   - Corneal ulcer
   - Endophthalmitis
   - Trauma
   - Factitious.
- *Painless*
   - Central retinal vein thrombosis
   - Retinal artery occlusion
   - Optic neuritis
   - Detachment of the retina
   - Ischemic optic neuropathy (e.g. as a complication of temporal arteritis)
   - Vitreous hemorrhage (massive)
   - Exudative macular degeneration
   - Cerebrovascular accidents (CVA)
   - Factitious.

Chronic progressive vision loss is found in cataract, refractive error, macular degeneration (age-related), primary optic atrophy, chorioretinitis and open-angle glaucoma.

COLOR BLINDNESS

Three primary colors are red, green and blue. Congenital red or green color blindness is X-linked and almost exclusively found in male children. Green-blindness is the most common in clinical practice. Ideally color vision is tested by Ishihara's chart (pseudoisochromatic plates). The color vision assesses the function of the retinal cones and optic nerve. The causes are:
- *Congenital (hereditary)*
   - Partial—cannot recognize primary colors
   - Total—cannot recognize any color and sees everything gray.

- ***Acquired***
  - Age-related macular disease
  - Optic nerve diseases
  - Toxic amblyopias, e.g. ethambutol or chloroquine-induced.

TUBULAR VISION (CONCENTRIC NARROWING OF FIELD OF VISION)

Classical tubular vision is found in hysteria or psychogenic field defect (tunnel vision); may also be seen in advanced retinitis pigmentosa and terminal glaucoma (*see* Chapter 26).

PERIPHERAL DEFECT IN VISUAL FIELD

- Retinitis pigmentosa (funnel vision)
- Chorioretinitis (blurring or gradual loss of vision)
- Psychogenic [tunnel vision; all other parameters—within normal limit (WNL)]
- Lesion in optic chiasma (bitemporal hemianopia)
- Lesion in optic tract (homonymous hemianopia)
- Lesion in visual cortex (homonymous hemianopia or quadrantopia).

THE PEARLS

In all the conditions described, try to refer the patient to an ophthalmologist and/or neurologist. The earlier the referral, the better is the outcome.

Nocturnal Enuresis

SYNONYM

Bed-wetting, sleep enuresis, self-wetting.

DEFINITION

Nocturnal enuresis is the involuntary voiding of micturition into clothes or in bed during sleep in the young (i.e. >5 years of age). It is one of the parasomnias like sleep-walking or sleep terrors. Bed-wetting is considered a normal feature of development before the age of 5 years; it usually improves at puberty and is rare in adults. Incidence rate is 1–3% in late adolescence and affection of males are more than females.

CLINICAL PRESENTATION OF ENURESIS

- Nocturnal only—occurs in first third of sleep, frequently during rapid eye movement (REM) sleep; usually recalls a dream with voiding
- Diurnal only—more in girls, voiding in early afternoon on school days mainly
- Combined nocturnal and diurnal enuresis.

CLINICAL ASSOCIATIONS

- Lack of toilet training, anxiety, fear, ↑ intake of water
- Epilepsy, mental subnormality, meningomyelocele, cauda equina lesion
- Urinary tract infections or UTI (urethritis, cystitis), epispadias, phimosis, meatal stenosis
- Threadworm infestation, neurovascular dysfunction.

MANAGEMENT

- Bladder training and behavioral therapy (alarm and pad technique, scheduled voiding to reduce voiding at night or arrange rewards for 'dry nights')
- Phimosis should be operated, if present
- Secondary enuresis is commonly due to emotional disturbances. UTI, urinary tract malformations, cauda equina lesions, sleep apnea or epilepsy → the cause should be corrected

- ***Pharmacotherapy***—desmopressin (0.2 mg, intranasally at bedtime), oxybutynin (5-10 mg, at bedtime), indomethacin suppositories, or imipramine (10-50 mg, at bedtime).

INCREASED FREQUENCY OF MICTURITION

Normally an adult with an average fluid intake evacuates his/her bladder approximately 4-5 times during daytime and once during night. If the micturition is more than this, it is known as increased frequency of micturition, which may be associated with increased or normal urine output.

The common associations noticed are as follows:
- UTI
- Urinary bladder—cystitis, small bladder (e.g. thimble bladder), bladder stone/tumor, cystocele in females
- Bladder neck—benign hypertrophy of prostate (BHP), uterine prolapse, lax internal urethral sphincter
- Urethra—urethritis, stricture of urethra, phimosis, pinhole meatus
- Psychogenic
- As a part of polyuria
- Pregnancy, and intra-abdominal tumor pressing over the urinary bladder.

Four common causes in clinical practice are UTI, BHP, calculus in urinary bladder and uterine prolapse.

IMPROPER URINARY STREAM

Improper urinary stream occurs when there is impairment in the smooth and free flow of urine.

For example, BHP is associated with nocturia, reduced size and force of urinary stream, straining to urinate and dribbling at the end; often these are associated with increased frequency, precipitancy and urgency.

The common causes of improper urinary stream are:
- ***Children:*** Phimosis, meatal stenosis, posterior urethral valve
- ***Adults:*** BHP, stricture of urethra (fork urine or bifid urine), UTI, bladder neck obstruction, vesical calculus, phimosis or bladder dysfunction due to neurological diseases (neurogenic bladder).

HESITANCY AND PRECIPITANCY

One has to remember that parasympathetic nerves (S2, 3, 4) are nerve of evacuation and sympathetic nerves (T10-L2) are nerve of filling of the urinary bladder.
- ***Hesitancy:*** Difficulty in initiating micturition in spite of presence of urge to do so
- ***Precipitancy:*** Inability to stop voiding of urine when desire for micturition occurs.

The common causes in clinical practice are:
- **Uninhibited bladder:** Found in frontal lobe tumours, parasagittal meningioma, dementia. There is urgency at low bladder volume (like a child) with sudden uncontrolled evacuation of urine. It is also known as **mental incontinence** (i.e. loss of social control of micturition).
- **Spinal bladder:** Incomplete lesion in spinal cord results in:
  - Hesitancy—due to involvement of facilitatory fibers, e.g. incomplete cord compression
  - Precipitancy—due to involvement of inhibitory fibers, e.g. multiple sclerosis
- **Disorders of urinary tract:** BHP, bladder neck obstruction.

TREATMENT

- Hesitancy—reassurance and not to exert undue stain
- Precipitancy—a condom catheter is applied in male patients. Surgical correction of the urinary tract, if needed.

NOCTURIA

Increased frequency of micturition at night and passing of more than one-third of the total daily output by night is nocturia. The common causes are:
- All polyuric states
- Edema-forming states (i.e. cirrhosis of liver, congestive cardiac failure)
- Diabetes mellitus
- BHP
- Salt-losing nephropathy
- Cystitis
- Vesico-ureteric reflux
- Autonomic dysfunction
- Insomnia even without renal disease
- Low bladder capacity (e.g. infection, tumor or stone).

Nocturia is usually assessed as pathological. Like tachypnea in respiratory disorders, nocturia may be an early manifestation of renal disorder or cardiac failure. Diabetes and BHP are very common causes.

URINARY INCONTINENCE

It is the inability to hold urine in the bladder or it is the involuntary urinary leak.

Types of Urinary Incontinence

- **Physiological:** Upto 3 years of age
- **Urge incontinence:** The person cannot hold the strong urge to void and soils his/her cloth if toilet facility is not available nearby. It is due to overactivity of detrusor muscle and commonly results from UTI, vesical calculus, or spinal cord compression.

- **Stress incontinence:** Urinary incontinence occurs after stress, e.g. coughing, sneezing or laughing (laughing-induced incontinence in young girls is known as giggle incontinence), and are commonly seen in multiparous women or after childbirth (due to obstetrical trauma). It is also noticed in males after prostatic surgery.
- **Overflow incontinence:** Commonly seen in acute transverse myelitis when the neural shock stage is over (retention of urine with overflow incontinence); may be seen in stricture of urethra or secondary to bladder neck obstruction. It is the urinary leak after chronic urinary retention.
- **True incontinence:** The urine leakage is constant (at any time and at any position) in vesico-vaginal fistula, or after pelvic surgery (acquired). Congenital causes are patent urachus or exstrophy of urinary bladder.
- **Psychogenic incontinence:** It is found in children in an attempt to draw attention.

Incontinence of urine is commonly seen in BHP (hesitancy, dribbling, ↑ frequency), UTI (pyrexia, dysuria, ↑ frequency), uterine prolapse (characteristically low volume bladder frequency), and weakness of pelvic floor muscles (stress incontinence).

ANURIA

Anuria is no urine output for 12 hours (some nephrologists define anuria as less than 50 mL urine output per day). Oliguria is less than 400 mL of urine output per day.

CAUSES OF LOW URINE OUTPUT

- **Oliguria:** Acute gastroenteritis, high fever, acute glomerulonephritis, congestive cardiac failure (decompensated), renal failure (acute and chronic), hypovolemia and shock, ***third space loss*** in acute peritonitis, acute pancreatitis and burn.
- **Anuria:**
  - *Prerenal*
    - Shock, sepsis (septicemia), hemorrhage (massive)
    - Dehydration due to any cause (e.g. acute gastroenteritis)
    - Crush syndrome
    - Burn (extensive)
    - Intravascular hemolysis, mismatched blood transfusion
    - Congestive cardiac failure
    - Acute pancreatitis.
  - *Renal*
    - Acute glomerulonephritis, rapidly progressive glomerulonephritis (RPGN)
    - Acute renal failure (ARF)
    - Acute papillary necrosis (diabetes, sickle cell disease, phenacetin-induced)
    - Diffuse cortical necrosis
    - Complete renal arterial and venous obstruction
    - Chronic renal failure (produces anuria terminally).

- *Post-renal*
  - Reflex anuria (calculus in one ureter may produce reflex obstruction of the other ureter)
  - Ligation of the ureters (accidental) or bilateral ureteric obstruction by clots, stone or crystals
  - Ureteric obstruction due to retroperitoneal fibrosis or malignant infiltration around the ureters.

Complete anuria (i.e. no urine by catheterization):
- Bilateral ureteric obstruction
- RPGN
- Diffuse cortical necrosis
- Bilateral renal artery stenosis.

POLYURIA

It is the urine output persistently above 3 L per day. The normal urine output for a healthy adult is approximately 1.5 L (400 mL–3 L) per day.

The common causes of polyuria are:
- Chronic renal failure
- Diabetes mellitus
- Diabetes insipidus
- Psychogenic polydipsia (compulsive water drinking)
- Use of diuretics in patients with edema
- Diuretic phase of ARF
- Hypercalcemic nephropathy
- Hypokalemic nephropathy
- *Solute diuresis*—glycosuria (diabetes mellitus), high protein tube feeding, infusion of mannitol
- Post-obstructive uropathy
- *Transient polyuria*—after epileptic seizure, paroxysmal atrial tachycardia, migraine or asthmatic attack, pregnancy, consumtion of alcohol or caffeine.

Hematuria is blood in the urine. Dysuria is pain or discomfort felt during micturition. Strangury is severe form of dysuria where there is painful passing of urine drop by drop with severe suprapubic pain. Chyluria is passage of milky urine.

THE PEARLS

Approximately 75% of children with enuresis have a first-degree relative with history of enuresis. Enuresis correlates with other maturational delays (e.g. language and motor skills) and social development. It is to be remembered that 1% of males aged 18 years may have history of enuresis, which produces a tremendous social embarrassment to the patient.

Drugs are effective in the treatment. An enuresis alarm is an effective intervention for nocturnal enuresis in children in the long run.

54

Pallor

DEFINITION

It is the waxy appearance of skin and mucous membrane. When the skin and mucous membrane lack the normal color/complexion and look pale, it is known as pallor.

PATHOGENESIS

In healthy patient, blood flows through capillaries and make the skin, mucus membrane and nails pink. Pallor depends on thickness and quality of skin, and quality and amount of blood in the capillaries. Thus in the presence of normal hemoglobin concentration, a person looks pale if he/she has thick skin and nail than an average individual. A person, who is having ↓ red blood cell (RBC) or ↓ hemoglobin, always looks pale. Pallor and anemia are not interchangeable terms; there are many causes of pallor and anemia is most common of them.

Pallor may be:
- *Temporary:* Intense emotion, fright, shock (due to vasoconstriction, associated with cold and clammy skin), hemorrhage
- *Persistent:* Anemia due to any cause or peripheral vasoconstriction (e.g. severe atopy, edematous part or myxedema).

Anemia denotes the color of the blood and itself a 'pathological' condition while pallor is a 'clinical' entity. A person without losing a drop of blood may become deadly pale (e.g. shock and collapse), and similarly a person looking severely pale may not be grossly anemic (e.g. Sheehan's syndrome). It is difficult to detect pallor in deeply pigmented individuals.

The observation of increasing pallor by friends or relatives may point towards early manifestation of progressive anemia or any other disease menifested by pallor.

The opposite term of pallor is plethora (e.g. polycythemia).

SITES TO BE LOOKED FOR ANEMIA

- Lower palpebral conjunctiva
- Tongue, especially the tip and the dorsum
- Soft palate
- Nail-beds (these are the windows of capillary network)
- Palms, soles and general skin surfaces.

Pallor due to anemia is best manifested in mucus membranes (e.g. mouth), conjunctiva and palmar creases. In a thick skinned person (in health), mucus membranes are not pale. ***False pallor*** may be due to anasarca (e.g. nephrotic syndrome), myxedema or thick skin, and is mainly menifested in skin (described below).

In healthy persons, palpebral conjunctiva is red, which appears pale pink in anemia; and may look totally white if anemia is severe.

CAUSES OF PALLOR WITHOUT ANEMIA

- Peripheral circulatory failure (e.g. low cardiac output in acute left ventricular failure) or shock (ashen-gray pallor) or vasoconstriction due to any cause
- Acute myocardial infarction
- Very tight aortic stenosis or mitral stenosis
- Myxedema (pallor > anemia)—pallor is due to vasoconstriction plus lemon-yellow tint due to carotenemia plus anemia
- Nephrotic syndrome
- Sheehan's syndrome or panhypopituitarism (due to ↓ skin pigment)
- Night workers
- Thick skin (e.g. scleroderma)
- Vasovagal attack, fear, exposure to cold, intense emotion, syncope due to any cause.

- Patients of subacute bacterial endocarditis have a pallor which is known as cafe-au-lait pallor (i.e. color of white coffee)
- A limb or part of a limb may look pale due to arterial spasm (e.g. Raynaud's phenomenon), exposure to cold, deprived of blood supply (e.g. ligature applied in snake bite), having edematous swelling (e.g. anasarca), or thick skin (e.g. scleroderma)
- So, pallor may be of two types:
  1. Pallor associated with anemia
  2. Pallor without anemia (described above).

THE PEARLS

The color of the face depends on oxyhemoglobin, reduced hemoglobin, melanin and carotene. Remember, pallor and anemia are not interchangeable terms. In clinical practice, the most common cause of pallor is anemia.

Pallor should always be investigated. A doctor should train his/her eyes to diagnose sallow (pale) yellow-brownish tinge of skin in chronic renal failure, blotting paper like pallor in hookworm anemia, or severe progressive pallor in ruptured ectopic pregnancy.

55

Parotid Swelling

STEPS TO DIAGNOSIS

- ***Unilateral:*** Parotid tumor [look for lower motor neuron (LMN) type VIIth nerve palsy], parotitis (painful and tender on palpation, history of pyrexia), or leukemic or lymphomatous deposits.
- ***Bilateral***
  - Mumps (commonly children with pyrexia and tender parotids) (Fig. 55.1)
  - Bacterial parotitis or suppurative parotitis (with history of poor oral hygiene, pyrexia ± hot and tender fluctuating swelling)
  - Chronic alcoholism (history of alcohol intake with flushed face)
  - Cirrhosis of liver (especially, alcoholic cirrhosis + look for other stigma like gynecomastia, Dupuytren's contracture, loss of body hair and features of portal hypertension)
  - Sjögren's syndrome (xerostomia + keratoconjunctivitis sicca + arthritis)
  - Sarcoidosis (uveoparotid fever or Heerfordt's syndrome → with facial palsy, may have generalized adenopathy, swelling of lacrimal glands, uveitis)

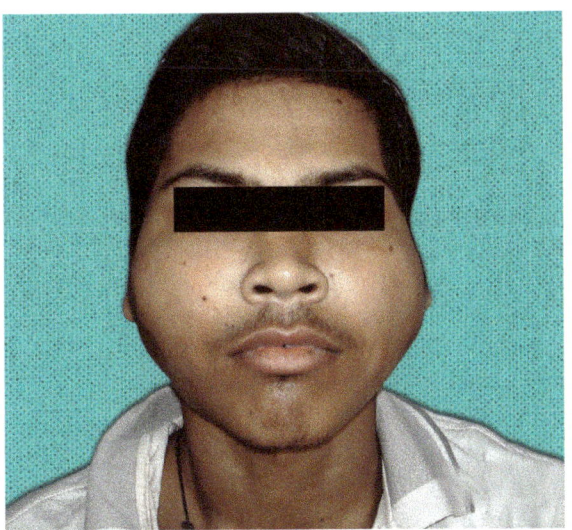

Fig. 55.1: Bilateral parotid swelling in mumps

- Drug-induced (***iodine mumps*** after intravenous pyelogram (IVP), phenylbutazone, guanethidine or bretylium → tender parotids)
- Amyloidosis (macroglossia with hepatosplenomegaly, malabsorption, nephrotic syndrome or lymphadenopathy)
- Metabolic—cirrhosis of liver, diabetes mellitus, chronic pancreatitis, hyperlipoproteinemias
- Endocrine—acromegaly, gonadal hypofunction
- Leukemic or lymphomatous deposits.

DIFFERENTIAL DIAGNOSIS OF PAROTID SWELLING

- Hypertrophy of masseter muscle
- Jaw tumors
- Lymphadenopathy (preauricular nodes mainly)
- Temporomandibular joint swelling (e.g. from rheumatoid arthritis)
- Dental abscess
- Infantile cortical hyperostosis (of mandible).

DRY EYES (XEROPHTHALMIA)

- Sjögren's syndrome (keratoconjunctivitis sicca)
- Stevens-Johnson syndrome
- Pemphigoid or burns
- Impaired lacrimal gland function
- Hypovitaminosis A (advanced stage)
- Anesthetic cornea
- Trachoma stage IV (due to severe scarring)
- Aging, lid scarring, chronic conjunctivitis.

DRY MOUTH (XEROSTOMIA)

- Transient—fear, anxiety, tension, high fever, dehydration, mouth breathing
- Psychogenic
- Drug-induced—diuretics, antihypertensives, parasympatholytics, psychotherapeutics (e.g. amitriptyline), levodopa
- Sjögren's syndrome, sarcoidosis, amyloidosis, human immunodeficiency virus (HIV) infection, graft-versus-host disease
- Irradiation for head and neck cancers, post-parotidectomy
- Diabetes mellitus, alcohol-intake—as a result of polyuria
- Old age (especially females).

Xerostomia (i.e. ↓ saliva production) may be complicated by halitosis, caries tooth and candidosis of oral cavity.

SIALORRHEA (PTYALISM OR HYPERSALIVATION)

It is the opposite of xerostomia and is seen in:
- Pregnancy
- Stomatitis, carcinoma of the tongue or mouth
- Schizophrenia
- Wilson's disease (drooling of saliva)
- Hydrophobia
- Bulbar palsy
- Postencephalitic parkinsonism
- Acid or alkali poisoning; arsenic, mercury and lead poisoning.

MIKULICZ'S SYNDROME

Long-standing, painless parotid swelling + lacrimal and other salivary adenitis + fever + uveitis, may occur in tuberculosis, Hodgkin's disease, leukemia or systemic lupus erythematosus (SLE), and is known as Mikulicz's syndrome.

DRUG-INDUCED SALIVARY GLAND SWELLING

- Guanethidine
- Bretylium
- Iodides
- Bethanidine
- Phenylbutazone
- Clonidine
- Lead, mercury
- Thiouracil.

> **THE PEARLS**
>
> In a patient of parotid swelling, always examine:
> - Other salivary glands, lacrimal glands
> - Lymph nodes all over the body, especially the glands in neck
> - Look for LMN type VIIth cranial nerve palsy
> - Do not wait for fluctuation as a sign for parotid abscess; incise and drain it as early as possible (also in breast and anorectal abscess, and hand infection).

56

Patch Tonsil

PATCH OR MEMBRANES SEEN OVER TONSILS

- Acute follicular tonsillitis
- Faucal diphtheria
- Thrush or candidial infection
- Agranulocytosis
- Acute lymphoblastic leukemia (ALL)
- Vincent's angina (spirochetes and fusiform bacilli)
- Infectious mononucleosis
- Milk card (in neonates and infants).

CLUE TO DIAGNOSIS

- History of (H/O) sore throat, odynophagia, fever, weakness, intake of drugs like carbimazole (i.e. developing agranulocytosis) should be enquired into
- Cervical lymphadenopathy (diphtheria, tonsillitis, infectious mononucleosis, ALL)
- Petechial rashes at the junction of hard and soft palate (infectious mononucleosis)
- Splenomegaly (ALL, infectious mononucleosis)
- Pyrexia (tonsillitis, diphtheria, ALL, infectious mononucleosis)
- Trismus (may be present in tonsillitis)
- Easily detachable membrane (all except diphtheria, where the membrane cannot be separated easily and it leaves a bleeding, raw surface after separation)
- Blood for total leukocyte count (TLC), differential leukocyte count (DLC) (leucocytosis/agranulocytosis), abnormal cells (leukemia), Monospot and Paul-Bunnell test (infectious mononucleosis).

PREDISPOSING CONDITIONS FOR ORAL CANDIDIASIS

- AIDS (acquired immune deficiency syndrome) or any immunodeficiency (Fig. 56.1)
- Diabetes mellitus
- Hematological malignancy
- Hypoparathyroidism
- Disseminated malignancy
- Immunosuppressive therapy with corticosteroids, anti-cancer chemotherapy

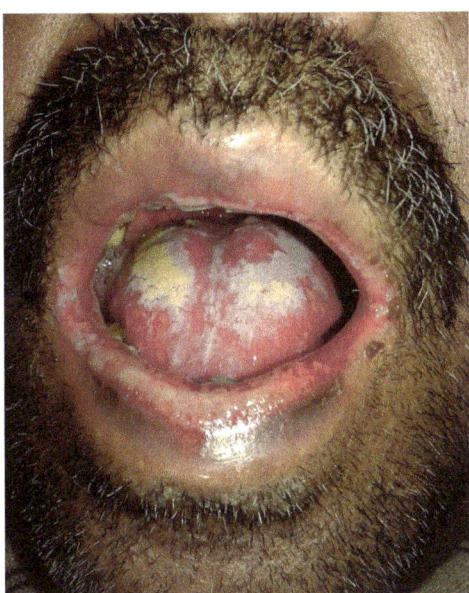

Fig. 56.1: White curd-like material in tongue with stomatitis in a patient of AIDS

- Antibiotic therapy, e.g. penicillins
- Neutropenia due to any cause (neutrophils are resposible for major host defence against *Candida*).

- Candidiasis is synonymous with **thrush** or **moniliasis**.
- Candidiasis is diagnosed by demonstration of ovoid cyst and hyphae in scrapings treated with potassium hydroxide (KOH) culture.

WHITE LESIONS IN ORAL CAVITY

- Candidiasis (seen in very young and the very old with above-mentioned predisposing factors; white curd-like material, which are easily detachable when wiped off)
- Leukoderma (filmy opalescent-appearing mucosa; can be reverted to normal appearance if stretched)
- Leukoplakia (white lesion, which cannot be scraped off; premalignant)
- Hairy leukoplakia [shaggy white surface which can not be wiped off; seen in HIV (human immunodeficiency virus) or Epstein-Barr virus infection]
- Lichen planus (linear, reticular, slightly raised striae; skin is also involved)
- Discoid lupus erythematosus (DLE), which resembles lichen planus
- Darier's disease (keratosis follicularis; white papules on dorsal tongue, alveolar mucosa, and gingiva; autosomal dominant)

- ***Miscellaneous:*** Chemical injury, nicotine stomatitis (white palate with red papules), white sponge nevus (thick, white, corrugated folds in buccal mucosa; benign condition), and squamous cell carcinoma (last but not the least).

THE PEARLS

Patch tonsil is usually due to various infections of which diphtheria is one, which may turn into a fatal outcome. Agranulocytosis and ALL are to be diagnosed as soon as possible.

If a white lesion is seen within the oral cavity, it is the duty of the physician to exclude any immunodeficiency.

57
Photosensitivity

PHOTOSENSITIVE DISEASES

- Solar urticaria
- Photoallergic reaction
- Systemic lupus erythematosus (SLE)
- Erythropoietic porphyria
- Porphyria cutanea tarda
- Pellagra, albinism (Fig. 57.1)
- Kwashiorkor
- Carcinoid syndrome
- Hartnup disease
- Xeroderma pigmentosum
- Phenylketonuria
- Drug-induced (e.g. tetracyclines)
- Photoaging
- Polymorphous light eruption (PMLE)
- Basal cell carcinoma
- Pemphigus
- Actinic keratoses
- Actinic reticuloid
- Melanoma
- Phototoxic reaction.

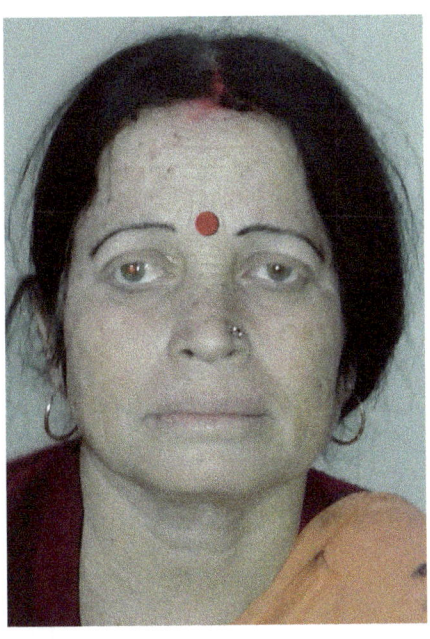

Fig. 57.1: Albinism. A congenital disorder manifested by complete or partial absence of pigment in skin, eyes and hair (here, the patient used black dye in scalp hair); the photosensitive skin can burn more easily from exposure to ultraviolet radiation

PHOTOSENSITIVE REACTIONS

- *Phototoxic (nonimmunologic) reaction*
  - Exaggerated sunburn reactions
  - Precipitated by tars, psoralens, plants (phytophotodermatitis) or phenothiazines
  - Erythema → peals off, edema, vesicles, bullae.
- *Photoallergic (immunologic) reaction*
  - Mimics contact dermatitis
  - Restricted to light-exposed areas (i.e. face, anterior 'V' of the chest, ears and back of the hands)
  - Common allergens are bithionol, buclosamide, plants like parthenium hysterophorus
  - Intensely pruritic eczematous dermatitis → lichenified.

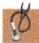

> Drug hypersensitivity, SLE and porphyria should be excluded in all photosensitive patients.

PHOTODERMATOSES

- Chronic actinic dermatitis
- Polymorphous light eruption
- Solar urticaria
- Phototoxicity and photoallergy
- Porphyrias.

PHOTOAGING

- A chronic effect of sun exposure
- Photodamaged skin consists of wrinkling, blotchiness, telangiectasia and a rough, irregular *weather-beaten* appearance (Fig. 57.2)
- It is also known as *dermatoheliosis*.

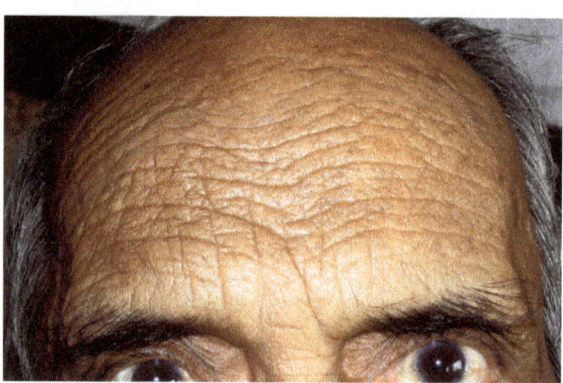

Fig. 57.2: Chronic photodamage (photoaging)—wrinkling and changes in photoexposed forehead skin are due to chronic damage from solar ultraviolet radiation

PHOTOTOXIC DRUGS

- Amiodarone
- Tetracyclines
- Sulfonamides
- Sulfonylureas
- Phenothiazines
- Psoralens
- Vinblastine
- 5-Fluorouracil
- Frusemide
- Retinoids
- Thiazides
- Dyes (methylene blue or Rose Bengal)
- Coal tar derivatives.

POLYMORPHOUS LIGHT ERUPTION (PMLE)

This is the most common type of photosensitivity after sunburn → usually transient and ignored by the person → gradually 'hardening' of skin occurs → ultimately pruritic erythematous papules form and coalesce into plaques in sun-exposed areas of forearms and trunk (may give rise to severely inflamed and edematous skin) → affection of face is mild → the diagnosis is done by skin biopsy and the treatment is aimed at use of sunscreens along with administration of artificial ultraviolet (UV) A and UV B rays for 2–3 weeks when maximum seasonal skin reaction occurs.

BUTTERFLY-LIKE ERYTHEMATOUS LESION IN FACE

- SLE (Fig. 57.3)
- Rosacea
- Malar flush
- Lupus vulgaris (most common form of skin tuberculosis)
- Leprosy (lepromatous)
- Dermatomyositis

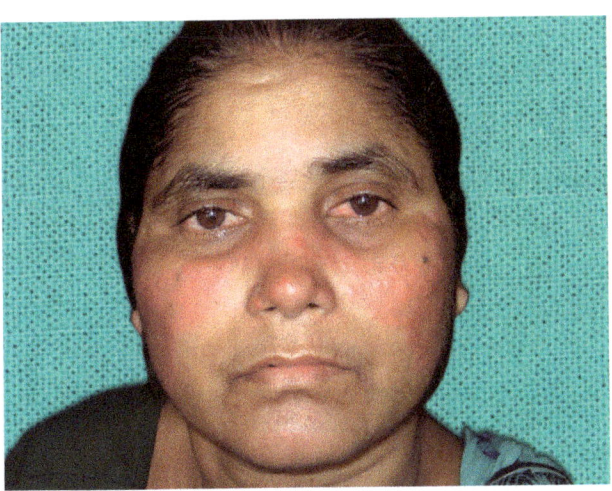

Fig. 57.3: A female patient of systemic lupus erythematosus with classical photosensitive "butterfly rash" in face

- Post kala-azar dermal leishmaniasis (PKDL)
- Pemphigus erythematosus
- Chloasma or melasma (mask of pregnancy)
- Photosensitive reaction (after intake of tetracycline or phenothiazines)
- PMLE
- Sarcoidosis (lupus pernio; rare).

> Butterfly rash in SLE is due to apoptosis of keratinized layer of skin exposed to sunlight/UV light.

SPECTRUM OF ULTRAVIOLET RAYS

Ultraviolet light is an electromagnetic radiation with three major segments (wavelengths between 10 and 400 nm)
1. **UV C:** Wavelengths 10–290 nm
   (does not reach the earth)
2. **UV B:** Wavelengths 290–320 nm
   (produces redness and erythema—the ***sunburn spectrum***)
3. **UV A:** Wavelengths 320–400 nm
   (very very less efficient than UV B in producing skin hyperemia)

Visible wavelengths 400–700 nm → the ***white light*** we see which breaks into VIBGYOR (V = violet, I = indigo, B = blue, G = green, Y = yellow, O = orange, R = red) while passing through a prism.

Wavelengths > 700 nm → ***infrared rays*** (primarily evoke heat).

> The UV radiation can cause skin diseases (e.g. these are mutagenic and carcinogenic) and may also be used to treat certain dermatological ailments in necessity.

PHOTOCHEMOTHERAPY

- PUVA: (Psoralens + UV A) therapy are used in:
  - Psoriasis
  - Vitiligo
  - Eosinophilic fasciitis
  - Cutaneous T-cell lymphoma.
- PUVB: (Psoralens + UV B) therapy are used for remission in psoriasis.

THE PEARLS

The sun gives the beneficial effect of warmth and synthesis of vitamin D, though acute and chronic sun exposure may have some deleterious effects (e.g. photosensitive skin diseases). The initial management of those conditions are avoidance of exposure to sunlight and use of sun-block cream. Then specific investigations are targeted to have a pin-point diagnosis.

Polycythemia

SYNONYMS

Dusky cyanosis or ruddy cyanosis.

DEFINITION

Polycythemia (often used interchangeably with erythrocytosis) is an increase in hemoglobin, packed cell volume (PCV) and red cell count.

Polycythemia may be divided into absolute (true increase in red cell mass) or relative (↓ in plasma volume with normal red cell mass) erythrocytosis. Absolute erythrocytosis is due to primary polycythemia (i.e. polycythemia vera) and secondary polycythemia (i.e. anoxia, neoplasms).

CLINICAL FEATURES

- Facial plethora
- Suffused conjunctiva (Fig. 58.1)
- ↑ redness of lower palpebral conjunctiva
- Oral mucus membrane turns dusky-red (i.e. congested)
- Ruddy complexion (Fig. 58.1)
- Palmar erythema.

SITES TO BE LOOKED FOR

- Lower palpebral conjunctiva
- Tongue
- Soft palate
- Nail-beds
- Palms, soles and general skin surfaces
- Face.

DIFFERENTIAL DIAGNOSIS OF PLETHORIC FACE

- Polycythemia
- Chronic alcoholism
- Cushing's syndrome

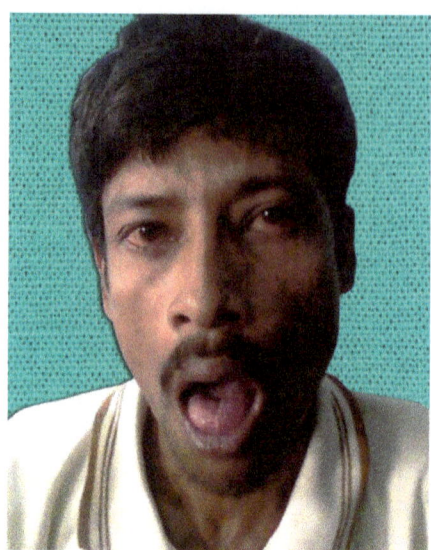

Fig. 58.1: A patient of Fallot's tetralogy complicated by cyanosis, polycythemia (suffused conjunctiva) and respiratory distress

- Chronic cor pulmonale
- SVC (superior vena caval) syndrome
- Carcinoid syndrome.

DIFFERENTIAL DIAGNOSIS OF POLYCYTHEMIA

- Smoking (secondary to ↑ carboxyhemoglobin)
- Hypoxemia (secondary polycythemia due to living in high altitudes, pulmonary fibrosis, or congenital heart disease with right-to-left shunts)
- Erythropoietin-producing states (polycystic kidney diseases, neoplasms described below)
- Stress polycythemia (Gaisbock's syndrome)
- Hemoglobinopathies associated with high oxygen affinity.

FEATURES OF POLYCYTHEMIA VERA

- ↑ Red cell mass
- Arterial O_2 saturation ≥ 92%
- Splenomegaly (75% cases)
- ↑ Platelets (> 4 lacs/mm^3)
- ↑ WBC (white blood cell > 12000/mm^3)
- ↑ LAP (leukocyte alkaline phosphatase > 100) score
- ↑ Serum vitamin B_{12} level (> 900 pg/mL).

ERYTHROPOIETIN STATUS

- Polycythemia vera: ↓ erythropoietin (EP)
- Secondary erthrocytosis, e.g. hypoxia, neoplasms: ↑ EP.

NEOPLASMS ASSOCIATED WITH POLYCYTHEMIA

- Renal cell carcinoma
- Hepatocellular carcinoma
- Uterine leiomyoma
- Cerebellar hemangioblastoma
- Ovarian carcinoma
- Pheochromocytoma.

GAISBOCK'S SYNDROME

- It is also known as **relative, apparent** or **spurious polycythemia**.
- Originally thought to be stress-induced → decreased plasma volume with normal red cell volume.
- However, spurious polycythemia is more common than polycythemia vera and is seen in middle-aged men who are obese, smokers and hypertensive (probably diuretic therapy reduces the plasma volume).
- May present with acute myocardial infarction (AMI) or cerebral infarction.
- Treated by venesection; cessation of smoking.

OUTSTANDING CLINICAL FEATURE OF POLYCYTHEMIA VERA WHICH DIFFERENTIATES IT FROM OTHERS

Splenomegaly.

MOST COMMON CAUSE OF POLYCYTHEMIA IN A CITY HOSPITAL

Chronic obstructive pulmonary disease (COPD).

HYPERVISCOSITY SYNDROME

Causes

- Multiple myeloma
- Polycythemia vera
- Chronic myeloid leukemia (CML)
- Essential thrombocythemia
- Myeloid metaplasia
- Waldenström's macroglobulinemia
- Malignancy-induced (e.g. untreated acute leukemia).

Features

- Visual disturbances (mild vision loss to abrupt blindness)
- Gum or nose bleeding
- Thrombotic episodes [cerebrovascular accident (CVA), acute MI, peripheral vascular disease, mesenteric/hepatic vein thrombosis]
- Pruritus (especially after a hot bath in polycythemia vera)
- Raynaud's phenomenon
- Peptic ulcer disease
- Neurological features, e.g. fatigue, malaise, dizziness, headache, fluctuating consciousness, transient paresis
- Congestive cardiac failure
- Peripheral cyanosis.

Ophthalmoscopy (Hyperviscosity Syndrome)

- Engorgement of retinal veins
- Vessel tortuosity
- Constriction at arteriovenous crossings
- Areas of beading (vascular segmentation) and dilatation of small venules ('string of sausages' appearance)
- Hemorrhages and exudates.

Treatment

- Basic disease
- Plasmapheresis
- Leukapheresis.

TREATMENT OF POLYCYTHEMIA VERA

- Phlebotomy (venesection) to keep the hematocrit <45% in men and <42% in women
- Hydroxyurea; busulfan
- Radioactive P32—its use is nowadays avoided because it may be leukemogenic
- Baby aspirin (100 mg/day) to prevent thrombotic complications
- Allupurinol (to treat hyperuricemia) and antihistaminics (for pruritus).

THE PEARLS

Polycythemia is an important window in clinical medicine like anemia, cyanosis and jaundice. Polycythemia vera (a myeloproliferative disorder characterized mainly by ↑ in RBC mass) is not very common. For a clinician, diagnostic pearls remain in lungs [pulmonary fibrosis, chronic obstructive pulmonary disease (COPD)], heart (congenital heart diseases) or abdomen (splenomegaly in polycythemia vera). Many a time, the patient complains of red vision in polycythemia vera.

Note: Yellow vision or xanthopsia in digitalis toxicity, and blue vision after use of sildenafil.

Like anemia, polycythemia is not a disease (except polycythemia vera) but denotes manifestation of some disease, and thus a cause must be searched for.

Pruritus

BASIC PATHOPHYSIOLOGY

Pruritus is the unpleasant and irritating cutaneous sensation with intense desire to itch or scratch. It is a harmless but annoying symptom.

There are no end organs in the body specified for itching. The itch-receptors lie in the papillary layer of the dermis. The sensation of poorly-localized itching is principally carried by unmyelinated, slowly-conducting 'C' group of fibers to the central pool present in the spinal cord → posterior roots of the spinal nerves → thalamus → sensory area of gyrus postcentralis of the cortex. The well-localized itch is conducted by myelinated, rapidly conducting delta 'A' fibers.

Itching receptors are stimulated by several exogenous and endogenous stimuli, e.g. histamine, bradykinin, prostaglandins, eicosanoids, opioid peptides, proteases, bile salt, platelet activating factors, etc. Inadequate lipid production (leads to lack of moisturizing effect of skin) resulting in xerosis, and certain psychological factors (e.g. extreme emotional stress) may provoke itching.

PRINCIPAL CAUSES

- ***Local (i.e. itchy lesion in skin)***
  - Scabies (Fig. 59.1)
  - Dermatitis herpetiformis

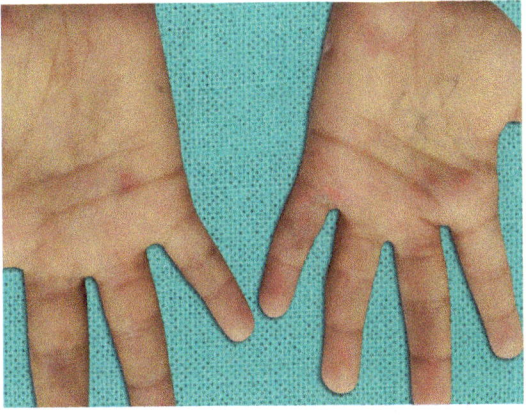

Fig. 59.1: Scabies with papules (itchy and red) and pustules

- Lichen planus
- Atopic dermatitis
- Psoriasis
- Pediculosis pubis
- Xerosis (dry skin)
- Seborrheic dermatitis
- Urticaria
- Contact dermatitis
- Fungal infection (e.g. ringworm)
- Pityriasis rosea
- Lichen simplex chronicus
- Allergic contact dermatitis, asteatotic eczema
- Pompholyx
- Drug eruption
- Insect bite.

■ ***Systemic (i.e. internal causes)***
- Obstructive jaundice (Fig. 59.2), hepatitis B or C infection
- Diabetes mellitus
- Chronic renal failure
- Lymphoma (especially, Hodgkin's disease), leukemias
- Multiple myeloma
- Polycythemia vera
- Iron deficiency anemia
- Systemic mastocytosis

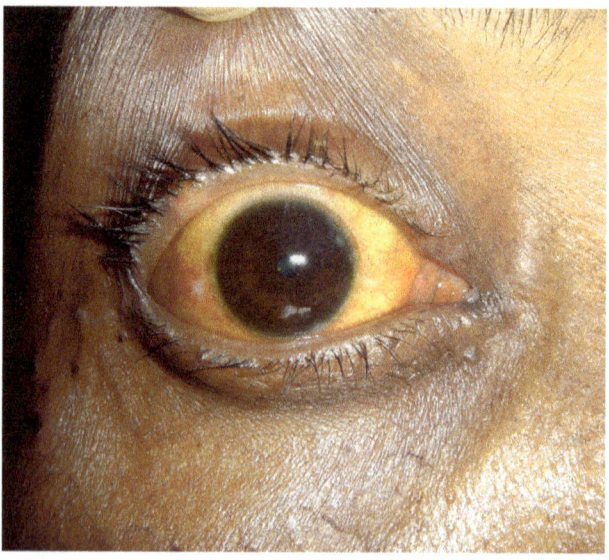

Fig. 59.2: A patient of obstructive jaundice with subconjunctival hemorrhage who is having intense pruritus

- Carcinoid syndrome
- Multiple sclerosis
- Intestinal parasitic infestations
- Pregnancy (last trimester)
- Malignancy (internal)
- Thyrotoxicosis or myxedema
- Neuropsychiatric disorders—delusions of parasitosis, neurosis
- Senile pruritus
- AIDS (acquired immune deficiency syndrome)
- Hyperhidrosis (↑ sweating—may be seen in an obese patient)
- ***Drug-induced:*** Aspirin, opiates, quinidine, phenothiazines, ultraviolet A radiation.

In Hodgkin's disease and primary biliary cirrhosis, pruritus may be the first symptom.

PRURITUS DISTURBING SLEEP

Persistent and irresistably severe pruritus is often paroxysmal in character, and awakens the patient from sleep as soon as pain is induced by scratching (also called paroxysmal pruritus).

Severe itching in lichen simplex chronicus, atopic dermatitis, dermatitis herpetiformis, pediculosis corporis, uremic pruritus, subacute prurigo, prurigo nodularis may interfere with patient's sleep. Usually, neither psychogenic nor senile pruritus leads to a loss of sleep.

AQUAGENIC PRURITUS

Sometimes, itching is evoked by contact with water of any temperature. The common situations are:
- Polycythemia vera (especially after a warm bath)
- Hypereosinophilic syndrome
- Myelodysplastic syndromes
- Juvenile xanthogranuloma
- Fungal infections.

Often a positive family history is obtained from the patient. There is ↑ degeneration of mast cells, and ↑ concentrations of histamine and acetylcholine which are liberated after contact with water. In polycythemia-induced pruritus aspirin, PUVA (psoralen with ultraviolet A) and therapy with interferon alfa-2b are tried.

PRURITUS ANI

Very often pruritus is concentrated in anal and perianal region (chiefly nocturnal) with little or no pruritus elsewhere. It is a social embarrassment for the patient. Possible etiology could be:
- Pinworm (*Enterobius vermicularis*) infestation, especially in children; other intestinal parasites; scabies
- Allergic contact dermatitis [from local anesthetic used in suppositories for hemorrhoids, cathartics; failure to cleanse the area adequately after defecation (poor anal hygiene/perfumed toilet paper); spicy foods/citrous foods or colchicine.
- Anal tags, fissure, fistula, rectal prolapse; diarrhea or anal incontinence
- Anal warts, condylomata lata (syphilis), anal granuloma, lymphogranuloma venereum (LGV); herpes simplex virus or human papillomavirus
- Perianal candidiasis (from diabetes mellitus)
- Seborrheic dermatitis
- Lichen planus
- Psoriasis
- Fungal pruritus ani, erythrasma of groin and perianal region
- Anal neurodermatitis (characterized by paroxysm of violent itching leading to tearing and bleeding).
- As a part of pruritus due to systemic causes.

Proper cleansing of local area and treatment of specific etiology (e.g. diabetes, parasites or hemorrhoids) are done. Topical pramoxine hydrochloride (nonsteroidal topical anesthetic) with hydrocortisone is tried.

RECTAL PAIN (OR PERIANAL PAIN)

- Anal fissure
- Thrombosed hemorrhoids
- Anorectal abscess
- Rectal carcinoma
- Pelvic inflammatory disease
- Prostatitis
- Compression/inflammation of sacral nerves
- Impaction of faeces/foreign bodies
- Proctitis (radiation, ulcerative, sexually-transmitted)
- **Miscellaneous:** Proctalgia fugax (severe, sharp, stabbing, episodic rectal and sacroccygeal pain, probably due to cramp of levator ani muscle), coccygodynia (fleeting pain in rectum or coccyx, often related to sitting, but not with defecation), fecal impaction, foreign bodies.

PRURITUS VULVAE

Think of:
- Vaginitis *(Candida albicans, Trichomonas vaginalis)*—most common
- Chronic cervicitis, carcinoma of cervix
- Contact dermatitis (nylon, detergent, contraceptive gels, scent)
- Lichen sclerosus of vulva, lichen planus, psoriasis
- Scabies, pediculosis and pinworms
- As a part of generalized pruritus
- ***Physiological:*** lack of cleanliness, menstruation, pregnancy, menopause, senility.

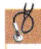

> In intense itching, always try to exclude diabetes mellitus, lymphoma, leukemia and anxiety states in a case of pruritus vulvae.

SUGGESTED WORK-UP FOR CHRONIC (> 2 WEEKS) GENERALIZED PRURITUS

1. Thorough history with psychoanalysis
2. Meticulous clinical examination
3. Blood for total leukocyte count (TLC), differential leukocyte count (DLC), erthrocyte sedimentation rate (ESR), fasting sugar level
4. Chest roentgenography
5. Thyroid, renal and liver function tests
6. Hepatitis B and C serology
7. Screening for internal malignancy [computed tomography/magnetic resonance imaging (CT/MRI) scan, tumor markers].

TREATMENT MODALITIES OF PRURITUS

Treatment of primary cause (e.g. cholestyramine in cholestasis), PUVA therapy in uremia/mastocytosis/chronic liver diseases, antihistaminics, H_2-receptor antagonists (e.g. in polycythemia, mastocytosis), ondansetron, benzodiazepines, corticosteroids (beginning with 1 mg/kg with tapering over 2–3 weeks), topical emollient cream (e.g. calamine lotion, petrolatum or any lubricant cream at bedtime), aspirin; acupuncture, mechanical vibratory stimulation, transcutaneous electrical nerve stimulation may be beneficial in some patients.

Nowadays anti-*Helicobacter pylori* treatment, terbutaline or montelukast are tried in nagging cases.

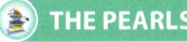
THE PEARLS

The causes of pruritus are diverse, and thus its management demands the etiological treatment. Itching the skin in mild pruritus may give a painful pleasure but severe and recalcitrant pruritus is a nightmare to the patient. Severe pruritus is often diagnosed clinically by scratch marks in the skin along with shiny nails. Many a time pruritus is a sign of internal malignancy.

Ptosis

DEFINITION

Drooping of one or both upper eyelid. The term ptosis is derived from the Greek word meaning 'to fall'.

MECHANISM

The upper eyelid muscles are levator palpebrae superioris (LPS), supplied by IIIrd cranial nerve) and Müller's muscle (supplied by sympathetic trunk). Paralysis of either of the nerves gives rise to ptosis. In LPS palsy, there is complete ptosis whereas in Müller's muscle palsy, there is development of partial ptosis. In LPS weakness, on attempted elevation of upper eyelid there is compensatory, contraction of frontal belly of occipitofrontalis muscle, and thus increased furrowing in the forehead may be seen in any long-standing ptosis. In orbicularis oculi paralysis (VIIth cranial nerve palsy), there may be apparent diminution of palpebral fissure but ptosis is never present.

TYPES

- Blepharoptosis
- Mechanical
- Aponeurotic
- Myogenic
- Neurogenic
- Congenital
- Acquired
- Complete
- Partial

DESCRIPTION

- **Blepharoptosis:** Unilateral or bilateral, may be congenital dysgenesis of the LPS or from abnormal insertion of aponeurosis of LPS into the eyelid. A history of eye surgery, old trauma, contact lens, or a family history of ptosis should be sought for. Inspection of old photographs may help to diagnose an acquired ptosis.
- **Mechanical:** Excessive weight [e.g. edema of the upper eyelid, tumors or dermatochalasis (redundancy of eyelid skin and subcutaneous fat, commonly seen in elderly)] and conjunctival scarring are two chief causes.
- **Aponeurotic:** As a result of restricted transmission of force from LPS muscle to the upper eyelid, and is due to acquired dehiscence or stretching of the aponeurotic

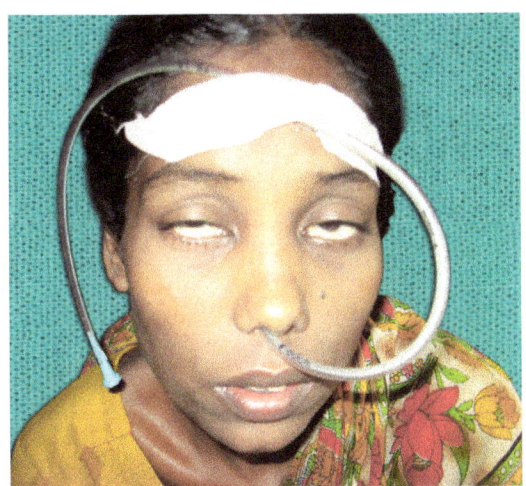

Fig. 60.1: Bilateral partial ptosis in myasthenia gravis (Ryle's tube introduced to combat nasal regurgitation)

tendon, which connects the LPS muscle to the tarsal plate. It occurs commonly in older patients due to loss of connective tissue elasticity and is seen after cataract surgery, blunt orbital trauma or sequela of eyelid swelling from infection.
- *Myogenic:* The causes are myasthenia gravis (Fig. 60.1), and different ocular and oculopharyngeal myopathies; myotonic dystrophy also produces ptosis.
- *Neurogenic:* Developed as a result of IIIrd cranial nerve (complete ptosis) or sympathetic palsy (partial ptosis).

DIFFERENT CAUSES

1. IIIrd cranial nerve (oculomotor) paralysis
2. Sympathetic paralysis (Horner's syndrome)
3. Tabes dorsalis (partial; not seen nowadays)
4. Myasthenia gravis (worsens as day progresses)
5. Myotonic dystrophy or ocular myopathy
6. Congenital
7. Snake bite (*Elapidae* group)
8. Botulism
9. Periodic paralysis
10. Hysterical
11. Edema or tumor of upper eyelid, enucleation of the eyeball
12. Temporal arteritis.

Congenital ptosis may be unilateral or bilateral. **Unilateral:** 1, 2, 6, 10, 11, 12; **bilateral:** 3, 4, 5, 6, 7, 8, 9, 10; unilateral ptosis is a recognized finding in cluster headache (a variety of migraine), syringobulbia and cavernous sinus thrombosis.

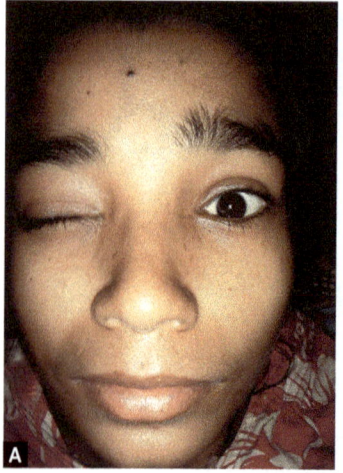
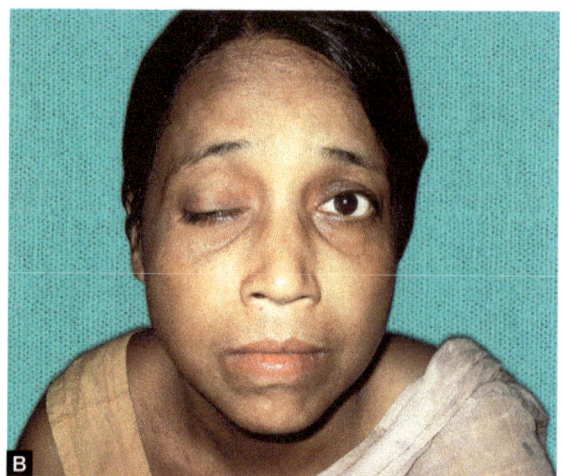

Figs 60.2A and B: Complete ptosis in right eye—patients with right sided IIIrd cranial nerve palsy. **A.** From intracranial space occupying lesion; **B.** From type 2 diabetes mellitus

HOW TO RECOGNIZE PARTIAL PTOSIS?

It is clinically evaluated by the narrowing of the palpebral fissure. By standing in front of the patient, the width of the palpebral fissure is measured in primary gaze. In partial ptosis, part of the eyeball is seen. Partial ptosis is characteristic of Horner's syndrome, recovering IIIrd nerve palsy, myasthenia gravis, myotonic dystrophy, congenital defect, tabes dorsalis and snake bite.

SOME FACTS

- *Congenital ptosis:* The horizontal wrinkling in the upper eyelid is absent (i.e. there is smoothness of upper eyelid); from birth.
- *Myasthenia gravis:* 'Fluctuating' ptosis and most prominent towards the end of the day (i.e. evening onwards); no alteration in pupillary reflex or size.
- *Horner's syndrome:* This syndrome produces partial ptosis which is also known as pseudoptosis, i.e. the ptosis is corrected on looking upwards voluntarily.
- *Hysterical:* Blepharospasm and hysterical ptosis (both are spastic ptosis) are associated with wrinkling of the eyelid and angle of the eye, and absent contraction of frontalis muscle.
- *Marcus-Gunn jaw-winking phenomenon:* Ptosis occurs on opening of the jaw as a result of anomalous communication between IIIrd and Vth cranial nerves.
- *Senile ptosis:* Senile atrophy of skin and subcutaneous tissue are commonly seen after cataract, glaucoma and retinal detachment surgeries.
- *Ptosis and pupil:*
  - Ptosis + dilated pupil → IIIrd nerve palsy
  - Ptosis + constricted pupil → Horner's syndrome

- Ptosis + normal-size pupil (i.e. pupil-sparing) → myasthenia gravis, myotonic dystrophy, botulism (in majority), snake bite, congenital variety, hysterical, and rarely in ischemia or infarction of IIIrd nerve (i.e. vasculitis, migraine or diabetes mellitus).

COMPONENTS OF THIRD NERVE PALSY

- Complete ptosis
- Lateral squint
- Fixed and dilated pupil.

COMPONENTS OF HORNER'S SYNDROME

- Pseudoptosis
- Miosis (constriction of the pupil)
- Anhidrosis (of ipsilateral half of face and neck, front and back of upper chest, arm)
- Enophthalmos
- Loss of ciliospinal reflex.

Note: Exophthalmos in one eye may mislead the clinician by putting a diagnosis of ptosis (partial) in the other eye; the pupillary size in the other eye helps in that situation to determine whether the ptosis is true or false (i.e. pupillary size and reaction remain normal in false ptosis).

Other than ptosis and pseudoptosis, 'narrow palpebral fissure' is seen in enophthalmos and blepharospasm.

THE PEARLS

Oculomotor palsy and Horner's syndrome are two common causes of ptosis. Oculomotor palsy is characterized by complete ptosis (Fig. 60.2) (on elevating the drooped eyelid, patient may complain of diplopia), dilated pupil, squint and extraocular muscle palsy; while Horner's syndrome (sympathetic paralysis) is manifested by partial ptosis, constricted pupil, absence of squint and intact extraocular muscles. Wrinkling of forehead happens to be present in long-standing ptosis.

Pupil-sparing oculomotor nerve palsy has specific causes (see text above). Ptosis is a serious complaint by the patient, which needs immediate attention.

Purpuric Spots

CLASSIFY HEMORRHAGIC SPOTS

- ***Petechiae:*** 1–2 mm in diameter (pinhead-size or tiny)
- ***Purpura:*** 3–5 mm in diameter
- ***Ecchymosis/bruise:*** Large purpura (>5 mm)
- ***Suggillation:*** >20 mm in diameter
- ***Hematoma:*** Large hemorrhages in the skin with surface elevation.

- Hemorrhagic spots never blanch on compression as they contain extravasated blood
- Hemorrhagic spots are collectively known as purpuric spots.

MECHANISMS

Purpuric spots are produced due to thrombocytopenia and/or vessel wall abnormalities and/or platelet function defect.

- Petechiae/purpura → bleeding from small capillaries into skin, mucus membrane or retina (Fig. 61.1)

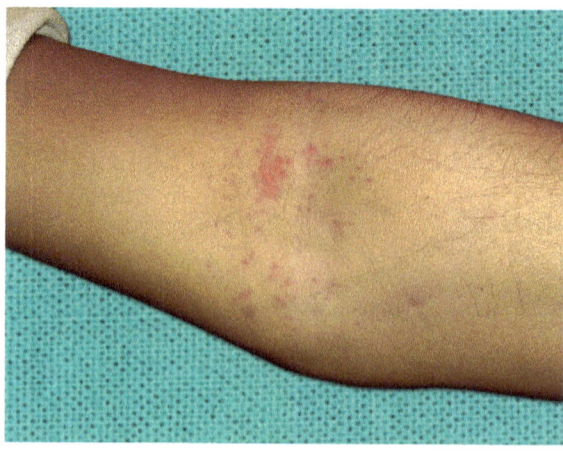

Fig. 61.1: Petechiae/purpura in the junction of arm and forearm, seen in immune thrombocytopenic purpura (ITP)

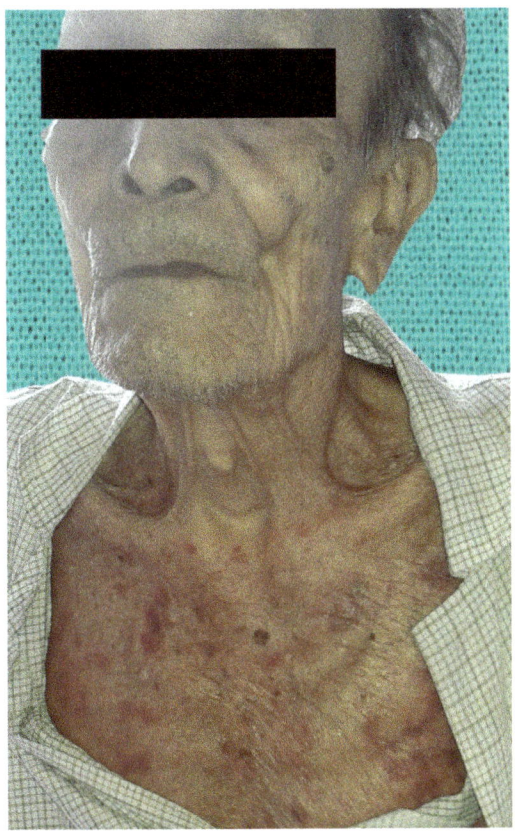

Fig. 61.2: Subcutaneous hemorrhages (ecchymoses) over the chest wall of an aged person, probably as a result of increased fragility of blood vessels due to senility

- Ecchymoses/bruises → bleeding from vessels which are larger than capillaries; suggillations or hematomas are commonly associated with bleeding disorders or coagulopathy (Fig. 61.2).

COMMON SITES

Commonly legs are involved. Purpuric rashes may be seen over buttocks too.

CLINICAL EXAMINATIONS

- Anemia
- Oral cavity and whole of the body surface (skin)
- Lymph nodes, all over the body
- Sternal tenderness
- Liver and spleen
- Ophthalmoscopy.

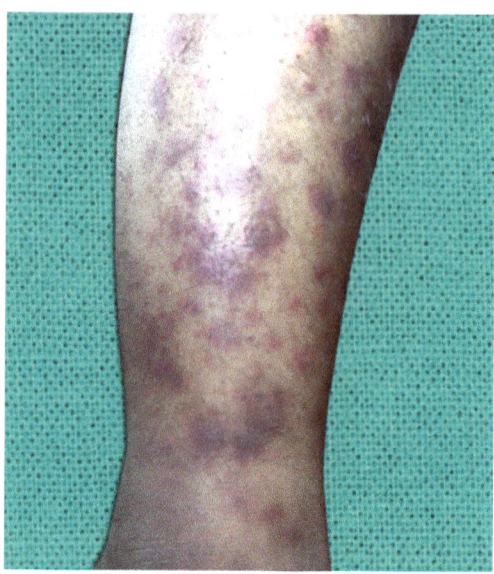

Fig. 61.3: Purpuric spots over leg in septicemia

PALPABLE PURPURA

Usually purpura are flat (i.e. from thrombocytopenia) but palpable purpura are raised from skin surface, often pruritic, and present over buttocks and extensor surfaces bilaterally. They are commonly due to vasculitis (e.g. Henoch-Schönlein purpura or IgA vasculitis, leukocytoclastic vasculitis) or infected emboli (e.g. meningococcemia, septicemia) (Fig. 61.3).

PURPURA WITH SPLENOMEGALY

- Acute leukemias (Fig. 61.4A)
- Lymphoma
- Systemic lupus erythematosus (SLE)
- Idiopathic thrombocytopenic purpura (ITP) (Fig. 61.4B) → spleen is palable in 10% cases only
- Blast crisis of chronic myeloid leukemia (CML) and rarely chronic lymphocytic leukemia (CLL)
- Subacute bacterial endocarditis (SBE)
- Myelofibrosis
- Hypersplenism.

CRITICAL PLATELET COUNT

It is $20,000/mm^3$ (recently, hematologists opined it as $10,000/mm^3$). Below this level, spontaneous hemorrhage in any vital organ may endanger the life of the patient. The patient requires temporary support with platelet or fresh blood transfusion.

Chapter 61 Purpuric Spots

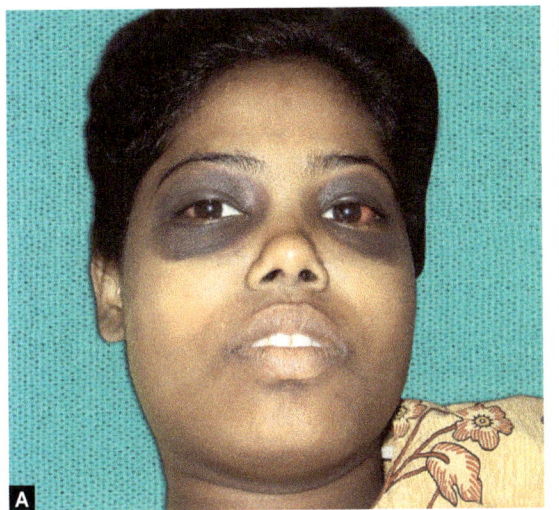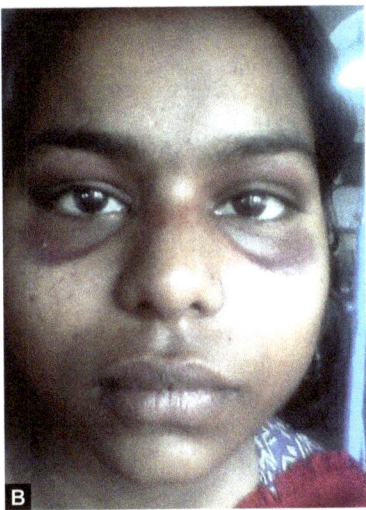

Figs 61.4A and B: Periorbital ecchymosis (panda eyes or racoon eyes like post-head injury) in patients with bleeding manifestations; **A.** Acute leukemia; **B.** Idiopathic thrombocytopenic purpura

HISTORY

- Bleeding gum, epistaxis, menorrhagia or hematuria
- Joint pain and/or swelling
- Drug intake (sulphonamide, penicillin, aspirin, quinine, heparin, etc. may have side effects as thrombocytopenia).

QUALITY OF PURPURIC RASH

- Thrombocytopenia/thrombasthenia → legs commonly; flat purpura
- Vessel wall abnormalities/vasculitis → may involve buttocks; commonly urticarial (i.e. raised and itchy).

HOW TO SUSPECT INTERNAL BLEEDING?

- Shock and peripheral circulatory failure
- Pallor
- Tachycardia and hypotension
- Internal organs
  - Chest (hemothorax)
  - Cardiovascular system (cardiac tamponade)
  - Central nervous system (neck rigidity, subhyaloid hemorrhage)
  - Retroperitoneum (Cullen's sign and/or Grey Turner's sign)
  - Gastrointestinal tract (distended and tender abdomen; rebound tenderness+)
  - Intramuscular (swelling of thigh in fracture femur).

CAUSES OF PURPURA

- Thrombocytopenia or platelet functional defects
- Meningococcemia, echo or coxsackie infection, septicemia
- Henoch-Schönlein purpura
- Hereditary hemorrhagic telangiectasis
- Purpura simplex (devil's pinches)
- Harmolytic-uremic syndrome
- Paraproteinemias
- Scurvy
- Rocky Mountain spotted fever (RMSF)
- Disseminated intravascular coagulation (DIC)
- Cryoglobulinemia
- Vasculitis
- Drugs–sulfonamide, penicillin
- Hyperglobulinemic purpura
- Cushing's syndrome
- Uremia.

Except 1st bullet, others are causes of non-thrombocytopenic purpura.

BLEEDING DISORDERS

Bleeding disorders are usually due to one of the following:
- Coagulation disorders (e.g. hemophilia)
- Platelet disorders (number and/or function defect) or von Willebrand factor defects
- Vessel wall abnormalities (common in old age).

The bleeding time (BT) and clotting time (CT) in thrombocytopenia is ↑ BT and normal CT; in coagulation disorders, it is normal BT with ↑ CT; in vessel wall abnormalities BT and CT both remain normal; and the platelet count remains normal in all except in thrombocytopenic purpura.

LIVEDO RETICULARIS

It is the cyanotic mottlings of skin with a fishnet appearance, and is usually seen in:
- Antiphospholipid syndrome (most common cause)
- Atheroembolism (left atrial myxoma, cholesterol emboli, SBE)
- Leucocytoclastic vasculitis (hypersensitivity vasculitis)
- Cryoglobulinemia
- Thrombocythemia or polycythemia
- Pancreatitis, SLE, dermatomyositis
- Polyarteritis nodosa (chronic cases)
- Drugs (amantadine)
- Physiologic (cutis marmorata).

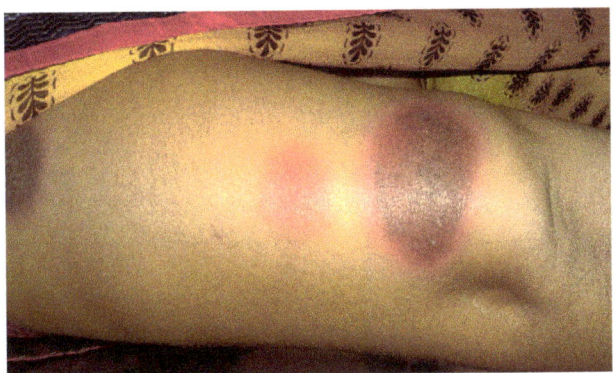

Fig. 61.5: Fixed drug eruption (FDR)—three annular erythematous, sharply-demarcated patches as a result of systemic exposure to sulpha drugs; these lesions normally resolve with hyperpigmentaion and may recur at the same site with re-exposure to the drug

Telangiectasia, spiders and fresh mosquito bite marks blanch on pressure as they are differential diagnosis of petechiae/purpura, which never blanches on pressure given by pinhead. Fixed drug eruption (FDR) is to be differentiated from ecchymosis (Fig. 61.5)

THE PEARLS

- Purpuric spots should be clinically differentiated from telangiectasia (small, dilated blood vessels visible on skin surface), mosquito bite marks, spider nevi, cherry angioma and drug rashes
- Bleeding from mucous membrane (gum), nose (epistaxis), skin (petechiae, purpura), per vaginum → platelet disorders
- Bleeding into joints, muscles → hemophilia (coagulation disorder)
- Bleeding from multiple sites → DIC
- Bleeding out of proportion to anemia → think of acute leukemias, aplastic anemia, coagulation disorders, anticoagulant therapy and SLE instead of simple thrombocytopenia where anemia is usually proportionate to bleeding
- Purpura without splenomegaly → think of aplastic anemia.

Purse-lip Respiration

WHAT IS THIS RESPIRATION?

It is breathing that consists of exhaling through tightly pressed lips and inhaling through nose with mouth closed. This technique can ease shortness of breath in few respiratory diseases (Fig. 62.1).

CONDITIONS ASSOCIATED

Chronic obstructive pulmonary diseases (COPD), i.e. where there is chronic obstruction to airflow due to chronic bronchitis, emphysema and chronic bronchiolitis.

WHY IS THERE PURSE-LIP RESPIRATION?

Pursing of lips during expiration helps the patient to maintain high intrabronchial pressure above that within the surrounding alveoli (alveoli are overinflated or

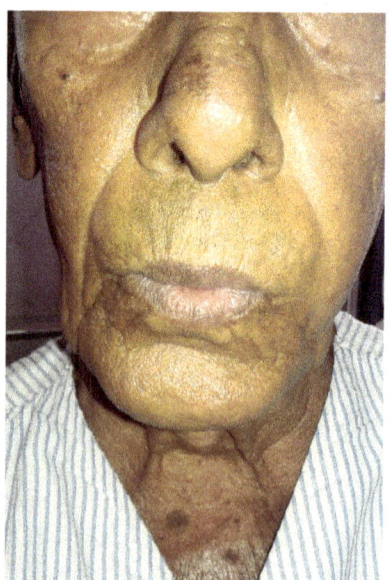

Fig. 62.1: Purse-lip respiration—exhaling through pursed lip while inhaling through nose to overcome shortness of breath

air-trapped in COPD patients) and thus helps to prevent the collapse of bronchial walls by overinflated alveoli.

BEDSIDE FINDINGS IN ADVANCED AIRFLOW OBSTRUCTION

- Dyspnea and even orthopnea (often with purse-lip respiration)
- Hyperactive accessory muscles of respiration
- Decrease in the length of trachea palpable above the suprasternal notch
- Tracheal tug, i.e. tracheal descent during inspiration
- Inspiratory excavation of the suprasternal notch and supraclavicular fossa
- Expiratory filling of neck veins
- Central cyanosis
- Intercostal suction
- Relative increase in antero-posterior diameter of the chest
- Wheezing.

Characteristic 'tripod' position (the patient sits with knee bending and flexed head placed in between knees) and Hoover's sign (paradoxical inward movement of rib cage with each inspiration) may be seen in advanced COPD.

AIR HUNGER

Deep sighing, rapid breathing at a regular rate and with a hissing sound (i.e. hyperpnea) is known as **Kussmaul's breathing** or air hunger. It is commonly seen in metabolic acidosis and may be called as 'acidotic breathing'. It is seen in:
- Ketoacidosis (diabetes, alcoholic)
- Uremia
- Lactic acidosis
- Sometimes in hepatic coma.

WHAT IS COR PULMONALE?

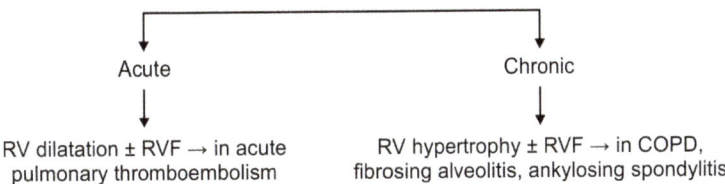

RVF = right ventricular failure; COPD = chronic obstructive pulmonary disease

SIGNS OF DETERIORATING PULMONARY FUNCTION (ACUTE SEVERE ASTHMA)

- Tachypnea, severe dyspnea (orthopnea) with wheezing
- Rising pulse rate
- Central cyanosis
- Inability to complete a sentence in one breath
- Progressive exhaustion
- Altered sensorium
- Profuse perspiration
- Pulsus paradoxus
- Silent chest
- Peak expiratory flow rate (PEFR) is <50% of predicted or patient's best.

MOUTH-BREATHING

- Nasal obstruction due to any cause, e.g. adenoids, nasopharyngeal fibroma, deviated nasal septum, antrochoanal polyp, mental subnormality, etc.
- It starts from childhood, and there is presence of:
  - High arched palate
  - Crowding of teeth
  - Underslung lower jaw and protrusion of upper jaw
  - Absence of nasolabial furrows.

HYPERVENTILATION

- Increase depth of respiration is hyperventilation (↑ rate + ↑ depth is **hyperpnea**; ↑ rate is **tachypnea**)
- Persistent hyperventilation is seen in:
  - Hysteria (young females mainly, if associated with 'hyperventilation syndrome', patient may complain of giddiness, tingling of extremities, black-out, weakness, palpitation; "main d'accoucheur" hand)
  - Anxiety neurosis, phobia, pain, panic reaction
  - Salicylate overdose
  - Pain anywhere in the body
  - Metabolic acidosis (diabetes mellitus, uremia)
  - Pyrexia
  - Fibrosing alveolitis, pneumothorax, bronchial asthma, pulmonary thromboembolism
  - Midbrain or pontine lesions.

SIGHING RESPIRATION

- Commonly seen in young females and children; functional in nature
- Deep inspiration → gap → forceful and deep expiration

- Occur in the presence of relatives or parents; never occurs during sleep or when left alone
- May have history of 'hyperventilation syndrome' → giddiness, black-out, tingling of extremities, circumoral numbness, palpitation, chest tightness with local tenderness elicited all over the chest, and features of tetany (carpopedal spasm).

GASPING RESPIRATION

Dying patients often take few deep, irregular and intermittent inspirations mimicking a 'fish out of water', is known as 'gasping' respiration. It is the terminal respiratory pattern of lower brainstem damage.

PERSISTENT HYPERCAPNEA

It is commonly seen in:
- COPD
- Hypercapnea with normal lung—metabolic alkalosis, primary alveolar hypoventilation, encephalitis
- Severe kyphoscoliosis, ankylosing spondylitis
- Myasthenia gravis, Guillain-Barré syndrome, poliomyelitis, motor neuron disease.

NOISY BREATHING

It is a labored breathing with snoring sound or associated with, wheezing or stridor (i.e. noisy).
- Upper respiratory tract infection, peritonsillar/retropharyngeal abscess, epiglottitis, tracheitis, bronchitis, bronchiolitis
- Bronchial asthma, angioedema, rhinitis or foreign body in respiratory tract
- Laryngeal webs, laryngotracheomalacia, cystic fibrosis, bronchiectasis or compression of airways from outside (e.g. huge goiter)
- Nasal polyp, hypertrophied adenoids/tonsils, vocal cord palsy.

BILATERAL POOR CHEST EXPANSION

Unilateral poor chest expansion is due to chest trauma, pleural effusion, pneumothorax, collapse/fibrosis/consolidation of lung. The causes of bilateral diminished movement of chest are different and they are:
- Emphysema (may lead to COPD)
- Diffuse interstitial fibrosis of lung
- Hydrothorax (bilateral)
- Ankylosing spondylitis
- Weak inspiratory muscles (e.g. myasthenia gravis, Guillain-Barré syndrome developing into respiratory paralysis)
- Obesity (producing hypoventilation syndrome).

RESPIRATORY PATTERNS IN COMA

- Post-hyperventilation apnea (periods of apnea coming after 5–10 deep breaths) indicates bifrontal disease.
- Cheyne–Stokes respiration (periods of apnea rhythmically alternates with periods of hyperpnea, i.e. a variety of periodic breathing) indicates supratentorial lesion, i.e. massive cerebral lesions, or seen in severe heart failure, renal failure, raised intracranial tension and narcotic poisoning.
- Central neurogenic hyperpnea (regular breathing with increased rate and depth) indicates midbrain-upper pontine lesion.
- Apneustic breathing (a pause of 2–3 seconds after full inspiration).
  or
  Biot's breathing (i.e. 3–4 respirations without waxing or waning, followed by a pause) indicates lower pontine lesion.
- Ataxic breathing (with chaotic rate, depth and rhythm) indicates medullary lesion.
- Hypoventilation (regular, rhythmic shallow breathing) may have lesion in brainstem.

THE PEARLS

In clinical medicine, 'respiration' is analyzed by rate, rhythm, type (abdominal or thoracic), depth, and breathing pattern. Different breathing patterns may give a clue to a particular clinical entity, e.g. purse-lip respiration in COPD, Kussmaul's breathing in diabetic ketoacidosis or gasping respiration in a moribund patient.

Rectal Bleeding

DEFINITION

It is the passage of bright red (i.e. fresh) blood per rectum during defecation. Blood in the stool may be present in three different forms:
1. Frank blood or hematochezia
2. Altered blood or melena
3. Invisible blood or occult blood (detected chemically at laboratory).

Visible blood per anum signifies bleeding from a source which is usually distal to ligament of Treitz, in comparison to melena where the bleeding site is proximal to ligament of Treitz.

- Frank blood per anum with or without stool is hematochezia
- Massive upper gastrointestinal (GI) bleed may give rise to bright or dark red (maroon) colored stool, if there is hurried peristalsis.

POSSIBLE ASSOCIATIONS

- **Anal:** Fissure, fistula, trauma, foreign body, carcinoma, prolapse of mucosa
- **Rectal:** Hemorrhoids, polyp, carcinoma, foreign body, proctitis (ulcerative/radiation), villous adenoma, solitary rectal ulcer
- **Colon:** Carcinoma (especially left colon), diverticular disease, angiodysplasia, dysentery (amebic/bacillary), colitis (ischemic/radiation/uremic/infectious), inflammatory bowel disease, irritant drug-induced
- **Small intestine:** Ischemic bowel disease (mesenteric embolism/thrombosis, vasculitis), Peutz-Jeghers syndrome, tuberculous enteritis, Crohn's disease, volvulus, intussusception, Henoch-Schönlein purpura, lymphoma/Kaposi's sarcoma, Meckel's diverticulitis, hereditary hemorrhagic telangiectasis, aortoenteric fistula
- **Miscellaneous:** Blood dyscrasias, anticoagulant therapy, uremia, hemangioma, endometriosis of rectum (rare), massive upper GI bleeding.

HOW TO MANAGE THIS PATIENT INITIALLY?

- Intravenous infusion + colloids
- Check hemoglobin, urine routine examination

BLACK STOOL IN CLINICAL PRACTICE

- Melena
- Ingestion of iron (as a hematinic) usually associated with hard stool
- Ingestion of bismuth (in anti-*Helicobacter pylori* treatment)
- Intake of licorice, charcoal (in the treatment of poisoning) or blackberries.

> Other than melena, all are non-sticky (pseudomelena).

CHARACTERISTICS OF MELENA STOOL

Melena is 'altered blood in stool' with features of:
- Black tarry stool (due to acid hematin); sticky too
- Offensive (acid hematin is altered by bacteria)
- Semisolid in consistency
- Red-colored fluid comes out from the stool after addition of water
- Usually associated with vertigo, dizziness or syncopal attack during defecation.

SEVEN COMMON CAUSES OF BRIGHT RED BLEEDING PER RECTUM

1. Bleeding hemorrhoids
2. Polyps
3. Diverticular disease
4. Colitis
5. Angiodysplasia of colon
6. Carcinoma (rectal or colonic)
7. Ischemic bowel disease.

Note: In the presence of severe diverticular disease, a polyp or carcinoma should always be excluded by colonoscopy as they can be the cause of bleeding. Hemorrhoids are so common that they should not be granted as the cause and effect of rectal bleeding in a particular patient → always search the above.

FROM BENCH TO BEDSIDE

- ***Anal fissure:*** Bright red-colored; clearly seperated from the feces → often seen only in toilet paper; associated with anal pain 'during and after defecation.'

- **Hemorrhoids:** Profuse bleeding → splash the toilet pan and/or continue 'following defecation.'
- **Colitis (e.g. ulcerative):** Associated with urgency of defecation → passage of liquid or semisolid bloody stool mixed with mucus and pus.

BLEEDING PER RECTUM WITH ACUTE ABDOMEN
- Mesenteric ischemia
- Ischemic colitis
- Necrotizing enterocolitis (NEC)
- Intussusception.

TENESMUS IN CLINICAL PRACTICE

It is the feeling of incomplete evacuation with a constant desire for defecation (often associated with rectal pain), and is commonly seen in:
- Infective colitis (e.g. amebic and bacillary dysentery)
- Rectal carcinoma
- Rectal prolapse
- Tumor of descending colon
- Irritable bowel syndrome (IBS)
- Acute proctitis
- Impacted feces
- Pelvic inflammatory disease.

Tenesmus (rectal) is the homologue of strangury (of micturition).

THE PEARLS

In a developing country like India, where the poor people use shabby and dark toilet, or go to open field for defecation, it is very difficult for them to diagnose 'rectal bleeding' on their own.

It is customary to inspect one's stool by his own or look for the toilet paper for signs of rectal bleeding. Many a time, it is profuse and needs immediate attention. One has to remember that hemorrhoids are benign but rectal malignancy may kill a person. So, early diagnosis of the etiology is always beneficial for the patient.

64

Recurrent Oral Ulcers

DEFINITION

Recurrent oral ulcers (ROUs) consist of repeated bouts of one/more, small/large, painless/painful ulcers occurring at intervals of days to a few months.

POSSIBLE ASSOCIATIONS

- ***Unknown:*** Aphthous ulcer (Fig. 64.1), periodic fever, tumor necrosis factor receptor-associated periodic syndrome.
- ***Infections:*** Herpes simplex virus (HSV type 1 mainly), HIV (human immunodeficiency virus), herpes zoster (in acute infective phase), CMV (cytomegalovirus) in immunocompromized host, coxsackie A (hand, foot and mouth disease).
- ***Rheumatic diseases:*** Behcet's disease (painful), systemic lupus erythematosus (SLE) [painless commonly (Fig. 64.2)] and discoid lupus erythematosus (DLE), reactive arthritis (Reiter's syndrome), Sweet's syndrome.
- ***Dermatological diseases:*** Erythema multiforme, toxic epidermal necrolysis, pemphigus vulgaris, lichen planus, bullous pemphigoid, dermatitis herpeteformis, epidermolysis bullosa.

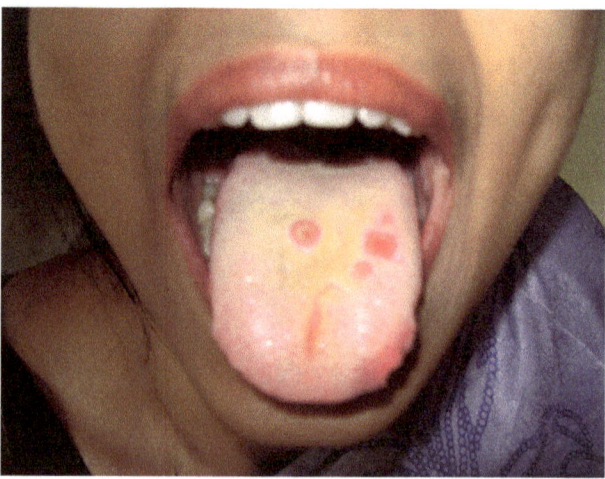

Fig. 64.1: Multiple, painful aphthous ulcers (recurrent) over tongue with fur around

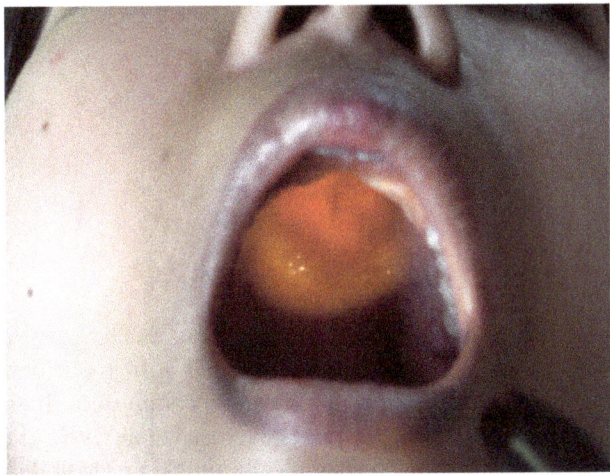

Fig. 64.2: Multiple, painless palatal ulcers (recurrent) in systemic lupus erythematosus (SLE)

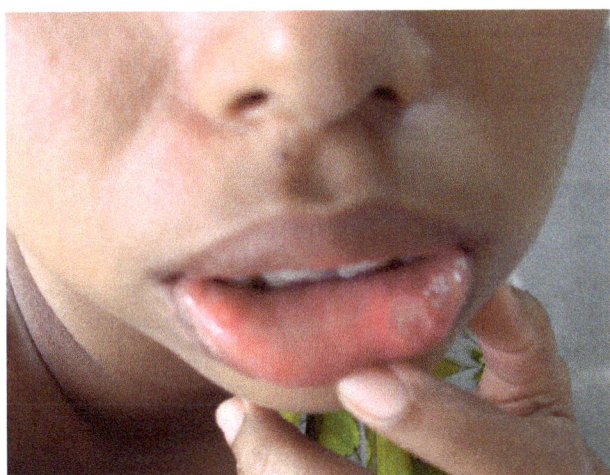

Fig. 64.3: Solitary painful ulcer in lip in acute myeloid leukemia

- ***Hematological diseases:*** Cyclic neutropenia, leukemia (Fig. 64.3), immunodeficiency disorders.
- ***Gastrointestinal diseases:*** Coeliac disease, inflammatory bowel diseases (IBD), i.e. ulcerative colitis and Crohn's disease.
- ***Traumatic:*** Laceration by sharp teeth, tooth brushing, ill-fitted dentures.
- ***Drugs:*** NSAIDs (nonsteroidal anti-inflammatory drugs), β-blockers, nicorandil, alendronate, gold salts, antimalarials, sodium lauryl sulfate (a component of toothpaste).

NOTABLE CAUSES

- Aphthous ulcer
- Celiac disease

- IBD
- Behçet's disease
- SLE
- Erythema multiforme
- Neutropenia (cyclic)
- Oral trauma
- Idiopathic.

RECURRENT APHTHOUS STOMATITIS (RAS)

These are also known as aphthae or canker sores. RAS is prevalent in women, < 40 years of age, whites, non-smokers, and people of high socioeconomic status. Probably, it is the most common cause of ROU in a community. These are recurring 'painful' ulcers of the mouth that are round or ovoid, shallow with a gray/white center, and have inflammatory halos. The ulcers typically appear first in childhood (may have a positive family history of RAS) and tend to abate around the third decade. The term 'RAS' should be reserved for recurrent ulcers confined to the mouth (labial or buccal mucosae, floor of the mouth, ventral surface or sides of the tongue), and are seen in the absence of any systemic disease. There is associated lymphadenopathy. However, ulcers that resemble RAS, can be found in systemic disorders like Behcet's syndrome, celiac disease or IBD, and immunodeficiency syndromes such as HIV infection or cyclic neutropenia.

Types

Minor and major type: **Minor** (80%) aphthous ulcers are < 10 mm in diameter, affect non-keratinized mucosae, and heal spontaneously within 10–14 days without scarring. Much less common are **major** aphthous ulcers—larger ulcers—often 1 cm or more in diameter, persists for weeks or months, and heal with scarring.

Various factors have been suggested to precipitate outbreaks of RAS in predisposed persons, including oral trauma, cessation of smoking, anxiety or stress, sensitivities to food preservatives, infections and hormonal changes related to the menstrual cycle.

EVALUATION OF RECURRENT ORAL ULCERS

- **History:** First attack/recurrent, oral trauma, stress, promiscuous sex, drug history.
- **Clinical examination:** Fever, joint pain/swelling, diarrhea, skin rash (butterfly-rash in face), urethritis, site of ulcer (palate—SLE, undersurface of tongue—probably aphthous ulcer).

INVESTIGATIONS

- Complete blood count
- Measurement of red-cell folate, serum vitamin B12, serum ferritin (especially, when findings suggest nutritional deficiency or hematologic disorder)

- Biopsy should be considered, if lasts for > 3 weeks
- Immunostaining is mandatory if a mucocutaneous disorder is suspected
- Serologic tests for rheumatologic diseases, e.g. rheumatoid factor, ANA (antinuclear antibodies), anti-dsDNA (double stranded DNA)
- Cultures or other specific tests for infectious agents (e.g. HSV, HIV, CMV)
- Evaluation of gastrointestinal diseases (e.g. studies of malabsorption, intestinal biopsy).

MANAGEMENT

Aphthous ulcer may affect as much as 20% of the population and often recalcitrant to treatment. Amount of pain is a matter of concern to the patient. Avoid oral trauma (e.g. hard toothbrush or foods such as toast) and acidic foods/drinks. Topical anesthetics (e.g. 0.15% benzydamine or 5% lidocaine gel) or protective bioadhesives (e.g. carmellose or cyanoacrylate) may be used four times daily for 2 weeks. Corticosteroids (1% triamcinolone paste, 2.5 mg hydrocortisone pellets or 0.05% fluocinonide in Orabase) may be used locally. Chlorhexidine gluconate (0.12–2%), triclosan or listerine mouthwash may be of some help; even tetracycline mouthrinse (contents of 100 mg doxycycline capsule dissolved in 10 mL of water) may also benefit patients. Amlexanox paste (5%) is a topical anti-inflammatory agent and early therapy with this drug may reduce size, pain and duration of aphthous ulcer. NSAID may be used, as and when pain is intolerable.

Major ulcers may be treated with systemic corticosteroid (30–60 mg prednisolone daily for 7 days, and tapered over the second week) and thalidomide [50–200 mg daily; especially for recurrent aphthae in AIDS (acquired immune deficiency syndrome patients)].

Other drugs like levamisole, colchicine, dapsone, azathioprine and pentoxifylline have also been tried in more refractory cases with variable effects.

POSSIBLE CAUSES OF INFLAMED (RED) PHARYNX ± TONSILS

- Viral pharyngitis (sore throat, odynophagia, pyrexia, inflamed fauces, cervical nodes +)
- Acute follicular tonsillitis (sore throat ++, odynophagia, pyrexia, swollen and patch tonsil, cervical nodes +)
- Agranulocytosis (sore throat, history of intake of offending drugs)
- Infectious mononucleosis (sore throat ++, petechial hemorrhages at the junction of soft and hard palate, pyrexia, cervical/generalized lymphadenopathy, palpable spleen)
- Meningitis [meningococcal (headache, vomiting, nuchal headache, sore throat, inflamed fauces ± purulent patches, neck rigidity)].

THE PEARLS

Always exclude oral carcinoma by repeated systemic examination (e.g. ipsilateral cervical adenopathy in an oral ulcer with induration/leukoplakia may indicate malignancy). Aphthous ulcer is benign per se but ulcers associated with vasculitis (e.g. Behçet's syndrome) are stubborn to treatment.

Red Urine

POSSIBILITIES

- Hematuria (most common cause)
- Hemoglobinuria
- Myoglobinuria
- Acute intermittent porphyria
- Drugs and vegetables, and others:
  - Phenolphthalein (in alkaline medium)
  - Rifampicin
  - Phenazopyridine
  - Clofazimine
  - Phenindione
  - Pigment of malignant melanoma
  - Beet roots, blackberries and vegetable dyes (e.g. food dye like acanthocyanins)
  - Phenol, thymol, senna, rhodamine B.

Dipstick-positive red urine are—hematuria, hemoglobinuria and myoglobinuria.

DIAGNOSIS

- ***Hematuria:*** Presence of blood in urine (often turbid) (Fig. 65.1). Microscopic examination of urine demonstrates plenty of RBCs (red blood cells) [normal urine contains not more than 3 RBCs/HPF (high power field) of uncentrifuged urine].
- ***Hemoglobinuria/myoglobinuria:*** Clear red or coca-cola colored urine. Special investigation like absorption spectroscopy confirms the constituents of urine sample as hemoglobin or myoglobin. When urine sediment gives a positive occult blood test, but no RBC are microscopically seen, myoglobinuria or hemoglobinuria is suspected. If the blood from these patients is kept in a test tube for few minutes, the supernatent serum will be reddish or pinkish in patients with myoglobinuria but the serum will be clear in patients suffering from hemoglobinuria.
- ***Porphyria:*** Freshly voided urine may be of normal colour but typical port-wine colour develops on standing because porphobilinogen polymerizes spontaneously to uroporphyrin and porphobilin. The confirmation of these products in urine is done by Watson-Schwartz test.

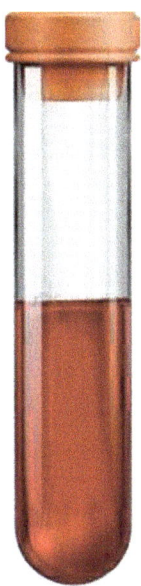

Fig. 65.1: Hematuria in a patient with papilloma of urinary bladder

- **Drugs and others:** Abstinence from intake of drugs will make the urine clear. Few drops of sodium hydroxide make the urine yellow, if it is blackberries or beet root-induced redness of urine.

- *Serratia marcescens* produces red urine and is known as red diaper syndrome.
- Collection of urine during menstruation and patients on anticoagulant therapy may falsely record RBC in urine.

COMMON CAUSES OF HEMOGLOBINURIA (INTRAVASCULAR HEMOLYSIS)

- **Acquired:** Incompatible transfusion, malaria (*Plasmodium falciparum*), clostridial infection, snake bite, systemic lupus erythematosus (SLE) or lymphoma-induced immune haemolytic anaemia, paroxysmal nocturnal hemoglobinuria (PNH), paroxysmal cold hemoglobinuria, methyldopa or penicillin-induced, septicemia, or extensive burn.
- **Hereditary:** Sickle cell disease, hemolytic crises, glucose-6-phosphate dehydrogenase (G6PD) deficiency, hereditary spherocytosis/elliptocytosis.

In hemoglobinuria, hemoglobin passes into urine (but no intact RBC is found).

LABORATORY FEATURES OF HEMOLYSIS

1. ↑ Serum bilirubin (unconjugated > conjugated; usually < 6 mg/dL)
2. ↑ Urinary urobilinogen
3. ↓ Plasma haptoglobin and ↓ hemopexin
4. Hemoglobinemia and hemoglobinuria
5. ↑ Methemalbumin in blood (detected by Schumm test)
6. ↑ Urinary hemosiderin
7. Fragmented RBCs in peripheral blood; may show spherocytes, target cells
8. Reticulocytosis
9. Hyperplastic bone marrow.

4 to 6 are classically seen in intravascular hemolysis.

CAUSES OF HEMATURIA

- **Renal:** Acute glomerulonephritis, papillary necrosis
- **Ureter:** Calculus, neoplasm
- **Bladder:** Cystitis, papilloma
- **Urethra:** Urethritis, trauma
- **Prostate:** Benign/malignant hypertrophy
- **Drugs:** Aspirin, anticoagulants, hexamine
- **Miscellaneous:** SLE, subacute bacterial endocarditis (SBE), leukemia, malignant hypertension, Henoch-Schönlein purpura (HSP), vasculitis, Weil's disease, renal ischemia, renal tuberculosis, Goodpasture's syndrome.

HARD DATA IN HEMATURIA

- **Renal disease:** Associated with significant proteinuria and RBC casts.
- **Infection:** Presence of pyuria.
- **Painless or painful:** Infection, calculus, papillary necrosis and trauma are associated with pain. **Painless hematuria** is classically seen in hypernephroma, tuberculosis of the kidney, sometimes in papilloma of urinary bladder, polycystic kidney, SLE, SBE, IgA nephropathy, hypertension, acute glomerulonephritis and acute cortical necrosis.
- **Timing of hematuria:**
  - Initial part—lesion in urethra
  - Terminal part—lesion in bladder
  - Uniformly distributed and mixed—usually renal or ureteric lesion but may occur in bladder lesion.
- **Microscopic hematuria:** When the urine color is normal and presence of RBCs are detectable only under light microscopic examination, it is designated as microscopic hematuria. The common associations are:

- Urinary tract infection (UTI)
- SBE
- Drug-induced (e.g. anticoagulants)
- SLE
- Acute glomerulonephritis
- Calculus in the urinary tract.

COMMON MEDICAL CAUSES OF HEMATURIA

- Acute glomerulonephritis
- SBE (usually microscopic hematuria)
- Malignant hypertension
- Snake bite (Viperidae group)
- HSP or other coagulation disorders
- Weil's disease
- Anticoagulant therapy
- Renal tuberculosis
- Papillary necrosis (diabetes mellitus, sickle cell disease, analgesic-induced)
- SLE (e.g. vasculitis).

MYOGLOBINURIA

- Severe muscle trauma (crush injury)
- Hyperthermia
- Polymyositis/dermatomyositis
- Carbon monoxide poisoning
- Drugs toxicity, e.g. nicotinic acid or amphetamine
- Acute myocardial infarction (AMI)
- Hypothyroidism
- Muscle ischemia
- Rhabdomyolysis (heat stroke, crush injury, severe exercise, seizures, alcohol-induced toxicity, influenza-induced, arterial insufficiency, ↓ K, ↓ PO_4 or G6PD ↓)
- Phosphorylase deficiency (hereditary myoglobinuria).

TREATMENT (HEMATURIA)

- Reassurance. The patient may require tranquilizer
- Plenty of fluid to be taken to flush the crystals and clots
- Treatment of specific etiology
- Renal colic may be alleviated by antispasmodic-analgesic
- **Blood transfusion** in profound hematuria
- Referral to surgeon, if necessary.

THE PEARLS

Red urine in a patient gives rise to tremendous anxiety and worry. Drug and dietary history are very important. Routine examination of urine under microscope is often rewarding. As some of the patients with red urine may land in malignancy (e.g. papilloma of urinary bladder), an immediate attention is needed by the attending doctor.

66
Rings around Cornea

DIFFERENTIAL DIAGNOSIS OF RINGS OR PIGMENTATION AT LIMBUS

- Kayser-Fleischer ring (K-F ring)
- Arcus senilis or arcus juvenilis
- Band keratopathy
- Argyrosis (dark-brown discoloration at limbus or of conjunctiva due to prolonged use of silver nitrate preparation as eye drop or as a result of working with silver dust)
- Cystinosis (deposition of cystine crystals)
- Chloroquine crystals after long-continued use, e.g. discoid lupus erythematosus (DLE).

> Blood-staining ring in severe hyphema and deposition of melanin pigment in high myopia are not uncommon.

KAYSER-FLEISCHER RING

- Golden-brown pigment of copper deposited in the Descemet's membrane layer of cornea in a patient suffering from Wilson's disease
- Seen at limbus; broaded superiorly and inferiorly than laterally and medially; the superior pole is affected first
- May be seen in naked-eye examination but confirmation with slit-lamp examination by an ophthalmologist is a must
- Clinical hallmark of Wilson's disease, and is present in >99% patients with neurologic or psychiatric form of the disease:
- Eyes in Wilson's disease—look for
  - Jaundice
  - K-F ring
  - Sunflower cataract
- K-F ring never hampers vision
- K-F like ring is seen in:
  - Cryptogenic cirrhosis

- Prolonged cholestasis, e.g. primary biliary cirrhosis
- Long-standing intrahepatic cholestasis in childhood.

WILSON'S DISEASE

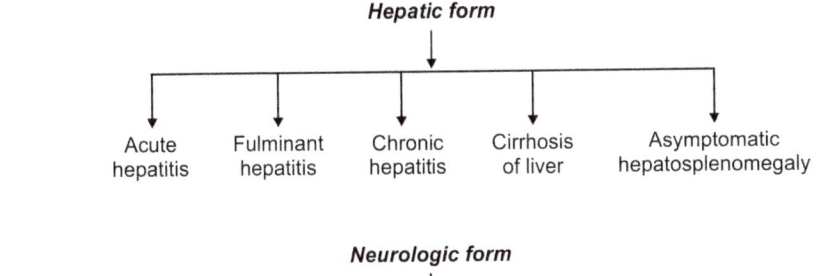

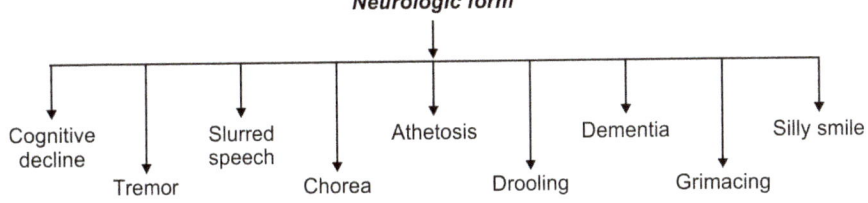

Diagnosis

- Ceruloplasmin in serum (< 20 mg/dL)
- K-F ring (Fig. 66.1)
- Copper in liver biopsy > 200 µg/g of dry weight of liver
  Confirmation: 1 + 2, or 1 + 3.

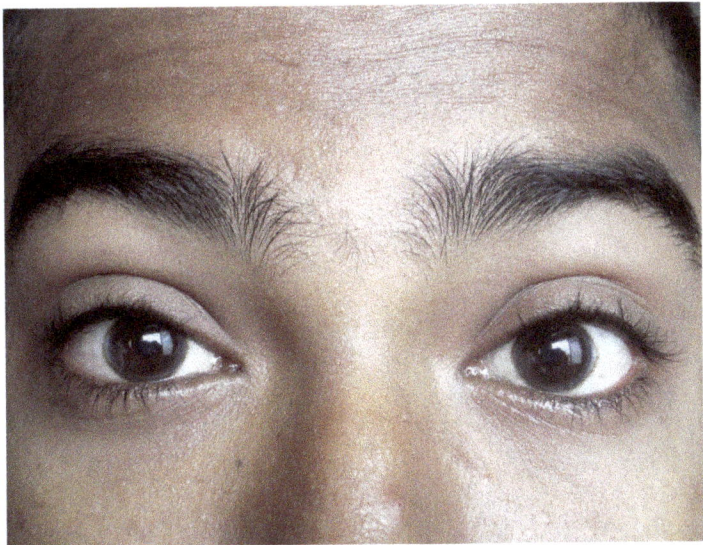

Fig. 66.1: Kayser-Fleischer (K-F) ring at limbus of both eyes in Wilson's disease in an young patient

Drugs used in Wilson's Disease

- D-penicillamine (1–1.5 g/day) with pyridoxine supplementation (25 mg/day)
- Elemental zinc as acetate (50 mg thrice daily)
- Trientine dihydrochloride (1.2–1.8 g/day)
- Potassium iodide (20 mg, qds)
- Cobalt chloride
- Tetrathiomolybdate

D-penicillamine is the mainstay of treatment. As it is a toxic drug, elemental zinc is now the therapy of choice by most of the clinicians.

ARCUS SENILIS (ARCUS CORNEAE) (FIG. 66.2)

- In aged persons (usually > 50 years); starts in lower pole and gradually affects the upper pole
- Grayish-white circular ring, may be partial or complete
- Just within limbus, so a clear area of cornea remains within the arcus and the limbus
- Represents deposition of cholesterol and phospholipid mainly in the substantia propria layer of cornea; search for xanthelasma around the eyes
- Virtually of no significance in elderly people (as like gray hair in scalp) but if present in less than 50 years *(arcus juvenilis)*, may be associated with atherosclerosis, systemic hypertension, ischemic heart disease (IHD), diabetes mellitus, myocardial infarction or stroke.

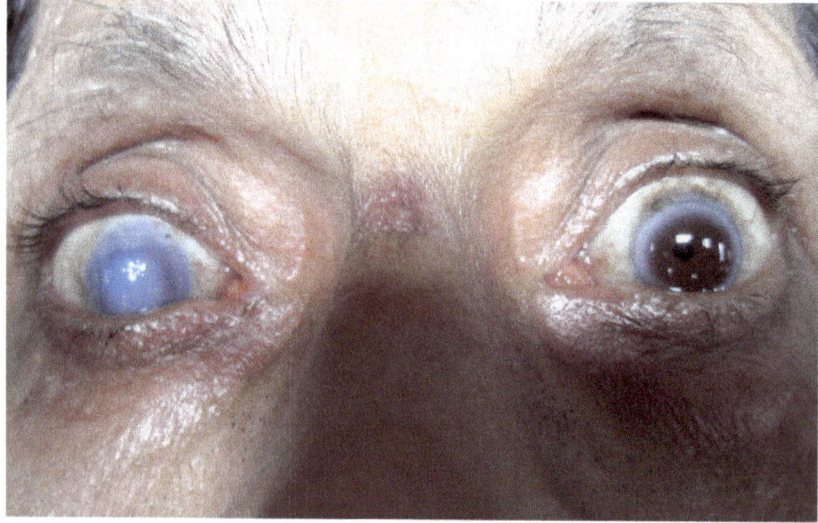

Fig. 66.2: Right eye with corneal opacity along with cataract, and arcus senilis in left eye of an aged person

BAND KERATOPATHY

- Corneal calcification, usually at the lateral and medial margins of cornea
- Seen in long-standing hypercalcemia, e.g. hyperparathyroidism.

THE PEARLS

Rings around cornea is commonly due to 5 'C', e.g. copper, cholesterol, calcium, cystine and chloroquine. Among all, K-F ring demands major attention. A patient of Wilson's disease with neuropsychiatric manifestations must have K-F ring in cornea. Arcus senilis is common and may indirectly points towards atherosclerosis. Anyway, pigmentation or rings at limbus does not hamper vision.

67

Shake Hands with the Patient

CLUE TO DIAGNOSIS

- The first physical contact with the doctor diagnoses is the dominant hand, i.e. the handedness of the patient
- A determined grip or soft, careless handshake often reflects the personality of the patient (Fig. 67.1)
- Weak grip-strength—weakness of small muscles of the hand, weakness of long flexor muscles or diseases of joints (i.e. to diagnose neurological or musculoskeletal diseases)
- Warm and moist hand—thyrotoxicosis, type II respiratory failure; pyrexia, palmar erythema and Paget's disease may give rise to warm hands (Fig. 67.2)

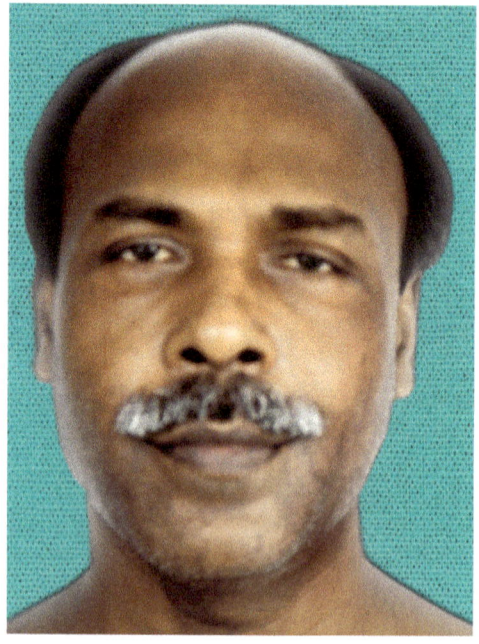

Fig. 67.1: Frontal baldness and bilateral partial ptosis in myotonic dystrophy (unable to relax the grip of handshake)

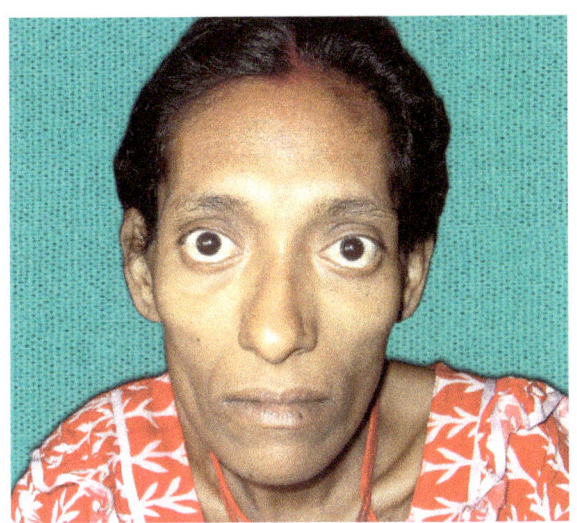

Fig. 67.2: Thyrotoxicosis with exophthalmos (warm and moist hand)

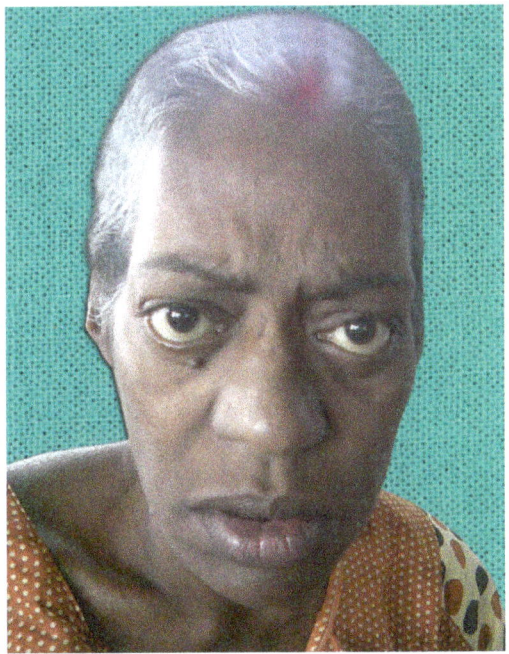

Fig. 67.3: Acromegaly with apparent exopthalmos (moist and doughy handshake)

- Cold and moist hand—anxiety neurosis; hypothermia and Raynaud's phenomenon produce only coldness of hands
- Cold and dry hand—myxedema
- Moist and doughy handshake—acromegaly (Fig. 67.3)

- Shake hand producing pain—rheumatoid arthritis
- Rough and thick palm—phrenoderma (vitamin A or essential fatty acid deficiency), tylosis (hyperkeratosis of palm often associated with carcinoma of the esophagus), arsenic poisoning, verruca vulgaris and psoriasis (palmar)
- Unable to relax the grip—myotonia dystrophica (Fig. 67.1)
- Digital throbbing—may point towards aortic incompetence
- Tremor—specially coarse tremor like flapping tremor (milkmaid's grip)
- Warmth, sincerety and personality—shake hand with both the hands.

- Face → mirror of the mind
- Hand → directed by the mind.

HANDS IN THYROTOXICOSIS

- Moist hand
- Warm palm
- Tremor (fine)
- Tachycardia
- Palmar erythema
- Plummer's nail (separation of distal margin of the nail from nail-bed)
- Clubbing (thyroid acropachy)
- Hyperpigmentation and vitiligo, rarely
- Spider nevi, rarely.

HANDS IN CIRRHOSIS OF LIVER

- Palmar erythema
- Leukonychia
- Clubbing, especially in biliary cirrhosis
- Jaundice
- Spider nevi
- Bleeding manifestations, e.g. petechiae, purpura, ecchymosis
- Flapping tremor in hepatic precoma
- Dupuytren's contracture in alcoholic cirrhosis
- Diffuse pigmentation on dorsum of hands.

WARM PALMS

- Pyrexia
- Type II respiratory failure, especially from chronic obstructive pulmonary disease (COPD)
- Thyrotoxicosis
- Palmar erythema (blanches on pressure)
- Paget's disease.

Note: Type II respiratory failure (combined hypercapnea and hypoxia)

- *Features of hypercapnea:* Headache, drowsiness, confusion/coma, flapping tremor, warm extremities, muscles twitching, water-hammer pulse, capillary pulsation, ↑ BP, papilledema and chemosis of the conjunctiva.
- *Features of hypoxia:* Restlessness, confusion, central cyanosis, tachycardia, ↓ BP, cardiac arrhythmias, convulsions, coma.

BP = blood pressure

Most common cause of respiratory failure is chronic bronchitis.

THE PEARLS

The first handshake with the patient builds up the first step in doctor-patient relationship. Many a time, examination of the hand gives a lot of information and helps to reach the final diagnosis. Examination of the hand is similarly important as the 'face reading' in clinical medicine.

Sneezing, Yawning and Snoring

SNEEZING

Act

Deep inspiration → violent and forceful expulsion of air through nose and mouth due to irritation of nostrils → give rise to a characteristic sound (sneeze). Sneezing is controlled by a reflex through trigeminal and vagus nerves.

Mechanism

Stimuli (dust, dirt, other irritant foreign body)
↓
Irritates the nasal endings of the trigeminal nerve present in nasal mucosa
↓
Sensory impulses are transmitted
↓
Sneezing.

Causes in Clinical Practice

- **Local:** Acute coryza (common cold), nasal allergy (allergic rhinitis), hay fever, foreign body in nose, irritant gases like tear gas/chlorine/phosgene/fumes from cooking oil, nasal polyp, or from pets/pollens/mold
- **Systemic:** Prodromal stage of measles/chickenpox/influenza/whooping cough
- **Miscellaneous:** Neurosis, hysteria, aspirin/iodide-induced, voluntary induction, change of environmental temperature, withdrawal state in opium addict.

> **THE PEARLS**
> - Essentially a protective reflex similar to cough and a helpful compensatory mechanism to clean the nasal cavity of foreign bodies or irritant gases.
> - Sneezing may be voluntary or involuntary; voluntary sneeze can be induced with a wisp of cloth/cotton/paper by touching the nasal mucosa or septum to find pleasure out of it.
> - Change of temperature may induce sneezing in some persons having hyperalgesia of nasal mucosa.
> - Bouts of sneezing, especially on waking in the morning may be an indicator of hay fever.
> - Strong sunlight may stimulate trigeminal nerve endings resulting in sneezing.

Contd…

Contd...

- During sneezing, eyes close involuntarily.
- In some of the places in India, sneezing is regarded as a social taboo where it is an indicator of a bad sign if the characteristic sound is heard before a journey or initiation of an act.
- It is believed that people sneezes between 30 and 35 miles/hour, and the droplets can spread in a 5-foot radius.
- Antiallergics often give magic relief.
- Sneezing is also known as **sternutation**

YAWNING

Act

Tonic contraction of facial and pharyngeal muscles → a deep inspiration follows → dilatation of pharynx associated with depression of tongue with mandible → air goes inside lungs → often seen along with stretching of arms as when waking from sleep (pandiculation).

Mechanism

Stimuli (boredom, feeling sleepy, seeing other person to yawn)
↓
Center in brain is probably at basal ganglia
↓
Yawning.

Causes in Clinical Practice

Very little is known about its etiology. Yawning is basically physiological but few pathological causes may give rise to yawning like,
 Following attacks of encephalitis
 Posterior fossa tumor
- Lower brainstem lesion (yawning, vomiting and hiccough)
- Seizure disorders (e.g. epilepsy)
- Opium addict (when effect of opium ceases).

> **THE PEARLS**
> - Treatment of yawning is not required.
> - Increases venous return to the heart; closed pulmonary alveoli are also opened up.
> - Sense of smell is very high during the act of yawning, probably because of the entry of large amount of air within the nasopharynx.
> - Regarded as a **negative body language** if happens to occur in an interview table or in the classroom.
> - Paralysed arm in **pandiculation** may be stretched when no voluntary movement is possible.
> - Yawning may be provoked on sight or sound of someone else's yawn. No valid explanation is known for the contagious nature of yawning though it is well known (probably a mode of social communication).

SNORING

Act

It is a disorder of sleep which is due to vibration by turbulent airflow of soft tissue above larynx. Three potential areas may be responsible for obstruction, e.g. nose, palate and/or, hypopharynx.

Management

- Thorough Ear, Nose and Throat (ENT) check-up
- Weight reduction
- Repair of deviated nasal septum or nasal polyps, if present
- Sleep **nasendoscopy** to identify the source of vibration
- ***Surgery:*** Uvulopalatopharyngoplasty, softening or shortening of soft palate via laser surgery
- Dental prosthesis at night (to hold the mandible forward) for hypopharyngeal snorers
- Continuous positive airway pressure (CPAP) via mask in selected cases.

THE PEARLS
- Approximately 40% of middle-aged men and 20% of middle-aged women snore.
- Common in obese people .
- Snoring has association with obstructive sleep apnea (OSA) syndrome. Simple snorers can develop sleep apnea after ingestion of alcohol.
- Habitual snorers have a higher incidene of pulmonary hypertension.
- ***Epworth questionnaire*** (e.g. how likely are you to doze off or fall asleep) differentiate sleep apnea from simple snoring.
- Habitual, non-positional and heroic snorers are easily identified in the family, and are avoided by others during sleeping hours.

69

Splinter Hemorrhage

POSSIBLE CAUSES

These are linear longitudinal hemorrhages under the nail and are also known as splinter hemorrhage or Horder's line. They are found in:
- Trauma (most common)
- Acute leukemias
- Scurvy
- Subacute bacterial endocarditis (SBE)
- Systemic vasculitis
- Rheumatoid arthritis
- Psoriasis
- Trichinosis.

WHAT IS VASCULITIS?

It is a heterogeneous group of conditions with necrotizing inflammation of the blood vessels. Endothelial edema and proliferation with hemorrhage contribute to the occlusion of vascular lumen, which results in subsequent ischemic changes along with organ damage.

CLASSIFICATION FOLLOWED GLOBALLY

- *Large-vessel vasculitis:* Giant cell arteritis (temporal arteritis) and Takayasu's arteritis (aortic arch syndrome or pulseless disease).
- *Medium-sized vessel vasculitis:* Polyarteritis nodosa (PAN) and Kawasaki disease (mucocutaneous lymph node syndrome).
- *Small-vessel vasculitis of arterioles, capillaries and venules:* Wegener's granulomatosis (or granulomatosis with polyangiitis), microscopic polyangiitis, Churg-Strauss syndrome (CSS), leukocytoclastic vasculitis (hypersensitivity vasculitis), Henoch-Schönlein purpura (HSP or IgA vasculitis) and essential mixed cryoglobulinemia.

- This is the most accepted classification (Chapel Hill consensus Conference Classification, 1994) though 'overlap' is not uncommon.
- Systemic lupus erythematosus (SLE), Behcet's disease, scleroderma, polymyositis or dermatomyositis, rheumatoid arthritis, subacute bacterial endocarditis (SBE) and paraneoplastic syndromes are also associated with vasculitis.
- The above classification has been revised in 2012 to improve the existing nomenclature.

DIFFERENT DERMATOLOGICAL MANIFESTATIONS OF VASCULITIS

- Large arteries—digital gangrene (Fig. 69.1)
- Small arteries
  - Palpable purpura
  - Urticarial rashes (tender)
  - Morbilliform eruptions (look like measles rashes)
  - Maculopapular eruptions
  - Subcutaneous nodules
- Arterioles and very small arteries
  - Digital infarction (pitted scars) (*See* Fig. 9.2)
  - Digital ulceration (Figs 69.2 and 9.2)
  - Nail-fold thrombi
  - Splinter hemorrhage

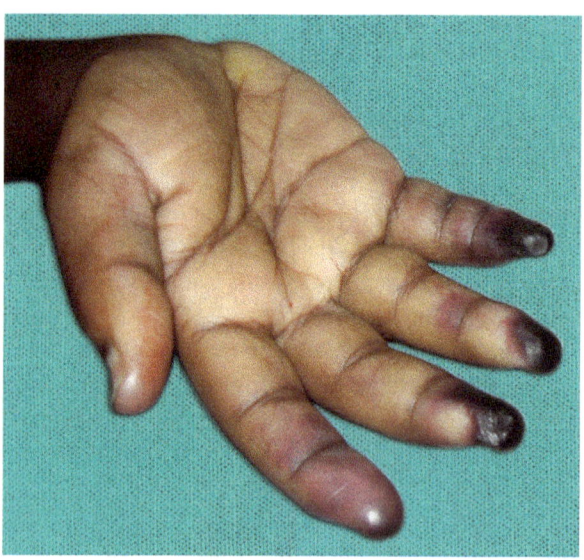

Fig. 69.1: Digital gangrene in tips of fingers in systemic vasculitis

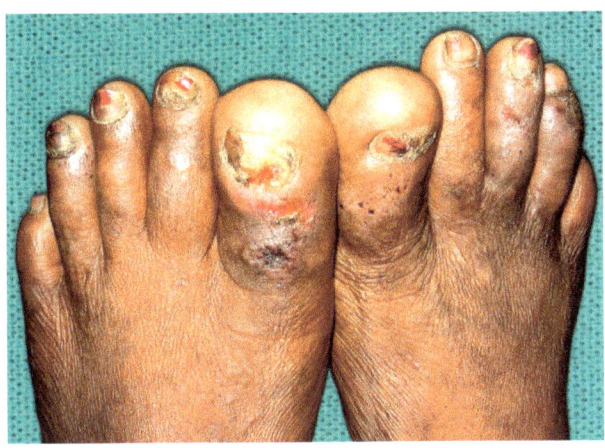

Fig. 69.2: Periungual erythema, nail dystrophy, swelling of the toes and digital ulceration in vasculitis

- Vesicular/bullous lesion
- Raynaud's phenomenon
- Pulp atrophy
- Necrotic ulcer.

DRUGS COMMONLY RESPONSIBLE FOR VASCULITIS

- Allopurinol
- Thiazides
- Propylthiouracil
- Carbimazole, methimazole
- Penicillins, minocycline, azithromycin, sulfonamides
- Montelukast, pranlukast
- Cocaine, morphine
- Phenytoin, gold
- Hydralazine.

Usually manifested as palpable purpura but may give rise to urticarial lesions, ulcerations and hemorrhagic blisters.

CUTANEOUS VERSUS SYSTEMIC VASCULITIS

- ***Predominantly cutaneous vasculitis:*** Usual presentation as palpable purpura, tender urticaria, bullous ulcers or splinter hemorrhages, commonly distributed over legs; buttocks and arms may be affected. The salient features are:
  - Absence of systemic involvement

- Small vessel leucocytoclastic vasculitis (numerous disrupted polymorphs at the site of damaged vessel) are caused by drugs, infection, inflammatory disease, malignancy or idiopathic
- Negative serology
- Course—variable, may be chronic and recurrent
- Confirmed by skin biopsy
- A better prognosis than systemic variety.
- **Systemic vasculitis**
  - Organ-specific clinical features (e.g. kidney—hypertension and renal failure; nerves—mononeuritis multiplex; gastrointestinal (GI) tract— bowel infarction)
  - Obviously, the prognosis is poor.

WHEN DO YOU SUSPECT VASCULITIS IN A PATIENT?

Presence of one or more findings described below should make the clinician suspicious. They are:
- Pyrexia of unknown origin, loss of weight
- Unexplained cerebrovascular accident (CVA) or coronary heart disease (CHD) events in the young
- Acute onset of mononeuropathy, e.g. wrist drop or foot drop
- Unexplained retinal vascular changes of acute onset without having diabetes mellitus or hypertension
- Occlusive arterial diseases or systemic hypertension in the young
- Unexplained proteinuria with or without casts
- Palpable purpura, splinter hemorrhage, erythema nodosum (Fig. 69.3), necrotic ulcer (Fig. 69.4) or Raynaud's phenomenon (*see* Fig. 9.1)
- Claudication of jaw
- Sudden monocular blindness in elderly with persistent headache
- Multiple organ dysfunction
- Unexplained chest X-ray with pulmonary nodular or cavitary lesions.

CLINICAL PEARLS TO DIAGNOSE VASCULITIS AT BEDSIDE

- Absent radial pulse or difficulty in obtaining blood pressure (BP)—Takayasu's arteritis; small nodules in the course of an artery—PAN.
- Visual loss, jaw claudication—giant cell arteritis (GCA)
- Hypertension—PAN and Takayasu's arteritis (renovascular), Wegener's granulomatosis (WG) and microscopic polyangiitis (MP) cause glomerular hypertension
- Mononeuritis multiplex—PAN, WG, CSS
- Sinus involvement—WG, MP
- Asthma—CSS; pulmonary involvement other than asthma are common in WG and MP
- Testicular tenderness—PAN

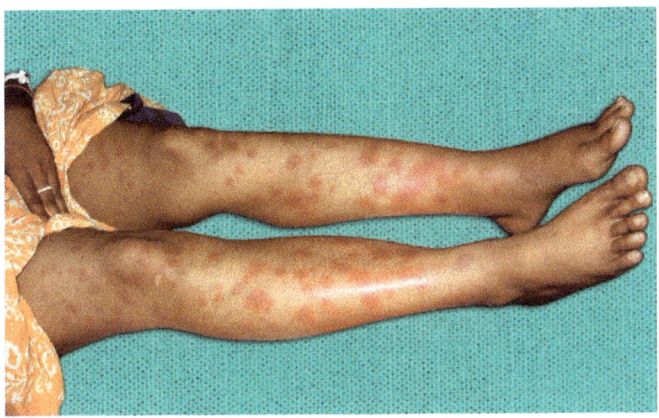

Fig. 69.3: Panniculitis (multiple erythema nodosum)

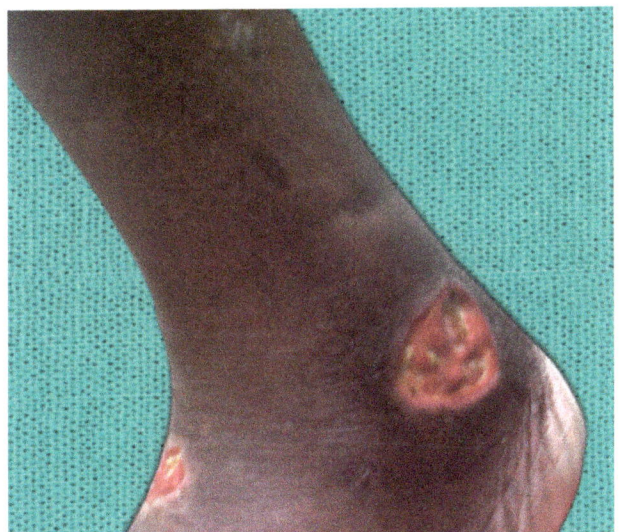

Fig. 69.4: Two punched-out, non-healing vasculitic ulcers in leg

- Bloody diarrhea—HSP
- Pulmonary-renal syndromes mimicking SLE and Goodpasture's syndrome in WG and MP.

VASCULITIS MIMICKERS (PSEUDOVASCULITIS)

Presence of one or more of the following will make the clinician suspicious of pseudovasculitis like extremes of age, usually with very high pyrexia, immunocompromised patient, appearance of new heart murmur (e.g. SBE), necrosis of lower extremity (e.g. cholesterol emboli), prior diagnosis of malignant disease, history of use of recreational drugs [(e.g. cocaine), human immunodeficiency virus

(HIV), hepatitis B virus (HBV)] or high-risk sexual activity, and acute onset with rapid deterioration of symptoms. The common vasculitis mimickers are:
- Septicemia
- Antiphospholipid antibody syndrome
- Bacterial endocarditis
- Thrombotic thrombocytopenic purpura (TTP)
- Lymphomas
- Ergot overdose/poisoning
- Viral infections, e.g. HBV, hepatitis C virus (HCV), HIV, cytomegalovirus (CMV)
- Cholesterol emboli syndrome
- Atrial myxoma
- Disseminated intravascular coagulation (DIC)
- Hypertensive arteriopathy
- Sarcoidosis.

Infections, thrombosis and neoplasia commonly mimic vasculitis.

DIAGNOSTIC WORK-UP FOR VASCULITIS

- *History and clinical examination* with special reference to peripheral pulses, discrepancies in BP, small nodules in the course of an artery, arterial bruit, different dermatological manifestations mentioned above, breath sound with adventitious sounds, etc.
- *Laboratory investigations* (done to confirm the diagnosis and to assess the extent of organ damage):
  - **Complete hemogram:** Majority have normocytic-normochromic anemia, leucocytosis (eosinophilia in CSS), ↑ erythrocyte sedimentation rate (ESR), ↑ C-reactive protein (CRP); usually the platelet count remains normal.
  - **Urine analysis:** Commonly having proteinuria, hematuria and red blood cell casts. Large-vessel vasculitis does not usually affect kidney.
  - **Serum proteins:**
    ↑ gamma-globulin of IgG type in majority [in HSP and WG, the gamma-globulin is immunoglobin A (IgA) type]
    ↑ IgE level in CSS
    ↓ complement level in SLE, cryoglobulinemia, polyarteritis nodosa.
  - Antinuclear antibody (ANA) test with anti-double stranded deoxyribonucleic acid (dsDNA) (SLE) or anti-topoisomerase 1 (scleroderma) or anti-Ro/La assay (Sjogren's syndrome).
  - Antineutrophil cytoplasmic antibodies (ANCA):
    - *C-ANCA ('c' stands for cytoplasmic):* Antibodies are directed against proteinase-3 (PR-3) and are commonly found in WG.
    - *P-ANCA ('p' stands for perinuclear):* Antibodies are directed against myeloperoxidase enzyme (MPO). They are commonly found in microscopic pol-

yangiitis, CSS, crescentic glomerulonephritis, inflammatory bowel disease, primary sclerosing cholangitis, classic polyarteritis nodosa, autoimmune chronic active hepatitis, primary biliary cirrhosis.
  - *'A' or x-ANCA ('A' stands for atypical):* It is a mixed pattern of fluorescence (i.e. cytoplasmic plus perinuclear). It is found in drug-induced vasculitis where the autoantibodies are directed against lactoferrin and elastase.
- *Selective organ biopsy:* It remains the gold standard for diagnosis of vasculitis. Full thickness biopsy should be taken from the involved site to diagnose cutaneous vasculitis. Usually, the histology shows vessel wall inflammation with perivascular involvement with or without leukocytoclasis. Renal biopsy is commonly performed.
- *Miscellaneous:*
  - Liver function panel
  - Renal function panel
  - Chest X-ray
  - CT (computed tomography) and MRI (magnetic resonance imaging) scan of thorax
  - Echocardiography (to rule out left ventricular dysfunction)
  - Serology for HBV, HCV, HIV, CMV, etc.
  - Pulmonary function tests which are useful in detecting stenosis of the airways (e.g. Wegener's granulomatosis).
- *Angiography:* It is helpful in diagnosing large and medium-vessel vasculitis. Polyarteritis nodosa may reveal multiple aneurysmal lesions.

- **ANCA**-Positive vasculitis are—Wegener's granulomatosis, microscopic polyangiitis and Churg-Strauss syndrome.
- **Treatment of vasculitis:** Cutaneous vaculitis may be self-limiting and may not require any treatment. Systemic vasculitis is treated with corticosteroid, usually in combination with immunosuppressive drugs.

SUBEPIDERMAL BLISTERS

Cutaneous blisters are known as vesicle (<0.5 cm) or bullae (>0.5 cm), and the common blistering diseases are:
- Bullous drug reaction
- Bullous pemphigoid
- Toxic epidermal necrolysis
- Dermatitis herpeteformis
- Epidermolysis bullosa
- Linear IgA disease
- Leukocytoclastic vasculitis
- Burns
- Porphyria cutanea tarda

- Acute graft-versus-host reaction
- Pressure necrosis
- Insect bite reaction
- Amyloidosis.

THE PEARLS

Vasculitis is a fatal disease and should be treated urgently as soon as diagnosis is confirmed, before the onset of organ damage.

Vasculitis should be differentiated from vasculitis mimickers (pseudovasculitis) to prevent the unnecessary use of immunosuppressants in vasculitis mimickers. A high index of suspicion, many a time, clinches the diagnosis of vasculitis. This type of patients are better dealt by a rheumatologist.

70

Spoon-shaped Nails

KOILONYCHIA (SPOON-SHAPED NAILS)

- Koilos means hollow
- Onikh means nail.

Method of Examination

Keep the patient's fingers at your eye level and look tangentially as done in clinical examination of clubbing. Observe as well as palpate the nails for spooning. The nails are soft, thin and brittle as well.

Clue to Diagnosis

- Iron deficiency anemia (Fig. 70.1) (most common cause; search for anemia, glossitis, angular stomatitis, cheilosis; enquire for dysphagia especially in middle aged women → Plummer-Vinson syndrome or Paterson-Kelly syndrome → endoscopic finding of *post-cricoid web* which is a premalignant condition) → meticulous history taking regarding chronic blood loss like menorrhagia, bleeding piles, melaena, nonsteroidal anti-inflammatory drug (NSAID) therapy; dietary history.

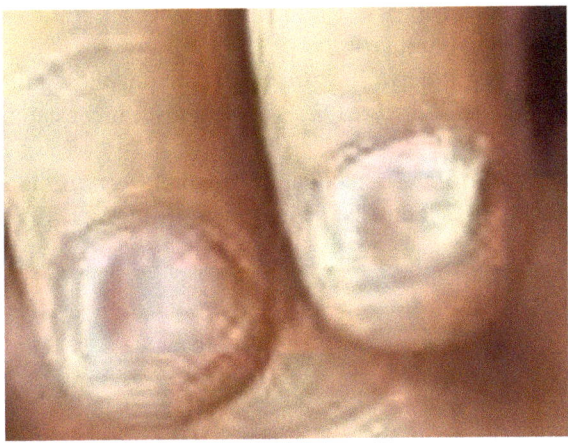

Fig. 70.1: Koilonychia in iron deficiency anemia

- Idiopathic or familial (examine the other members of the family) → autosomal dominant inheritance.
- Onycholysis (enquire for occupation like washer-woman; a person living in a high altitude may have onycholysis and koilonychia → i.e. from trauma).
- Overuse of solvent (e.g. nail varnish remover) or detergents for a long period.
- Very rarely in thyrotoxicosis (look for exophthalmos, tremor and tachycardia).

Stages of Koilonychia

- ***First stage:*** Stage of brittleness → nails are brittle and rough
- ***Second stage:*** Stage of flattening (platonychia) → nails are flat and thin, and there is absence of longitudinal ridges
- ***Third stage:*** Stage of spooning → nails are concave

- There is loss of normal convexity of nails
- The diagnosis of iron deficiency anemia is incomplete without an indication of its cause.

INVESTIGATIONS IN IRON DEFICIENCY ANEMIA

- ***Blood:*** Peripheral blood smear examination shows → ↓hemoglobin (Hb%), anisocytosis, poikilocytosis, occasionally target cells, microcytic-hypochromic anemia [central pallor of red blood cell (RBC) is considerably increased]. RDW (red cell distribution width) is more in iron deficiency anemia.
  ↓ Mean corpuscular hemoglobin (MCH), ↓ mean corpuscular hemoglobin concentration (MCHC), ↓ mean corpuscular volume (MCV)
  ↓ Serum iron (normal value: 70-140 µg/dL)
  ↓ Serum ferritin (normal value: 30–300 ng/mL)
  ↑ Total iron-binding capacity (TIBC) (normal value: 270-335 µg/dL)
- ***Stool:*** Occult blood present
  Hookworm ova present (chance finding)
- ***Per rectal and per vaginal examination:*** Carcinoma, piles or fibroid
- ***Upper and lower gastrointestinal endoscopy:*** Peptic ulcer, carcinoma of stomach or colon
- ***Bone marrow examination:*** Usually not necessary; ↑ erythroblasts in later stages of maturation with deficient Hb formation; staining reveals ↓ of storage iron (hemosiderin)

PITTING NAILS

- Psoriasis (thimble pitting)
- Eczema
- Alopecia areata
- Trauma.

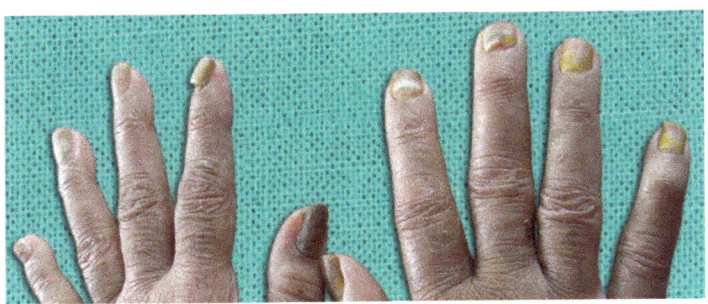

Fig. 70.2: Onycholysis in psoriasis; nail in left index finger is almost separated

ONYCHOLYSIS

- Candidiasis (onychomycosis)
- Ringworm infections
- Psoriasis (Fig. 70.2)
- Trauma
- Lichen planus
- Thyrotoxicosis (Plummer's nail)
- Chronic paronychia.

PLATONYCHIA (FLAT NAIL)

- Hereditary
- Iron deficiency anemia.

BITTEN NAILS

Persons with anxious personality.

SHINY NAILS

An indirect evidence of pruritus.

ONYCHODYSTROPHY

- Fungal infections
- Repeated trauma
- Reactive arthritis (Reiter's syndrome).

THE PEARLS

A simple clinical finding koilonychia becomes precious when an early gastrointestinal tract carcinoma presents with pallor (i.e. iron deficiency anemia evidenced by positive occult blood in stool), where the diagnosis comes out by meticulous clinical examination, and thereby prolongs the life of the patient by early detection of malignancy.

71 Sternal (Bone) Tenderness

BONES EXAMINED FOR DETECTION OF TENDERNESS
- Sternum
- Vertebrae
- Skull (forehead)
- Shin bone
- Ribs
- Wrists, ankles, pelvic bones, etc.

STERNAL TENDERNESS

Press the upper part of the body of sternum with ball of the right thumb for 2–3 seconds (Fig. 71.1). In the presence of sternal tenderness, the patient winces with pain (makes facial grimace) or complains of pain verbally.
- Clue to diagnosis in the presence of sternal tenderness
  - Acute leukemias [acute myeloid leukemia (AML) and acute lymphoblastic leukemia (ALL)]
  - Chronic myeloid leukemia (CML)

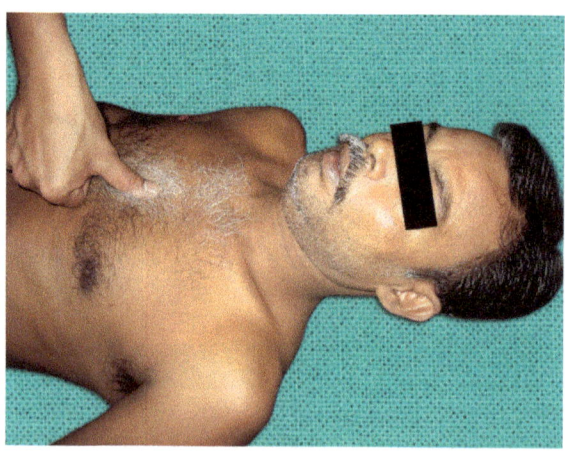

Fig. 71.1: Detection of sternal tenderness by pressing the upper part of body of sternum with ball of the right thumb

- Severe anemia due to any cause, e.g. thalassemia, chronic kala-azar
- Multiple myeloma
- Post-sternal puncture
→ So, look for hemorrhagic spots, splenomegaly, pallor, benzene seal over sternum.

Bone tenderness is also present in osteomyelitis, rickets and osteomalacia, Paget's disease of bone, osteosarcoma and fracture.

Mechanisms Responsible

In leukemias:
- Proliferation as well as hypercellularity of marrow
- Thinning/flattening of inner and outer layer of sternum.

Presternal Edema (Fig. 71.2)

It is a rare clinical entity and is found in:
- As part and parcel of anasarca
- Mumps (Gellis sign)
- Caries teeth with root abscess.

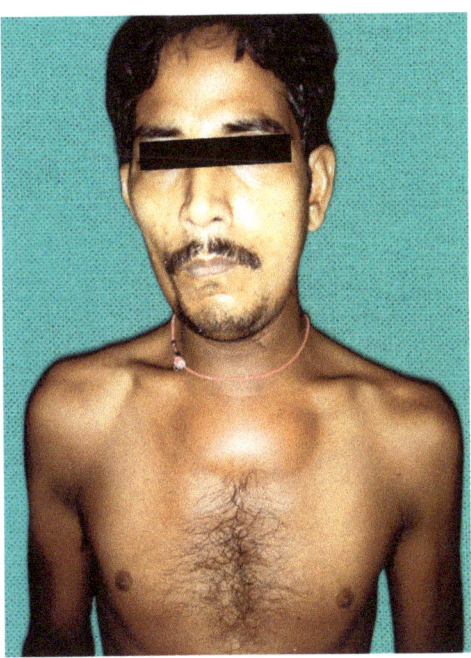

Fig. 71.2: Presternal edema from dental abscess (sometimes seen in cases of mumps)

TENDERNESS IN VERTEBRAE

- Press each spine of vertebral column one after another and enquire about tenderness (from trauma, caries spine, secondary deposits, multiple myeloma)
- Look for any kyphosis (smooth bending with convexity backwards)—osteoporosis with crush fracture
- Gibbus (acute angulation in the spine)—caries spine (tuberculosis)
- If multiple vertebrae are involved, think of secondary deposits.

TENDERNESS IN RIBS

- Trauma
- Multiple myeloma
- Cough fracture (i.e. resulting from violent cough, especially in older persons)
- Secondaries with pathological fracture.

TENDERNESS IN SKULL

- Trauma
- Multiple myeloma
- Secondary deposits
- Chronic hemolytic anemia (e.g. sickle cell anemia).
- Giant cell arteritis (scalp tenderness)

THE PEARLS

A definite bony tenderness (without history of trauma) always indicates some underlying pathology, which needs immediate care.

A positive sternal tenderness is a very important and unmistakable bedside sign for leukemia.

72

Sudden Cardiac Death

DEFINITION

It is the non-traumatic and unexplained death in a previously well person due to cardiac causes, which generally occurs within 1 hour of the onset of symptoms.

Patients at risk of sudden cardiac death (SCD) may have prodromal symptoms like chest pain, palpitations, shortness of breath, dizziness or fatigue. Patients at risk are those who have history of smoking, hypertension, diabetes, obesity, dyslipidemia, syncope, previous history of cardiac arrest or family history of SCD.

FACTS

- The major causes (80%) are due to coronary artery diseases (CAD), 10–15% are due to cardiomyopathies and 5% as a result of valvular heart disease.
- Sudden cardiac death is a direct consequence of cardiac arrest, which is potentially reversible if treated promptly. **Cardiac arrest** is due to ventricular fibrillation, pulseless ventricular tachycardia, cardiac asystole or electromechanical dissociation.
- Sudden death can be due to cardiac or non-cardiac causes (see below).
- Most common cause implemented is ventricular fibrillation in the setting of CAD.
- *Ventricular fibrillation:* A chaotic ventricular rhythm, is almost always the terminal rhythm in a case of SCD. As both organized electrical activity and ventricular depolarization do not occur, the patients have neither palpable pulse nor recordable blood pressure (BP).
- Patients with cardiac arrest require immediate cardiopulmonary resuscitation (CPR).
- Patients surviving cardiac arrest, an automatic implantable cardioverter defibrillator (AICD) is often required to prevent further cardiac arrest in future. Antiarrhythmic drugs like amiodarone may be used but are less effective than AICD.

CAUSES OF SUDDEN CARDIAC DEATH

- *Coronary artery disease:* Acute myocardial infarction (AMI), following coronary artery by-pass surgery, congenital anomaly of coronary arteries, coronary spasm, coronary arteritis, embolism of coronary artery or chronic ischemic heart disease (IHD)

- **Non-coronary artery disease:** Hypertrophic cardiomyopathy, dilated cardiomyopathy, myocarditis, congenital long QT syndrome, aortic stenosis, mitral valve prolapse, ball valve thrombus obstructing mitral valve, Fallot's tetralogy or transposition of great vessels, ventricular septal defect/patent ductus arteriosus (VSD/PDA).

SUDDEN CARDIAC DEATH IN YOUNG ATHLETES

- Hypertrophic cardiomyopathy
- Myocarditis
- Coronary artery anomalies
- Ruptured aortic aneurysm (e.g. Marfan's syndrome)
- Trauma (cerebral, cardiac, abdominal)
- Arrhythmias
- Aortic stenosis
- Heat stroke
- Bronchial asthma.

NON-CARDIAC CAUSES OF SUDDEN CARDIAC DEATH

- Pulmonary thromboembolism
- Dissection of the aorta
- Cerebrovascular accidents (e.g. cerebral hemorrhage)
- Anaphylaxis
- Acute adrenal failure
- Malignant hyperpyrexia (during or after anesthesia)
- Poisoning (e.g. cyanide)
- Foreign body in trachea
- Intravenous (IV) injections of a drug in hypersensitive subject
- Accidents (automobile, fall from a height, sudden blow in face).

FIVE MODES (5C'S) OF DEATH

1. Coronary artery disease (CAD)
2. Cerebrovascular accidents (CVA)
3. Casualty
4. Carcinoma
5. Chronic obstructive pulmonary disease (COPD)

THE PEARLS

In many countries (e.g. USA), SCD is the most common cause of natural death. SCD is responsible for one-half of total number of cardiovascular deaths.

Strategy for preventing SCD are divided into primary and secondary. **Primary prevention** refers to identify individuals at specific risk of development of SCD and institute preventive strategies. **Secondary prevention** refers to prevention of recurrent cardiac arrest or death in individuals who have survived previous cardiac arrest.

73

Swollen Legs

CLUE TO DIAGNOSIS

- Pedal edema
  - Congestive cardiac failure (CCF) (initially noticed at the end of days' work)
  - Nutritional edema (e.g. malnutrition or protein-losing enteropathy) → look for leukonychia and poor muscle mass
  - Varicose veins (examine for varicosities in standing position; enquire for occupation, which requires prolonged erect posture like tram driver, traffic police or security guards)
  - Deep vein thrombosis (DVT) [pain + tenderness in thigh or calf, positive Homan's sign; history of (H/O) prolonged immobilization or in a post-operative patient → look for recent onset varicosities] (Fig. 73.1)
  - Abdominal mass → tumor, cyst or pregnancy
  - Cirrhosis of liver (ascites, palmar erythema, scanty pubic hairs, spider nevi, splenomegaly, superficial abdominal veins) (Fig. 73.2)
  - Nephrotic syndrome (moon face, white striae, scrotal edema, periorbital puffiness, leukonychia) (Fig. 73.3)
  - Cyclical edema (female > male; temporal relationship with menstrual cycles)

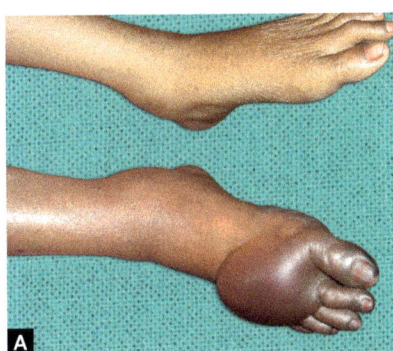 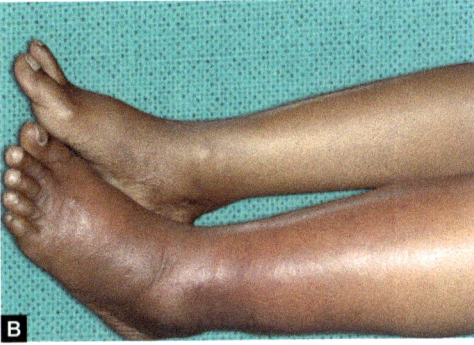

Fig. 73.1: Deep vein thrombosis. **A.** Cellulitis, erythema, ecchymosis, blister and gangrene formation in right leg secondary to iliofemoral venous thrombosis; **B.** Erythematous solid edema in left leg

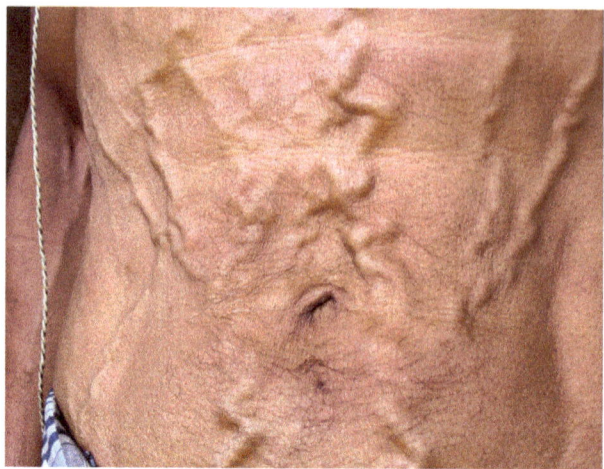

Fig. 73.2: Venous collaterals in portal hypertension with blood flowing away from the umbilicus in cirrhosis of liver

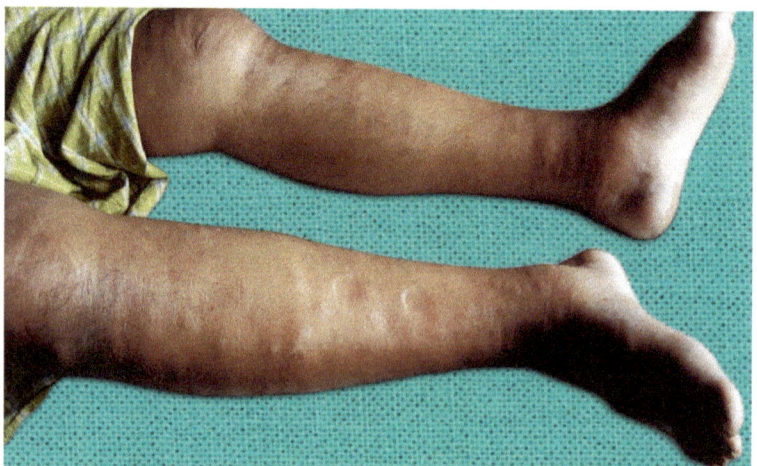

Fig. 73.3: Bilateral pedal pitting edema in membranous nephropathy (nephrotic syndrome)

- Drug-induced [H/O fludrocortisone, amlodipine/nifedipine, estrogens, nonsteroidal anti-inflammatory drug (NSAID) or corticosteroid consumption]
- ***Miscellaneous:*** Pericardial effusion/constrictive pericarditis (examine the neck veins), irradiation, myxedema, filariasis or lymphedema, pregnancy, retroperitoneal fibrosis, inferior vena caval (IVC) obstruction (Fig. 73.4), trauma, insect bite, hemangioma or lymphangioma.
- Calf hematoma (H/O trauma, hemophilia)
- Cellulitis (H/O diabetes mellitus, trauma, infection or any bite) → fever + pain + tenderness. Cellulitis is the spreading inflammation of skin and subcutaneous tissue with local pain, swelling and erythema (Fig. 73.5).

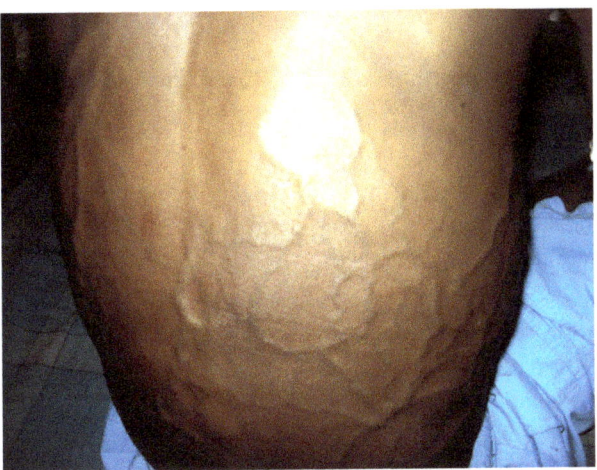

Fig. 73.4: Dilated and tortuous veins at back as a result of inferior vena caval obstruction with venous flow from below upwards in a patient of Budd-Chiari syndrome

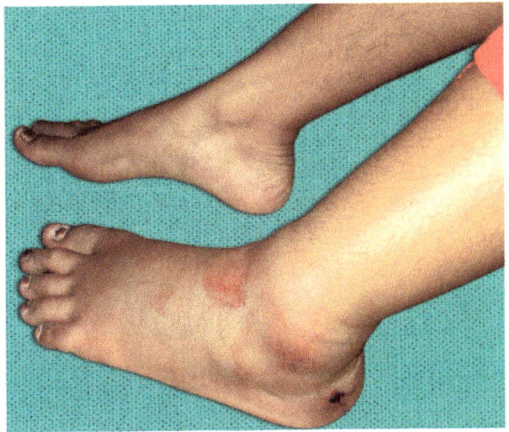

Fig. 73.5: Unilateral pedal edema as a result of snake bite; bite mark is seen in the back of left foot

BILATERAL INVOLVEMENT

CCF, nutritional edema, cirrhosis of liver, nephrotic syndrome, drug-induced, cyclical edema, IVC obstruction.

UNILATERAL INVOLVEMENT

DVT, cellulitis, popliteal cyst/gastrocnemius/Baker's cyst rupture, venous insufficiency, lymphedema (carcinoma, lymphoma, filariasis, retroperitoneal fibrosis), diabetic foot, hemiplegic side, postphlebitic syndrome.

ACUTELY SWOLLEN LEG

DVT, cellulitis, trauma or fracture, arterial occlusion, arthritis or insect bite.

POPLITEAL SWELLING

- DVT
- Ruptured Baker's cyst (from rheumatoid arthritis)
- Trauma (contusion/fracture)
- Popliteal abscess
- Ruptured tendon
- Ruptured varicose vein
- Phlebitis (superficial)
- Aneurysm of popliteal artery
- Miscellaneous—osteomyelitis, osteosarcoma, fibrosarcoma, hemangioma or lymphangioma.

PAINFUL LEGS

- DVT/thrombophlebitis
- Lymphangitis
- Cellulitis (i.e. infection)
- Trauma → fracture
- Arthritis of knee, ankle, tarsal joints
- Lymphatic obstruction, e.g. malignancy of pelvic organs, filariasis (Fig. 73.6)
- Vasculitis (i.e. ischemia)
- Crops of erythema nodosum (*see* Fig. 69.3)
- Buerger's disease

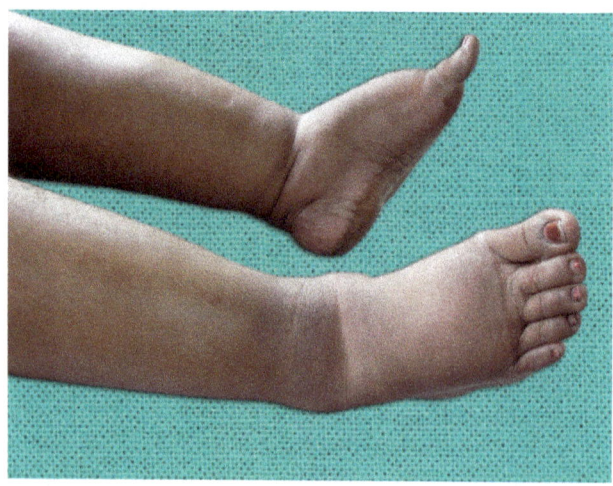

Fig. 73.6: Swollen legs from filariasis with non-pitting edema

- Phlegmasia alba dolens (swollen, white leg especially in relation to DVT/pregnancy)
- Diabetic foot.

FACIAL PUFFINESS (SWELLING)

- Familial
- Myxedema
- Cushing's syndrome (primary, or secondary to prolonged corticosteroid therapy)
- Angioneurotic edema (chiefly the lips and eyelids)
- Hypoproteinemia → nephrotic syndrome, acute nephritis, severe anemia, protein-energy malnutrition
- CCF, pericardial effusion, constrictive pericarditis
- Superior mediastinal syndrome or superior vena caval (SVC) syndrome (Figs 73.7 and 73.8)
- Trichinosis (due to infected pork ingestion)—edema of the eyelids are common
- Facial cellulitis
- Subcutaneous emphysema of face, extending from chest
- Infection by Marburg and Ebola viruses

- Facial swelling may also be due to anasarca, cellulitis, dental abscess, sinusitis (maxillary), preauricular lymphadenitis or bilateral parotid swelling.
- **Conjunctival edema** is common in hypoalbuminemia, Graves' disease, Weil's disease, SVC syndrome and fluid overload.
- **Eyelid edema** is commonly seen in nephrotic syndrome, acute glomerulonephritis, anaphylaxis, hypoproteinemia, myxoedema, dermatomyositis, blepharitis, trichinosis, right heart failure, cavernous sinus thrombosis and fracture of base of the skull.

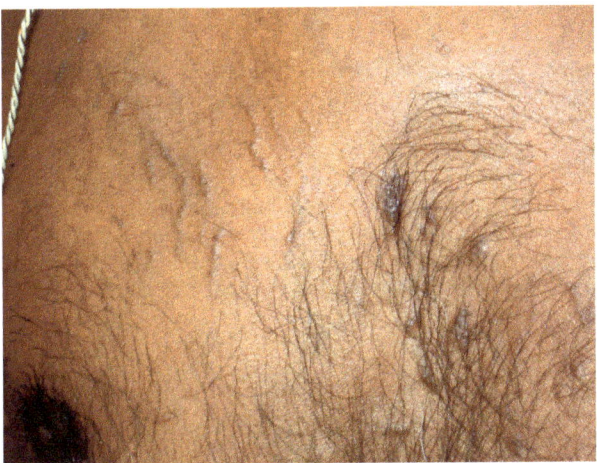

Fig. 73.7: Dilated superficial veins and venules over anterior chest wall in superior vena caval obstruction with venous flow from above downwards

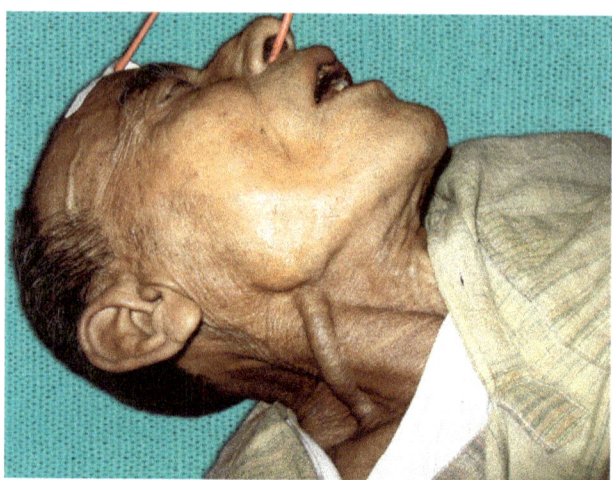

Fig. 73.8: Hugely distended external jugular vein in early superior mediastinal syndrome from brochogenic carcinoma (patient having haemoptysis)

RECURRENT SWELLING OF FACE AND LIMBS

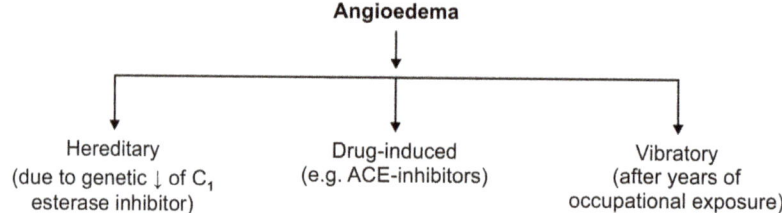

Note: ACE inhibitor—angiotensin-converting-enzyme inhibitor

- It is hypersensitive allergic edema involving the deeper layer of skin. It is a solid edema associated with itching (hereditary variety→no itching), which usually last for a few hours. It is commonly localized in tongue, lips, face, eyelids, etc. The swelling develops rapidly and is pale-pink in color. It may threaten life if larynx (i.e. laryngeal edema) or tongue is involved.
- Drugs should be stopped in drug-induced angioedema. The patients are usually non-responsive to treatment in hereditary form but cyproheptadine, danazol, hydroxyzine, epsilon-aminocaproic acid or fresh frozen plasma may be beneficial. The patients may complain of recurrent abdominal pain too. Other than angioedema, patients with **CCF, nephrotic syndrome, severe anemia or cyclical edema** may complain of recurrent swelling of face and/or limbs.

PRETHROMBOTIC DISORDERS IN RECURRENT DVT (PROCOAGULANT STATES)

- ***Inherited***
  - Antithrombin III ↓

- Protein C or S ↓
- Hyperhomocysteinemia
- Dysfibrinogenemia
- ↑ release of plasminogen activator inhibitor (PAI-1)
- Defective release of plasminogen activator
- Activated protein C resistance
- Factor V Leiden
- Prothrombin mutations.

- **Acquired**
  - Metastatic tumor
  - Extensive trauma/major surgery
  - Myeloproliferative disorders
  - Chronic congestive cardiac failure
  - Behcet's syndrome
  - Oral contraceptive pills (OCP) or L-asparaginase-induced
  - Hyperviscosity states
  - Antiphospholipid syndrome
  - Pregnancy and puerperium.

DEEP VEIN THROMBOSIS (FIG. 73.1)

The patient presents with pain or tight feeling in the calf with swelling, redness and non-pitting edema of ankle or legs. The common sites of DVT are calf muscle veins, popliteal, femoral and iliac veins. The local part feels warm and Homan's sign (induction of calf pain on dorsiflexion of foot) is often present → non-specific sign, may be positive in all inflammatory lesions in the calf (dangerous, because of risk of pulmonary embolism).

Predisposing factors (procoagulant states) are described above; moreover, post-acute myocardial infarction (AMI), CCF, varicose veins, prostatectomy patients, and cerebrovascular accident (CVA) patients are prone to develop DVT. Obesity, long air travel or prolonged immobility (bed rest > 4 days) are important provocating factors.

- **Phlegmasia cerulea dolens:** Deoxygenated hemoglobin in stagnant veins gives a cyanotic hue
- **Phlegmasia alba dolens:** Markedly edematons leg in DVT leads to ↑ in interstitial pressure exceeding capillary perfusion pressure → gives rise to pallor (i.e. alba or whiteness) of the limb. It is also seen in pregnancy.
- Clinical diagnosis of DVT is often unreliable; D-dimer level assay ↑ the sensitivity of diagnosis. B-mode venous compression, ultrasonography (USG) or Doppler ultrasound of lower limb vessels, impedence plethysmography and venography are diagnostic. The principal aim of diagnosis and treatment is to prevent pulmonary thromboembolism.
- Treatment is done by extremity elevation and bed rest. An elastic stocking may be used in the limb. Anticoagulation is started with low-molecular-weight heparin (i.e. LMWH) with a goal partial thromboplastin time (PTT) approximately twice

normal; warfarin is usually started (as 10 mg daily) after 5 days, overlapped with LMWH (e.g. enoxaparin) for at least 5 days, and then LMWH is stopped when the INR (international normalized ratio) is in target range (i.e. 2.5). Oral anticoagulation with warfarin is continued (maintenance dose as 3-9 mg, depending on INR) for 3-6 months with weekly checking of INR. LMWH do not require monitoring of coagulation factors and there is less chance of bleeding when compared to unfractioned heparin. NSAID may be used for pain and swelling of the limb.

Differential Diagnosis of Deep Vein Thrombosis (at Calf Muscles)
- Superficial thrombophlebitis
- Lymphangitis
- Cellulitis, abscess
- Hematoma
- Lymphedema
- Ruptured Baker's cyst
- Venous stasis
- Postphlebitic syndrome
- Soft tissue or muscle injury
- Achilles tendinitis.

WHAT IS SUPERFICIAL THROMBOPHLEBITIS?
It is an inflammatory thrombophlebitis in subcutaneous veins which is palpable as a tender cord with induration, redness, erythema and edema (along with ↑ temperature) of the overlying skin and subcutaneous tissue. The linear appearance is characteristic. Though low-grade pyrexia may be associated with, there is absence of significant swelling of the limb. The common causes of thrombophlebitis are as follows:
1. Intravenous (IV) cannulation is most common
2. Carcinoma of the pancreas
3. Infection (e.g. *Staphylococcus*)
4. Trauma to pre-existing varicose veins
5. Hypercoagulable states.

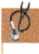

Points 2, 3 and 5 may give rise to *migratory thrombophlebitis*.

BEDSIDE FEATURES OF INCREASED EXTRACELLULAR VOLUME
Peripheral edema is produced by expansion of extracellular volume by at least 15% (i.e. 2 liter). The features are:
- Edema (face in the morning; sacral edema in bed-ridden patient)
- Pulmonary edema
- Pleural effusion
- Pericardial effusion
- Ascites

- Raised jugular venous pressure (JVP), gallop rhythm, cardiomegaly, basal crepitations and systemic hypertension (in few cases) are features of expansion of the blood volume.

THE PEARLS

'Edema' is accumulation of excessive amount of tissue fluid in the subcutaneous tissue (or serous sacs) due to increase in extravascular (interstitial) component of the extracellular fluid volume resulting in swelling of tissue. Other than edema, there are specific causes of face, leg, sacral area swelling. Remember, non-pitting edema (solid edema) is characteristic of myxedema, lymphedema, filariasis or angioedema. Swollen legs complained by the patient should draw immediate attention of a sensitive doctor.

Remember, superficial vein thrombosis is 'thrombophlebitis' and DVT is 'phlebothrombosis'. DVT is more dangerous for the patient.

74

Tongue: A Clue to many Diseases

INTRODUCTION

Tongue is composed of three elements—epithelium, muscles and glands.
1. *Epithelium* → stratified and non-cornified; two special structures are seen over the epithelium, i.e. the papillae and the taste bud. There are four types of papillae (minute projections over mucous membrane), e.g. filiform (major papillae in tongue), conical, fungiform (flat-rounded head) and circumvallate papillae (present at the back of the tongue).
2. *Muscles* → voluntary and cross-striated.
3. *Glands* → small and scattered throughout the tongue. These are mucous glands, serous glands, and lymph nodes (glands).

Discoloration of tongue is commonly associated with infections, deficiency disorders and metabolic diseases, and are important diagnostic clue in clinical medicine.

COLOR AND MORPHOLOGICAL CHANGES

- *Moist tongue:* Sialorrhea, heavy metal poisoning.
- *Dry tongue (also brown and a little furred):* Dehydration, mouth breathing, xerostomia, atropinization.
- *Pale tongue:* Anemia (severe).
- *Macroglossia and microglossia:* See Chapter 50.
- *Yellow tongue:* Intake of yellow colored food/sweets, jaundice (the undersurface).
- *Blue tongue:* Central cyanosis, meth- or sulfhemoglobinemia, intake of blue colored food/sweets (Fig. 74.1).
- *Bluish-red tongue:* Polycythemia.
- *Black tongue:* Addison's disease; after ingestion of liquorice, bismuth or charcoal.
- *Black hairy tongue:* Developed as a result of failure of keratin layer of the filiform papillae to desquamate normally. It is found in staining by tobacco, food, chromogenic organism, fungal infections and after use of penicillins/tetracyclines/antiseptic mouthwashes.
- *Magenta-colored tongue (a bit pinkish):* Riboflavin deficiency.
- *Furred tongue:* Heavy smokers, chronic debilitating disorders, acute tonsillitis, sore throat (i.e. painful conditions in mouth).

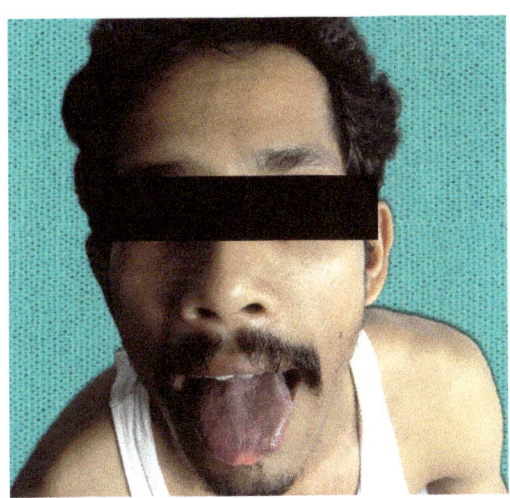

Fig. 74.1: Bluish-black tongue in methemoglobinemia

- **Geographic tongue (Fig. 74.2):** Denuded red patches ***wandering*** or ***migrating*** across the surface of the tongue due to rapid loss and regrowth of filiform papillae. The colour and features change from day to day creating a ***wandering rash***, which is an asymptomatic inflammatory condition. Though looks odd, it has no clinical significance and can be regarded as a variant of normal; may be familial. Though painless, the patient should be reassured.
- ***Strawberry and raspberry tongue:*** Hypertrophy of fungiform papillae with changes in filiform papillae, and are seen in scarlet fever.
- ***Blotting paper like pallor (with black pigmentation in the margins):*** Often seen in hookworm infestation.

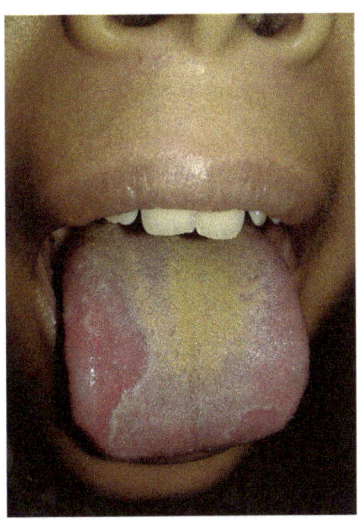

Fig. 74.2: Denuded 'migratory' patches in geographical tongue; of no clinical significance

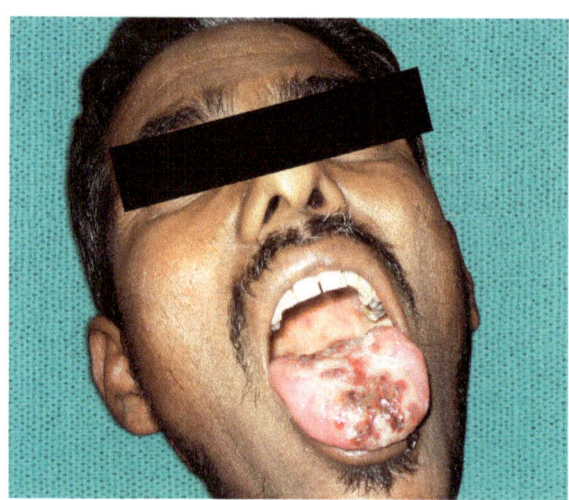

Fig. 74.3: Glossitis with superadded fungal infection and hemorrhage—a case in convalescence from viperidae snake bite

- ***Bald tongue:*** There is total loss or atrophy of papillae (i.e. pale and smooth tongue) and is classically seen in iron deficiency anemia, pernicious anemia, folic acid deficiency, tropical sprue and syphilis.
- ***Raw-beefy tongue:*** The tongue is red, swollen and painful; classically found in pellagra and vitamin B12 deficiency. This condition is associated with mucosal atrophy in the mouth and angular stomatitis.
- ***Angry-looking tongue:*** Central coating with red tip and margins; common in enteric fever (first week).
- ***Scrotal tongue:*** Deep horizontal fissures in the tongue where debris may collect; it is of no clinical significance.
- ***White patches on the tongue:*** Due to leukoplakia (a precancerous lesion), thrush [i.e. moniliasis due to immunodeficiency, diabetes mellitus, acquired immunodeficiency syndrome (AIDS), debilitated patients, immumosuppressive/corticosteroid treatment], other fungal infections, chronic superficial glossitis (Fig. 74.3), hairy leukoplakia (raised, painless, corrugated, poorly demarcated lesion mainly at the margins, which does not rub off and is found in AIDS due to Epstein-Barr virus infection). The lesion of thrush looks creamy-white curd-like patches which reveals a raw bleeding area when scraped (Fig. 74.4)
- ***Median rhomboid glossitis:*** It is a lozenge-shaped denuded area in the middle of the tongue posteriorly, itself a congenital abnormality. It should be differentiated from carcinoma of the tongue as it feels nodular.
- ***Bite mark in the tongue with hematoma around:*** Accidental bite during eating or convulsions.
- ***Flaccid tongue with rounded tip and the tongue rests on the floor of the mouth like a mushroom (grossly wasted), often with fasciculation:*** Seen in bulbar palsy.

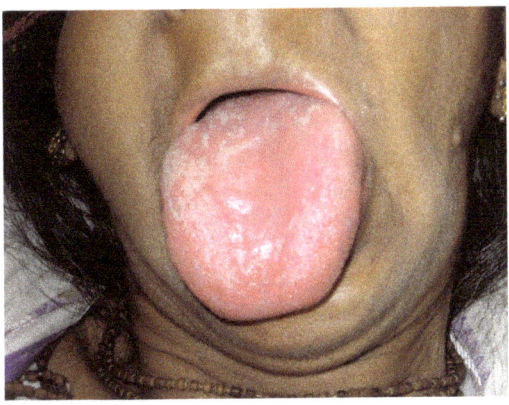

Fig. 74.4: Candidiasis (thrush) in tongue in a patient of diabetes mellitus

- **Spastic tongue with pointed tip (without any fasciculation):** Seen in pseudobulbar palsy.
- **Growth (cauliflower-like) in the tongue** is observed in squamous cell carcinoma (with halitosis).
- **Mushroom like tongue:** Sore tongue with white slough and is seen in corrosive (e.g. acid or alkali) poisoning (Fig. 74.5).
- **Horny tongue (crocodile tongue):** Tongue with cornification of mucosa and of no clinical value.
- **Dry, red tongue with atrophy of the papillae and fissures:** Seen in Sjögren's syndrome.
- **Ulcer in the tongue:** Aphthous ulcer (very painful, anywhere in tongue), frenal ulcer (in frenum), tuberculous ulcer (in dorsum), marginal ulcer (anywhere in tongue), snail-track ulcer (in dorsum and is seen in secondary syphilis), Behcet's disease (commonly painful), ulcers at tongue margins (by ill-fitted denture) may be present.

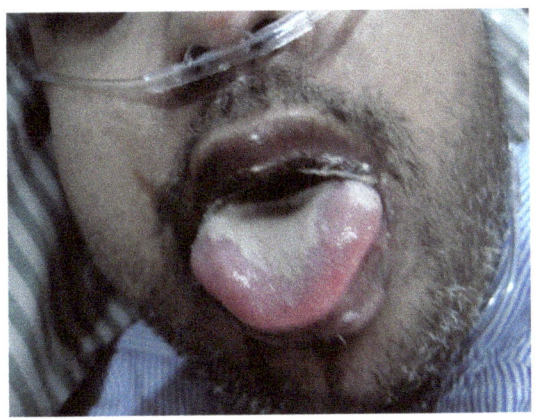

Fig. 74.5: Sore tongue with white slough over tongue in acid poisoning

- ***Shaggy, papillomatous dorsum*** due to hypertrophy of filiform papillae with blackish pigmentation found in Addison's disease and acanthosis nigricans.
- ***Miscellaneous:*** Lichen planus (glossy or glazed tongue), erythema multiforme (ulcers or blisters), pemphigus, pemphigoid, hereditary hemorrhagic telangiectasis (telangiectasia on the tongue) and Crohn's disease (raised, smooth, red nodules with hyperplastic ridges) may affect the tongue.

Tongue can also give clue to diagnosis if examined for movement [e.g. trombone tongue in general paresis of insane (GPI), Jack-in-the-box tongue in rheumatic chorea, or chewing tongue in athetosis], size (macro- or microglossia), deviation [i.e. tongue is deviated to opposite side or same side, respectively in upper motor neuron (UMN) type or lower motor neuron (LMN) type XIIth cranial nerve palsy], power of the tongue (in XIIth cranial nerve palsy), or taste sensation (by application of saccharin, salt, vinegar and quinine sequentially one by one for taste sensation of sweet, salt, sour and bitter ones respectively).

THE PEARLS

Tongue is one of the highest-rated window in clinical medicine. Though previously tongue was known as the mirror of gastrointestinal tract, it is now regarded as mirror of systemic dysfunction of all the systems in human body.

If the patient can not protrude the tongue after the question 'show me your tongue?' the possibilities come in mind are ankyloglossia (tongue-tie or short frenulum), XIIth cranial nerve palsy, carcinoma of the tongue or mental retardation.

However, tongue should always be examined in all conscious patients.

75

Weight Gain/Loss

WEIGHT GAIN

Acceptable range of body mass index (BMI) is 18.5–24.9 kg/m^2. When BMI $\geq$ 25 kg/m^2, it is defined as ***overweight*** and when $\geq$ 30 kg/m^2, it is designated as ***obesity***. Abdominal or truncal obesity is measured by ***waist-hip ratio***, which when > 1.0 in males and > 0.9 in females increase the morbidity and mortality risks. Weight gain is commonly due to:

- Sedentary life style with less physical activity, overeating or familial.
- Fluid overload [congestive cardiac failure (CCF), cirrhosis, nephrotic syndrome, hypoproteinemia, pregnancy].
- Obesity (Cushing's syndrome, hypothyroidism, Laurence-Moon-Biedl syndrome, Prader-Willi syndrome, hypothalamic disorders, e.g. Froelich's syndrome).
- Prolonged therapy with corticosteroids or estrogen (e.g. oral contraceptive pills).
- Anxiety disorder with compulsive eating.
- ***Miscellaneous:*** Insulinoma, hypogonadism, acromegaly, discontinuation of smoking, depression, craniopharyngioma.

Gain in weight is commonly associated with insulin resistance, diabetes mellitus, hypertension, osteoarthritis, atherosclerosis, dyslipidemia, cholelithiasis and sleep-apnea syndrome.

Clinical Diagnosis of Obesity

- Body weight > 20% than the upper limit of standard weight in relation to age and sex of the individual (body weight $\geq$ 10% is ***overweight***)
- BMI > 30 kg/m^2
- Skin thickness > 1 inch in inferior angle of scapula (male) or mid-triceps region (females), when measured by a special calliper (e.g. Harpenden or Schofield's calliper)
- Morbid obesity is 100% overweight (BMI $\geq$ 40) over the upper limit of standard weight.
- Obesity can be quantified by anthropometry (i.e. skinfold thickness), densitometry (underwater weight), computed tomography (CT) or magnetic resonance imaging (MRI) scan (measures mesenteric fat).

Appetite in Internal Medicine

- *Increase in appetite (polyphagia or hyperorexia)*
  - Diabetes, thyrotoxicosis, growth hormone excess (gigantism/acromegaly) (Fig. 75.1)
  - Malabsorption syndrome (e.g. sprue)
  - Binge eating, bulimia nervosa
  - Worm infestations.
- *Diminished appetite*
  - Depression, anorexia nervosa, boredom, emotional upset
  - Disseminated malignancy, tuberculosis, acute febrile illness, CCF, uremia
  - Hepatitis (acute viral), cholecystitis.

Drugs used in Treatment of Obesity

Phentermine, fenfluramine, sibutramine, orlistat (inhibitor of intestinal lipase), fluoxetine or sertraline (appetite suppressant), rimonabant (selective cannabinoid 1 receptor blocker), bulk preparation (e.g. guar gum), recombinant leptin, etc. Sibutramine and rimonabant have been withheld in some countries.

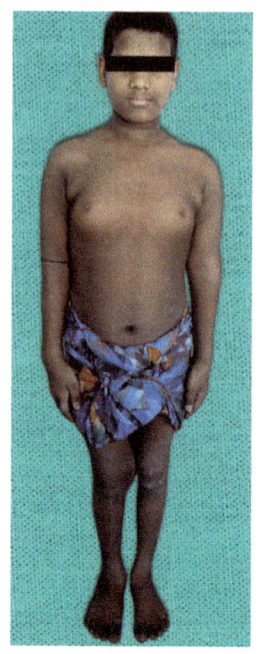

Fig. 75.1: A 9-year-old boy with gigantism (hypersecretion of growth hormone before puberty) and gynecomastia

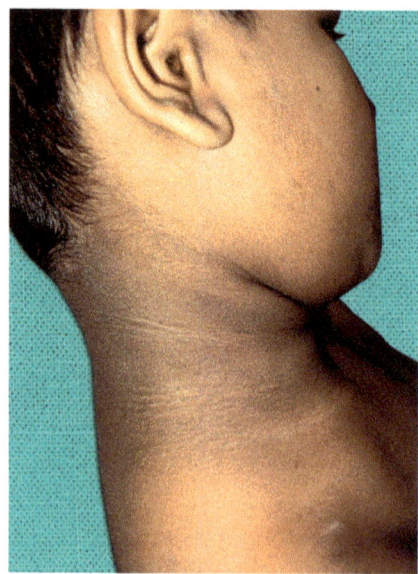

Fig. 75.2: Acanthosis nigricans (velvety thickening with hyperpigmentation) in an obese adolescent

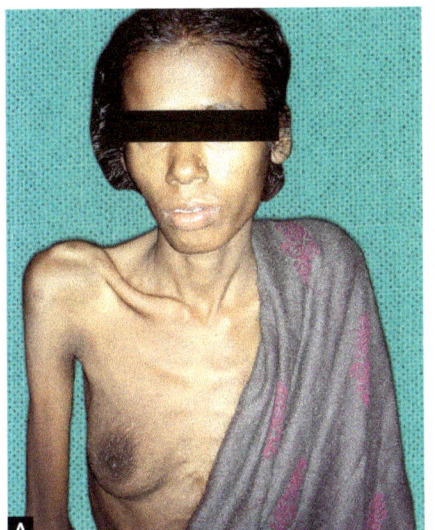 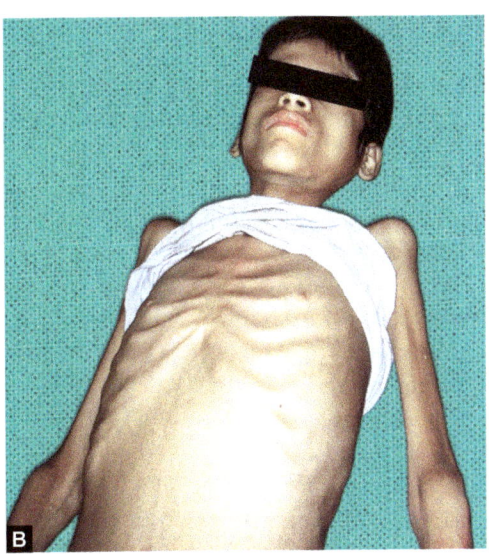

Figs 75.3: Emaciation **A.** All skin and bone as a result of pulmonary tuberculosis; **B.** Type 1 diabetes mellitus

WEIGHT LOSS

Generalized undernutrition, i.e. loss of total body fat and diminution of muscle bulk is known as ***emaciation*** (Fig. 75.3). Undernutrition with signs of vitamin, mineral and essential amino acid deficiency is designated as ***malnutrition***. ***Cachexia*** is a profound state of general ill-health and a combined manifestation of anorexia, anemia plus emaciation. Decrease in muscle mass is known as ***sarcopenia***. Weight loss is commonly due to:

- Chronic malnutrition (protein-energy malnutrition)
- Tuberculosis (Fig. 75.3A)
- Diabetes mellitus (especially new-onset) (Fig. 75.3B)
- Thyrotoxicosis
- Disseminated malignancy
- Acquired immunodeficiency syndrome (AIDS) (slim disease)
- Anorexia nervosa, severe depression
- Malabsorption syndrome
- Addison's disease, panhypopituitarism (e.g. Sheehan's syndrome), pheochromocytoma, hyperparathyroidism
- Collagen vascular diseases, e.g. systemic lupus erythematosus (SLE)
- Motor neuron disease
- Food faddism
- CCF (cardiac cachexia), chronic obstructive pulmonary disease (COPD), cirrhosis
- Drug-induced, e.g. metformin.

Relation of Weight Loss with Appetite

Weight loss + ↑ or normal appetite
- Diabetes mellitus (uncontrolled)
- Thyrotoxicosis
- Chronic kala-azar
- Malabsorption syndrome
- Pheochromocytoma
- Worm infestations in children.

Weight loss + ↓ appetite
- Malignancy (advanced)
- Tuberculosis (disseminated)
- Depression
- Addison's disease
- Anorexia nervosa
- Human immunodeficiency virus (HIV) infection.

Significant Weight Loss

When there is unexplained and unintentional weight loss of > 3 kg in the previous 6 months, it is known as ***significant weight loss***. It is very often associated with vitamin and nutrient deficiencies, higher surgical mortality rates, and proneness to acquire infections. Unintentional weight loss is associated with ↑ morbidity and mortality. Voluntary weight loss is seen in treatment of obesity, on anorexic drugs, models and gymnasts.

Screening Tests for Evaluation of Weight Loss

A loss of 5% of body weight in the preceding 6–12 months should prompt further evaluation:
- Complete blood count
- Liver and renal function tests
- Urine analysis
- Chest X-ray
- Glucose, electrolytes, calcium, thyroid-stimulating hormone (TSH)
- Cancer screening (e.g. tumor markers like CA-125 in ovarian carcinoma)
- Additional tests:
  - HIV
  - Upper and lower gastrointestinal (GI) endoscopy
  - Abdominal CT/MRI
  - High resolution computed tomography (HRCT) thorax

Remember: As 7000 kcal is the equivalent of 1 kg of human adipose tissue, a calorie deficit of 1000 kcal/day will produce a loss of weight approximately 1 kg/week. A variety of cytokines, e.g. tumor necrosis factor-alpha (TNF-α), interleukin-6 (IL-6), IL-1 and interferon-8 (IFN-8) can induce cachexia.

Chapter 75 Weight Gain/Loss

THE PEARLS

BMI (a measure of generalized obesity) is obtained by calculating a person's weight in kilograms and dividing it by the person's height in meter square (kg/m^2).

Obesity is classified into three types—android (↑ fat in waist, predominant in men), gynoid (↑ fat at hip or thigh, predominant in women) and truncal (↑ fat deposition on face, neck and upper trunk, e.g. Cushing's syndrome). **Apple-shaped obesity** (more fat in abdomen) is more harmful than **pear-shaped obesity** (more fat in hips and thighs); **apple-shaped obesity** is linked with diabetes, ischemic heart disease (IHD), hypertension, and ↑ lipids. Abdominal obesity (↑ fat deposition in abdominal viscera and omentum) is synonymous with visceral obesity.

Weight loss and weight gain both are, in the long run, similarly harmful to the patient, and should be investigated at the earliest.

76

Wheezing/Stridor

WHEEZING

Characteristics

- High-pitched musical sound heard from a distance
- Better heard in *expiratory phase*
- Indicates small airways obstruction
- Usually associated with rhonchi in the chest
- Constant wheezing may be audible in structural lesion of bronchus.

Wheezing is found in:
- Bronchial asthma (reversible wheezing)—most classical
- Chronic obstructive pulmonary disease (COPD) (irreversible wheezing)
- Interstitial lung disease
- Tropical eosinophilia
- Cardiac asthma
- Infections like pneumonia, bronchitis, bronchiolitis, epiglottitis
- Endobronchial disease (e.g. neoplasm)
- Airways obstruction (goiter, aneurysm, spasm, edema or hemorrhage, or foreign body aspiration)
- Carcinoid syndrome
- Gastroesophageal reflux disease (GERD) with aspiration.

STRIDOR

Characteristics

- Low-pitched crowing sound (loud) heard from a distance
- Better heard in *inspiratory phase*
- Indicates larger airways obstruction like larynx, trachea and major bronchus
- Very common in children
- Laryngeal stridor is a medical emergency and urgent respiratory support may be required.

Stridor is found in:
- Foreign body in larynx or trachea
- Laryngeal edema (anaphylaxis)

- Diphtheria, whooping cough
- Allergic (spasmodic) croup, i.e. acute laryngotracheobronchitis
- Acute epiglottitis
- Laryngeal obstruction (laryngomalacia, laryngeal webs, bilateral abductor paralysis of the vocal cord, tumor or foreign body)
- Mediastinal mass
- Vocal cord palsy due to recurrent laryngeal nerve paralysis (other features of recurrent laryngeal nerve palsy are bovine cough and hoarseness of voice)
- *Miscellaneous:* Hysterical, laryngismus stridulus in tetany (i.e. hypocalcemia), Cri-du-chat syndrome, Pierre Robin's syndrome, subglottic tracheal stenosis (e.g. Wegener's granulomatosis), tracheo-esophageal fistula.

CARDINAL SYMPTOMS OF RESPIRATORY SYSTEM

- Cough
- Expectoration
- Hemoptysis
- Chest pain
- Breathlessness
- Wheezing or stridor (audible sounds).

Note: Adventitious sounds in respiratory system are rhonchi, crepitations and pleural rub. The new terminology of rhonchi is ***wheezes***, which is always audible by a stethoscope; ***wheezing*** is an audible sound with naked ear, without the help of a stethoscope.

THE PEARLS

Wheezing or stridor is often first noticed by the bed-partner at night. Clinically, stridor is more dangerous than wheezing, and many a time it may lead to a medical emergency.

77 White Nails

SYNONYM

Leukonychia, Terry's nail

Impression: Hypoalbuminemia. The nail looks white with a ground-glass appearance without a lunula. It may be due to decreased vascularity and increased connective tissue within the nail-bed.

Conditions associated:
- Cirrhosis of liver
- Nephrotic syndrome
- Severe malnutrition
- Kwashiorkor
- Protein-losing enteropathy.

BLUE LUNULA (AZURE ARCS)

- Copper sulfate ($CuSO_4$) poisoning
- Wilson's disease
- After zidovudine therapy
- Ochronosis.

RED LUNULA

Congestive cardiac failure.

BROWN-BLACK NAIL

Hematoma underneath the nail, melanoma.

HALF-AND-HALF NAIL (PROXIMAL HALF IS WHITE WHILE THE DISTAL HALF IS PINK) OR LINDSAY NAIL

Chronic renal failure.

MEES' LINE: WHITE LINE OF 1–2 MM WIDTH ABOVE LUNULA

Arsenic poisoning.

BEAU'S LINE (TRANSVERSE RIDGES ON NAILS)

- Recovery from any febrile illness
- Zinc deficiency.

> Beau's line is the temporary interference of nail growth; usually self-limiting.

GREEN OR BLACK-GREEN NAIL

Pseudomonas infection.

YELLOW NAIL

Fungal infection, psoriasis, tobacco abuse, yellow nail syndrome, chronic infections (tuberculosis, sinusitis).

BLACKISH, YELLOW-GREEN NAIL

Yellow nail syndrome (lymphedema of extremities + pleural effusion + yellow dystrophic nails).

ONYCHOLYSIS (SEPARATION OF TERMINAL NAIL PLATE FROM UNDERLYING NAIL-BED)

Candidiasis, ringworm infection (Fig. 77.1), psoriasis, trauma, lichen planus, chronic paronychia, thyrotoxicosis (Plummer's nail).

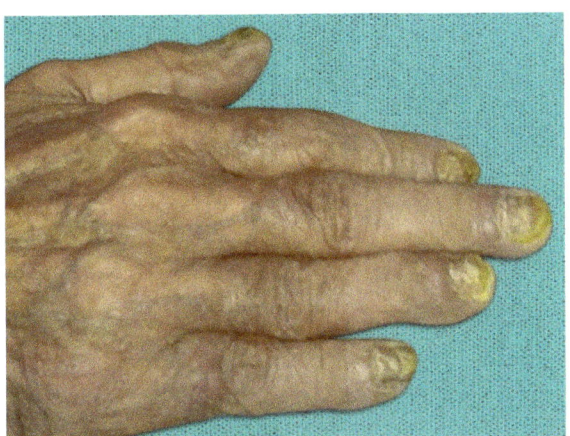

Fig. 77.1: Onychodystrophy due to fungal infections (onychomycosis or tinea unguium); the lesions may also be produced by psoriasis, chronic eczema, lichen planus and medications

ONYCHOMADESIS (SEPARATION OF PROXIMAL NAIL PLATE FROM UNDERLYING NAIL-BED)

- Trauma with hematoma underneath the nail
- Any period of severe illness; paronychia
- Malnutrition
- Pemphigus
- Kawasaki disease
- Hand, foot and mouth disease (in children).

ONYCHORRHEXIS (BRITTLE NAIL)

In older women, the nails of finger and toes may break easily and separate into horizontal strata (probably from repeated hydration and drying during cooking + mechanical + chemical trauma), and is known as onychorrehexis.

LONGITUDINAL RIDGES IN NAIL

- Lichen planus
- Alopecia areata
- Darier's disease.

MUEHRCK'E LINES

Paired white transverse bands due to hypoalbuminemia which disappears on pressure.

BLACK NAIL

Hair dyes, Peutz-Jeghers syndrome.

BROWN NAIL

Hydroquinone-induced.

ABSENT OR ATROPHY OF NAIL

Nail-patella syndrome, congenital ectodermal defect.

LONG NARROW NAIL

Hypopituitarism.

WIDER NAIL

Acromegaly.

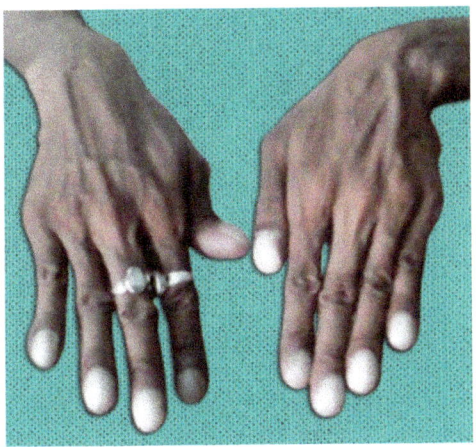

Fig. 77.2: Digital clubbing in congenital cyanotic heart disease

CONVEX NAIL

Clubbing (Fig. 77.2).

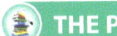 **THE PEARLS**

The nail consists of nail plate, nail matrix and nail-bed behind it. The nail plate is densely packed with keratin, hard and thus protects the finger tips. The fingernail is 0.3–0.5 mm thick and grows 0.1 mm/day, while the toenails grow slowly. The pink color of the nail is due to adjacent dermal capillaries.

The nails reflect many systemic diseases. It is also used in forensic sciences to identify an individual.

White (Milky) Urine

POSSIBILITIES

- **Chyluria** → as a result of passage of chylomicrons in urine.
- **Phosphaturia** → passing out of large amount of phosphates (amorphous or crystalline) in urine.
- **Lipiduria** → presence of fat droplets in urine.
- **Pseudochyluria** (milky or gold paint) → passage of large amount of protein, desquamated cells may turn the urine milky (on microscopic examination there is mixed cellularity with cholesterol excess).
- **Pyuria** → Urine is full of pus cells in urinary tract infection.

ETIOLOGY OF CHYLURIA

- **Blockage of lymph channels or thoracic duct by:**
  - **Parasites:** Filariasis, ascariasis, cysticercosis, Taenia and *Hymenolepis nana* infection.
  - **Non-parasitic:** Trauma to thoracic duct, tumors, obstruction of thoracic duct, pregnancy, tuberculosis, retroperitoneal fibrosis, congenital malformation of lymph channels or lymphangiectasia.
- Idiopathic.

Clue to Diagnosis

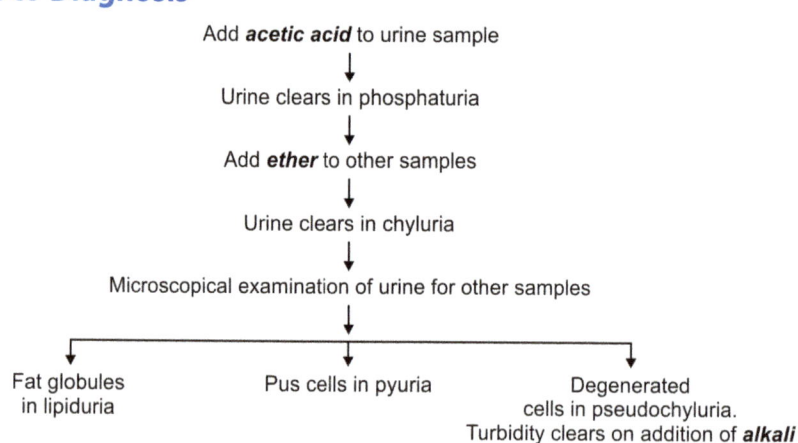

SPECIAL POINTS TO NOTE

- ***Chyluria:*** Most common cause is filariasis (e.g. *Wuchereria bancrofti*-induced), especially in India. A state of lymphatic hypertension with cavernous malformations of lymph channels at hilum of pelvis prevails which ultimately ruptures into the urinary passage (may be in the bladder or urethra too). The color of the urine is milky or creamy (Fig. 78.1), and the fat globules may be demonstrated microscopically by staining with Sudan III. Ether clears the turbidity in chyluria. Reassurance and treatment of the cause are the mainstay of management.
- ***Phosphaturia:*** Urine clears on addition of acetic acid. Oral aluminium hydroxide (antacid) may alleviate the problem.
- ***Lipiduria:*** Fat droplets usually float on the top of the urine or may be separated as a layer on top after ultracentrifugation. Lipid globules that do not contain cholesterol can be identified by adding Sudan III and seen under light microscope. Conditions associated with lipiduria are diabetes mellitus, nephrotic syndrome, eclampsia, fat embolism and arsenic poisoning.
- ***Pseudochyluria:*** Usually turbid urine as a result of large number of degenerated cells or tumor cells. Turbidity clears on addition of alkali.
- ***Pyuria:*** Large number of pus cells make the urine turbid and is commonly associated with pyelonephritis, cystitis or urethritis. Broad-spectrum antibiotics cure the ailment.

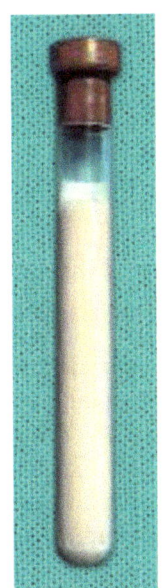

Fig. 78.1: White urine in chyluria

THE PEARLS

White urine passed by the patient is always a puzzle to the clinician. Clinical perspective of the patient gives a clue to diagnosis. Otherwise, microscopic examination of urine and/or addition of ether/acetic acid/alkali, many a time, solve the problem.

79 Winging of the Scapulae

WHAT IS MEANT BY WINGING OF THE SCAPULAE?

Winged scapula means the medial (inner) border of the scapula appears to be wing-like on the back. The scapula sticks out from the back because of malfunction of serratus anterior muscle. It can be partial or complete and leads to mechanical destabilization of the shoulder when raising the arm or doing a push-up type motion, which results in significant shoulder dysfunction and pain. It may be considered a normal posture in young children, but not older children and adults.

COMPLAINTS BY THE PATIENT

It can cause discomfort, decreased shoulder strength as well as range of motion and may create cosmetic deformity. The person may also have limited ability to raise his arm above his head, and thus may have difficulty in combing, removing or putting objects from the shelf.

The ***winging becomes more prominent*** if the patient pushes the outstretched arm against the wall or examiner's resistance in standing position.

CAUSES

- *Long thoracic nerve palsy or LTN palsy (nerve to serratus anterior):* The nerve originates from the cervical 5, 6 and 7 nerve roots, and innervates the serratus anterior muscle. This is the most common cause.
- *Spinal accessory or dorsal scapular nerve palsy/injury:* This gives rise to trapezius or rhomboid palsy respectively. These are uncommon causes.

ETIOLOGY

- *Long thoracic nerve palsy (or, as described above):* Traumatic (sports or whiplash injury, forceful manipulation of shoulder, mastectomy with dissection of axillary lymph nodes, electrical shock), non-traumatic (viral illness, radiculopathy) or idiopathic injury. Usually it produces unilateral winging.
- *Facioscapulohumeral muscular dystrophy (Landouzy-Dejerine type):* Usually bilateral (Fig. 79.1).
- Severe malnutrition associated with emaciation—usually bilateral.

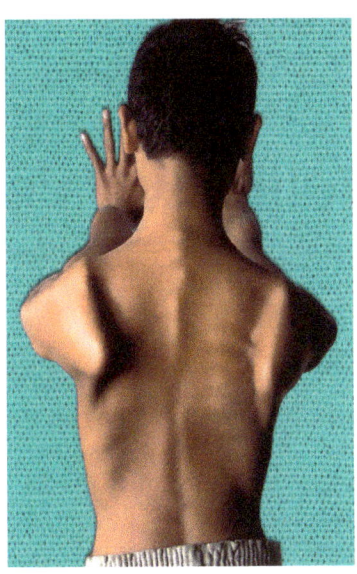

Fig. 79.1: Winging of the scapulae in a patient of facioscapulohumeral muscular dystrophy

- Injury to the upper trunk of the brachial plexus is commonly associated with the concomitant LTN injury. The long length of LTN provides some additional vulnerability to injury—usually unilateral.
- Associated with brachial neuritis (neuralgic amyotrophy), often following a viral infection or surgery. Pain and muscular weakness associated with muscular wasting around the shoulder are prominent features—usually unilateral.

MUSCLES MOSTLY AFFECTED IN WINGING OF THE SCAPULAE

Commonly serratus anterior and rarely trapezius.

MANAGEMENT

- ***Medical (conservative): Physiotherapy*** (rehabilitation and strengthening program consisting of ***winged scapular exercises***) and pain management are main modes of treatment. If symptoms continue to be severe for more than 3-6 months, surgery may be the next choice.
- ***Surgical:*** Options are scapulothoracic fusion, neurolysis ***(chordotomy)***, intercostal nerve transfer, ***arthrodesis*** (scapulodesis) or scapulothoracic fixation without arthrodesis (scapulopexy). Various combinations of fascial graft and/or transfer of adjacent muscles are being tried.

THE PEARLS

Always examine the neuromuscular system to exclude muscular dystrophy (especially, if there is bilateral winging). In unilateral winging, long thoracic nerve palsy is considered, which often needs surgical help.

80

Yellowish Palms/Soles

DIFFERENTIAL DIAGNOSIS

- Jaundice (sclera + mucus membrane + skin) → yellow (Fig. 80.1)
- Carotenemia (only the skin, mainly the forehead, nasolabial folds, and the palms and soles take a lemon-yellow tint) → carotenoderma
- Diffuse xanthomatosis (skin takes a yellowish-orange color; may have tuberous or palmar xanthoma, xanthelasma → lipid disorder)
- Quinacrine therapy (antimalarial, anti-giardia lamblia) → skin, eyes (only the regions of sclera exposed to light), urine are yellow
- Using turmeric for cooking/cosmetic purpose/taboo
- Acriflavine and picric acid ingestion → skin yellow, sclera normal.

Carotene, a lipid-soluble yellow pigment in the plasma, does not stain the conjunctiva and mucous membrane. However, the serum looks yellow in carotenemia.

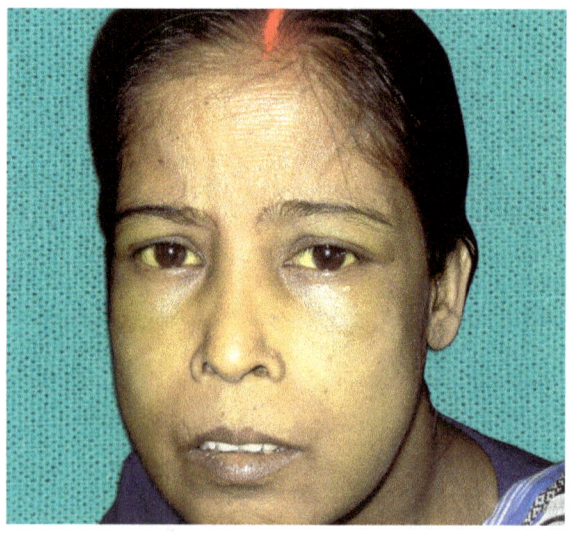

Fig. 80.1: Obstructive jaundice evidenced by deep yellow conjunctiva, greenish-yellow hue in skin and xanthelasma (underneath left eye)

WHAT IS LATENT JAUNDICE?

The normal serum bilirubin is 0.3–1.0 mg/dL. Clinical jaundice is evident when serum bilirubin is ≥3 mg/dL. Jaundice is latent, i.e. clinically non-evident (only detected by serum analysis) when the serum bilirubin level is in between 1 and 3 mg/dL.

CLUE TO DIAGNOSIS OF CAROTENEMIA

- Eating large quantities of carotene (vitamin A), carrots, mango, papaya, orange, squash and other colored fruits/vegetables
- *Hypothyroidism* → due to impaired metabolism of β-carotene in the liver
- Diabetes mellitus
- Receiving β-carotene therapy for erythropoietic porphyria
- Simmond's disease (panhypopituitarism)
- Anorexia nervosa (possible defect in conversion of carotene to vitamin A)
- Castrated male.

IS CAROTENEMIA INJURIOUS FOR HEALTH?

Except the cosmetic effect, excess carotene is non-injurious to health. Carotenemia does not develop into hypervitaminosis A.

XANTHOMA (FIG. 80.2)

- *Planus* → classical example is *xanthelasma* around the eyes (the upper eyelids more common than the lower) (Fig. 80.3). They are characteristically soft, yellowish and slightly raised from the surface, and are also seen in palmar creases, underneath the breast, chest or back. Xanthelasma is classically seen in conditions like:

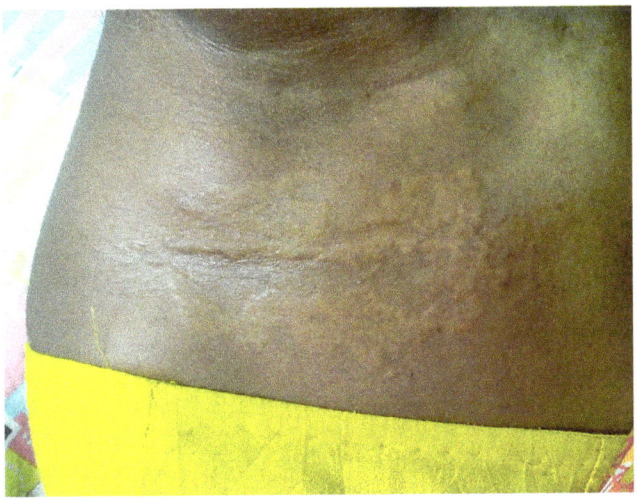

Fig. 80.2: Plane xanthoma over anterior chest wall in a female patient

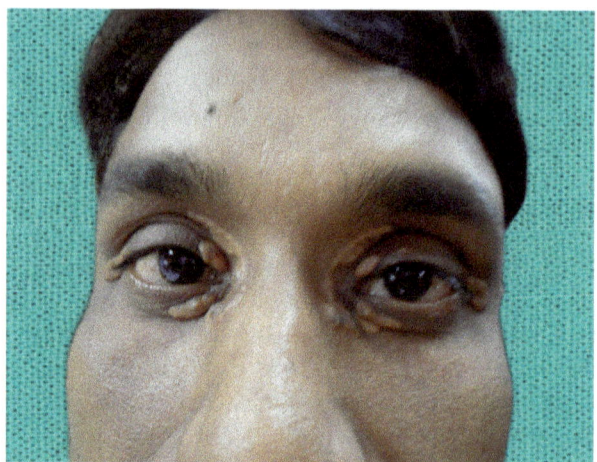

Fig. 80.3: Xanthelasma—sharply demarcated yellowish deposit of fat underneath the skin, usually on or around the eyelids; neither harmful nor painful

- Familial hypercholesterolemia
- Familial dysbetalipoproteinemia
- Diabetes mellitus
- Myxedema
- Prolonged cholestasis, e.g. primary biliary cirrhosis
- Nephrotic syndrome.
- ***Tuberus*** → commonly seen in extensor surface of elbow, knee, wrist, ankle and buttock.

Xanthomas are lesions which are characterized by accumulation of lipid-laden macrophages

TRIAD OF FAMILIAL HYPERCHOLESTEROLEMIA

- Tendon xanthoma
- Xanthelasma
- Arcus corneae.

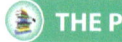 **THE PEARLS**

In the absence of jaundice, carotenemia is the most common cause of yellow hue of palms and sole. Sclera never turns yellow in carotenemia; probably, hypothyroidism is the most common etiology of this condition.

In a patient of xanthoma, always check the serum lipids, sugar level and thyroid hormones to come to an etiological diagnosis. Remember, few middle-aged or elderly people may have no lipid disorder though they have xanthelasma around the eyes.

Index

A

ABPI 186, 199
Aches, diffuse 80
Achilles tendonitis 151
Acrocyanosis 32
Acromegaly 107
Acroparesthesia 84, 186
Addison's disease 158, 206
Aerophagia 180
AIDS 18
Air hunger 255
Alkaptonuria 28
Alopecia 6
Alteration, facial contour 10
Amaurosis 216
Amblyopia 216
Amyloidosis 146, 147, 226
Anemia 21, 223, 289
ANCA 286
Angioedema 172, 302
Angular stomatitis 14
Anhidrosis 3
Anisocoria 105
Anuria 221
Aphthous stomatitis 264
Appetite 312, 314
Arcus corneae 272
Arcus senilis 100, 272
Argyrosis 270
Aseptic fever 16

B

Bags, under the eyes 101
Bald tongue 21
Band keratopathy 101, 270, 273
Bazin's disease 199
Bedsores 25
Belching 162, 182
Bell's palsy 10, 11, 108
Bitot's spot 101
Black urine 28

Black stool 29
Bleeding disorders 257
Bleeding, internal 251
Bleeding, rectum 259
Blepharospasm 102, 247
Blisters, subepidermal 287
Bow legs 53
Bradycardia 38
Breath, foul 132
Breathing, noisy 257
Bridge of the nose, depressed 71
Brushfield's spot 101
Bruxism 43
Bubo 137
Bull-neck 46
Butterfly rash, face 233

C

Cachexia 313
Calcanean spur 151
Calf pain 67
Calf swelling 68
Candidiasis 228, 229, 308
Cardiac arrest 295
Carotenemia 327
Carotidynia 121
Carpal tunnel syndrome 49
Cataract 101
Cellulitis 298
Chancroid 136
Cheilosis 156
Cheiroarthropathy 175
Chilblains 31
Chromhidrosis 4
Chronic fatigue syndrome 82
Chvostek's sign 69
Chyluria 222, 322, 323
Claudication 184
Claw foot 52
Claw hand 56
Coccygodynia 242
Color blindness 216

Compartment syndrome 152
Conjunctiva, chemosis 99
Conjunctival edema 301
Constipation 206
Coprolalia 58
Cor pulmonale 255
Corneal opacities 100
Cornea, rings around 270
Cough 60
Cough syncope 65
Cramp, leg 66
Cretinism 72, 109, 177
Cushing's syndrome 111, 113, 115, 165, 167

D

Day blindness 215
Day, sleepiness 44
Deep vein thrombosis 297, 300, 303
Defeminization 165
Dehydration 110
de Musset's sign 148
Dengue 17
Depressed, bridge of the nose 71
Dextrocardia 76
Dextroversion 77
Diagonal crease, ear 178
Diarrhea 206, 207
Diphtheria 228
Diplopia 85
Discolored teeth 88
Distension, abdomen 182
Down's syndrome 59, 72, 109
Drooling, saliva 211
Drop attacks 90
Dry mouth 226
Dry eyes 103, 226
Dyspepsia 180

E

Ears, low set 178
Ectodermal dysplasia 72
Ectopia lentis 101
Edema
  conjunctival 301
  eyelid 301
  facial 111, 112, 301
  pedal 297-300
  periorbital 111, 112
Elfin facies 115
Emaciation 313

Enophthalmos 102, 247
Enteric fever 17
Enthesopathy 190, 193
Epicanthic folds 101
Erb's sign 69
Erectile dysfunction 93
Eructation 162, 182
Erythromelalgia 31
Erythropoietin 236, 237
Exhaustion 124
Extracellular fluid 304
Eyes, clue to diagnosis 98
Eyes, dry 226
Eyes, pain 103, 122
Eyes, red 101

F

Facial contour, alteration 10
Facies 10, 106-119
Facial pain 120
Facial puffiness 301
Falls, in the elderly 91
Fatigue 82, 124
Fever 16-20
Fibromyalgia 83
Fingers, mutilated 54
Fits 91, 92
Flatulance 181
Fluorosis 88
Flushing, of face 113, 128
Foul breath 132
Frank's sign 178
Frontal bossing 73

G

Gain, weight 311
Gaisbock's syndrome 237
Gasping respiration 257
Genital discharge 137
Genital ulcer 135
Gingival bleeding 139, 142
Glossitis 15, 308
Granuloma inguinale 137
Gum hypertrophy 142
Gum pigmentation 143
Gumma 136

H

Hair, graying 168
Hair, types 166
Halitosis 132
Hands 173-175, 274-277, 326–328
Head-nodding 148
Head tilt 85, 148
Head retraction 149
Heel pad thickness 54
Heel pain 150
Hematuria 222, 266–269
Hemeralopia 215
Hemihypertrophy 12
Hemoglobinuria 266, 267
Hemolysis 266, 268
Hepatic face 110
Herpes genitalis 137
Herpes labialis 154
Herpes zoster 158–160
Hesitancy, urine 219
Heterotaxy 76
Hiccough 161
High-arched palate 74
Hirsutism 164
Hoarseness of voice 169
Homan's sign 297, 303
Horner's syndrome 245–247
Hutchinson's triad 72, 74
Hypercapnea 257, 277
Hypercholesterolemia 328
Hyperhidrosis 2
Hyperkeratosis, palms 173
Hypersomnia 44
Hypertelorism 101, 176
Hypertrichosis 165
Hyperventilation 256
Hyperviscosity syndrome 237, 238
Hypohidrosis 3
Hypotelorism 177
Hypoxia 277

I

Idioventricular rhythm 41
Impotence 93
Incontinence, urine 96, 220
Indigestion 180
Inequality, limb length 12

Infectious mononucleosis 16
Insomnia 44
Intermittent claudication 184
Iron deficiency anemia 21, 289

J

Jaccoud's arthritis 196
Jaundice 99, 326, 327
Joint pain 188
Joints, red hot 194

K

Kartagener's syndrome 78
Kawasaki disease 18
Kayser-Fleischer ring 100, 270–272
Knock-knees 53
Koilonychia 289, 290
Kussmaul's breathing 255

L

Lagophthalmos 102
Legs, painful 300
Legs, swollen 297
Leg ulceration 197
Leonine face 115
Leprosy 71, 115
Leukoplakia 23, 308
Limb length, inequality 12
Lipiduria 322, 323
Lipoid proteinosis 145, 146
Lips 15, 154, 156
Livedo reticularis 252
Lockjaw 200
Loose-jointedness 36
Loss, weight 313–315
Low set ears 178
Lumbar canal stenosis 184–186
Lump
    epigastrium 203
    face 123
    groin 138
    lymph node 46, 47, 206
    right iliac fossa 202
Lymphadenopathy 46–48
Lymphogranuloma venereum 137

M

Macroglossia 208
Madarosis 101, 107, 114, 208
Magenblase 181
Malar flush 113
Masked face 113
Measles 16
Melena 259, 260
Melanuria 28
Microglossia 210
Micrognathia 10
Micturition 219
Midline granuloma 72
Mikulicz's syndrome 227
Miliaria 4
Miosis 104
Mitral facies 114
Mongolism 59, 72, 109
Monoarthritis 188, 190, 194
Moon face 111
Mouth-breathing 256
Muscles, stiff 191
Myasthenia gravis 115, 124, 245-247
Mydriasis 104
Myoglobinuria 266, 269
Myokymia 101
Myotonia 68, 114, 276
Myxedema 114, 171, 301, 328

N

Nails, pitting 290
Nails, white 318
Nephritic/nephrotic face 112
Neuralgia
  brachial 325
  postherpetic 120
  trigeminal 120
Neurogenic claudication 184, 187
Night blindness 215
Night sweats 4
Nocturia 220
Nocturnal enuresis 218
Nodal rhythm 41
Non-ulcer dyspepsia 181
Nyctalopia 215
Nystagmus 101

O

Obesity 311, 312, 315
Ochronosis 28
Oculogyric crisis 114
Oculomotor palsy 245–247
Oliguria 221
Oliver's sign 170
Onycholysis 290, 291, 319
Onychomadesis 320
Onychorrhexis 320
Oral, pigmentation 158
Oral ulcers, recurrent 262
Osmidrosis 4
Osteosclerosis 89
Overweight 311

P

Pacemaker 40
Pain
  abdomen 204, 206, 207
  body 80
  bone 292, 294
  calf 67
  eyes 122
  face 120
  heel 82, 150
  joint 188
  leg 67, 300
  low back 81
  neck 80
  perianal 242
  shin 152
Palate, high-arched 74
Pallor 223
Palmar erythema 175
Palms 173–175, 276, 326
Parkinsonism 113, 114, 148
Parotid swelling 225
Patch
  tongue 23
  tonsil 228
Pellagra 22, 231
Periorbital edema 99, 111, 112
Perleche 15
Pernicious anemia 22
Pernio 31
Peroneal sign 69
Pes cavus 52

Petechiae 248
Pharynx, inflamed 265
Phosphaturia 322, 323
Photodermatoses 232
Photophobia 98
Photosensitivity 231
Phrenoderma 173, 276
Pica 21
Pigmentation, oral cavity 158
Pin-point pupil 105
Plantar fasciitis 151
Platynychia 290, 291
Plethoric face 113, 235
Polyarthritis 190, 194, 195
Polycythemia 114, 235
Polyphagia 312
Polyuria 222
Pompholyx 174
Popliteal, swelling 300
Porphyria 145, 147, 266
Postherpetic neuralgia 120
Prayer sign 175
Precipitancy, urine 219
Premature ejaculation 95
Presternal edema 293
Priapism 96
Procoagulant states 302
Proctalgia fugax 242
Prognathism 12, 107
Pruritus
  ani 242
  etiology 239
  vulvae 243
Pseudochyluria 322, 323
Pseudopelade 6, 8
Pseudoptosis 98, 247
Pseudoscleroderma 146
Pseudoseizures 92
Pseudovasculitis 285
Ptosis 244
Ptyalism 210, 227
Pupil 104, 105, 246, 247
Purpuric spots 248
Purse-lip respiration 254
PUVA therapy 234
Pyorrhea 132, 143
Pyrexia, unknown origin (PUO) 18, 19
Pyuria 322, 323

Q

QT-prolongation 296
Quinidine 162

R

Radio-femoral delay 42
Radio-radial delay 42
Raynaud's phenomenon 30–33
Rectal bleeding 259
Rectal pain 242
Red eyes 101
Red, hot joints 194
Red urine 266
Respiratory failure 276, 277
Retrograde ejaculation 96
Rhabdomyolysis 269
Rhagades 15, 113
Risus sardonicus 201
Rubella 17
Rumination 182

S

Sabre tibia 74
Saddle-nose deformity 72, 73
Sarcoidosis 72, 225
Sarcopenia 313
Scarlet fever 17
Sclera, blue 34, 100
Scleredema 146, 147
Scleroderma 31, 113, 145, 147, 282
Scleromalacia perforans 100
Scrotum, acute 205
Shake hands 274
Shingles 158–160
Short neck 55
Sialorrhea 210, 227
Sighing respiration 256
Sildenafil 95
Sinuses, abdomen 206
Sinus rhythm 41
Situs inversus 76
Sjögren's syndrome 103, 226
Skin, thickening 145
Sleep disorders 43
Smell 132
Sneezing 278
Snoring 280

Soft-tissue rheumatism 83
Sore mouth 157
Sore throat 157
Spatula test 200
Speech, disorder 58
Splinter hemorrhage 281
Spoon-shaped nails 289
Squint 85, 101, 247
Sternal tenderness 292
Stiff-man syndrome 200
Stool, black 29
Stooped posture 196
Strangury 222, 261
Stridor 316
Subconjunctival hemorrhage 99
Sudden cardiac death 295
Sweating 1
Sweat test 5
Swollen
   face 301, 302
   legs 297
Syncope 92
Syphilis 23, 72, 136
Systemic lupus erythematosus (SLE) 31, 112, 233, 264, 282

T

Tabes dorsalis 110, 245
Tachycardia 40
Teeth, discolored 88
Teeth chattering 43
Teeth grinding 43
Telogen effluvium 8
Temporal arteritis 122, 281
Temporomandibular arthritis 121
Tenderness, bone 292, 294
Tenesmus 261
Tetanus 200, 201
Tetany 68–70
Thalassemia 71, 73, 109
Thrombophlebitis 304
Thrush 228, 229, 308
Thyrotoxicosis 108, 274, 276
Tics 148
Tingling sensation 84, 186
Titubation 148
Tongue 21, 146, 208, 306
Tonsils 228, 265
Tourette syndrome 58

Toxic shock syndrome 17
Trichotillomania 8
Trigeminal neuralgia 120
Trismus 200
Trophic ulcer 26, 197
Tropical sprue 22
Tropical ulcer 197
Trousseau's sign 69
Tubular vision 103, 217
Typhus 18

U

Ulcer
   digital 32
   genital 135
   leg 197
   oral 262
Ultraviolet rays 234
Urethral discharge 137
Urine
   black 28
   color changes 29
   red 266
   white 322

V

Vasculitis 281–287
Vasospastic disorders 31
Vertigo 92
Virchow's gland 48
Virilization 164, 167
Vulvae, pruritus 243

W

Waist-hip ratio 311
Wegener's granulomatosis 72, 172, 281, 284, 286, 287
Weight gain 311, 312
Weight loss 313, 314
Wheezing 316
White lesions
   oral cavity 229
   tongue 23
   tonsil 228
White, nails 318
White, urine 322

Wilson's disease   270–272
Wind   181
Winging, scapulae   324

X

Xanthelasma   99, 327
Xanthoma   174, 326, 327
Xerophthalmia   103, 226
Xerostomia   226
X-ray, chest   78

Y

Yawning   279
Yellow, nails   319
Yellow, palms   326
Y-linked disorder   165

Z

Zinc deficiency   215
Zollinger-Ellison syndrome   128

EU GSPR Authorised Reprsentative
Logos Europe, 9 rue Nicolas Poussin
1700, La Rochelle, France
Phone: +33 (0) 6 67 93 73 78
E-mail: contact@logoseurope.eu

www.ingramcontent.com/pod-product-compliance
Ingram Content Group UK Ltd.
Pitfield, Milton Keynes, MK11 3LW, UK
UKHW021827140426
5217IPUK00016B/1248